ATTENTION DEFICIT DISORDER MISDIAGNOSIS:

**Approaching ADD from a
Brain Behavior/Neuropsychological
Perspective for
Assessment and Treatment**

ATTENTION DEFICIT DISORDER MISDIAGNOSIS

Approaching ADD from a Brain-Behavior/Neuropsychological Perspective for Assessment and Treatment

BARBARA C. FISHER, PH.D.

CRC Press

Boca Raton   Boston   New York   Washington, D.C.   London

Library of Congress Cataloging-in-Publication Data

Catalog information may be obtained from the Library of Congress.

© 1998 by CRC Press LLC
St. Lucie Press is an imprint of CRC Press LLC

No claim to original U.S. Government works
International Standard Book Number 1-57444-097-7
Printed in the United States of America 1 2 3 4 5 6 7 8 9 0
Printed on acid-free paper

Acknowledgments

Dr. Ross A. Beckley, my husband, co-director of United Psychological Services, Attention Deficit Disorder Clinic, was actually the first and only person to recognize this hidden attentional disorder in my son at the age of 6 years. His continual astuteness has remained a most treasured asset. Dr. Beckley, trained as an educator, specialist in learning disabilities, marriage and family psychologist, provided both his expertise and support in the completion of this book and is the co-author of a yet unpublished book for the lay population. Gail Jurczek, a professional writer, took the original manuscript and edited it, spending countless hours devoting herself to this task in an effort to bring knowledge to others about a rather overwhelming and misunderstood disorder. A special note of appreciation to my son, whom I learn from daily, together we developed numerous *home remedies* that have remained very successful coping mechanisms for addressing specific symptoms of Attention Deficit Disorder. Thanks is due to Terri and Greer who spent hours correlating references, Blythe, Jackie, and my family — father, mother, and Laura — who provided a continual support system when needed the most, and, finally, my dogs, Ralph and Alice, who kept me company during the early morning hours.

Preface

Professionals from psychology to neuropsychology and related, allied professions are responding to the question of overdiagnosing, the concern of overlapping symptoms of comorbid disorders, and the need for improved diagnostic measures that are uniform. While the explosion of Attention Deficit Disorder (ADD) has been positive in providing understanding to millions of confused children, adolescents, parents, and adults, it has been negative in the overall disagreement among professionals regarding diagnosis and treatment. Having observed all of the above from both a professional and personal viewpoint, this book represents my attempt to bring some clarity to the confusion, presenting in a logical, research-oriented approach my conclusions of the past 9 years of research and specialization in this area. I remain grateful to my forerunner, Dr. Russell Barkley, who first proposed viewing ADD from a neuropsychological perspective, and to Dr. Kenneth M. Heilman, the father of "neglect", who provided me with an understanding of an "inattention to the whole", which helped me to finally conceptualize my son's academic problems, and allowed for creative remediation of his difficulties and those of others.

Specific Goals of This Book

1. To provide a logical format to address ADD, the "phenomenon" that is being measured in so many different ways that the general population, including treating professionals, are hopelessly confused.
2. To separate Attention Deficit Disorder with hyperactivity (ADHD) from ADD, to explore the idea that the two subtypes exist, and are structurally and neurochemically quite different from one another.
3. To examine existing literature, reviewing the concepts in existence as a cohesive body in an attempt to make sense of the diverse research findings.

4. To understand the impact of comorbid or related disorders and the critical role they play in impacting treatment due to the interplay of the underlying psychological disorders and the symptoms of the attentional disorder. Treatment often will not succeed, due to underlying symptoms that have not been addressed and that emerge with the use of stimulant medication.

5. To explain the need for accurate assessment of ADD and underlying diagnosis. There is a great amount of misdiagnosis and non-diagnosis, due to the absence of a unified means of assessment, and the majority of present-day assessments do not address aspects of the disorder as it appears from a brain-behavior perspective.

6. To delineate the use of different treatment approaches that, to be successful, will be dependent on a total and accurate assessment.

7. To show how the whole-treatment approach identifies the need to approach the individual from a nutritional, clinical, neurological, and psychological perspective, and the need to develop coping mechanisms to address specific symptomatology. Treatment involves delineation of specific coping mechanisms, based on evaluation, re-training of the brain, and the use of medication and nutrition as they interact and counteract one another.

8. To answer the question why stimulants will or will not work, as well as their efficacy. The book addresses the idea of stimulants operating as augmenters of underlying disorders and the need to assess each individual reaction to arrive at the best treatment approach. We are currently in the process of delineating a pattern of comorbid disorders that are increasingly prevalent in our clinical practice. ADD without hyperactivity, the Overfocused Subtype denotes a more fragile, physically and emotionally reactive and vulnerable population from which emerges such diagnoses as Obsessive Compulsive Disorder, Borderline Personality Disorder, Depression, and Anxiety. Tourette's syndrome and/or a type of seizure activation presents as emotional, angry, and aggressive outbursts in the child population (exacerbated by stimulant medication). In the adult population this group is more vulnerable to the development of hypertension, sleep apnea, narcolepsy, and subsequent short-term memory losses. Accurate diagnoses serves to identify these issues and to provide treatment before further progressive impact to brain functioning occurs.

ADD is an extremely complex disorder that is in need of equally complex management and diagnosis for treatment.

Dr. Barbara C. Fisher

About the Author

Dr. Barbara C. Fisher is a fully licensed Ph.D. psychologist specializing in neuropsychology for the last 19 years. She approaches Attention Deficit Disorder (ADD) from a brain-behavior point of view and utilizes her knowledge of the brain and neuroanatomy to understand, diagnose, and explain specific symptoms of this disorder. Dr. Fisher with her husband, Dr. Ross A. Beckley have been addressing the attention deficit population for the last 10 years. They are the co-owners of United Psychological Services, Attention Deficit Disorder Clinic, located in Clinton Township, Michigan and a satellite office in Lansing.

Dr. Fisher is skilled in isolating and identifying the underlying co-morbid or co-associated disorders that frequently accompany an attentional disorder. She is aware of the latest research and thus is able to differentiate symptoms to allow for an extremely accurate diagnosis. Not only is she able to differentiate and separate the two subtypes of ADD, ADD without hyperactivity and Attention Deficit Disorder with hyperactivity (ADHD), but she is also able to define other existing disorders that would contribute to the creation of problems when attempting treatment. She finds that symptoms from these undiagnosed underlying disorders frequently contribute to the side effects which occur when using a stimulant medication.

It is Dr. Fisher's belief that ADD represents a very complex syndrome which requires very specific diagnosis, identifying not only the specific attentional symptoms but also the other accompanying issues. The idea is to approach treatment from a whole perspective, using not only medication, but also, and more importantly, coping mechanisms to address the specific problems as well as to understand the emotional issues that may prevent the child, adolescent, or adult from working to their full potential.

Dr. Fisher is the co-author of the book, *We Are Not Getting Older, We Are Just Coming of Age*. She also co-owns and operates the Tillie M. Fisher Home, an adult foster-care unit and is currently specializing in the aged population. Using neuropsychological evaluation and addressing ages from 5 to 96 years, she specializes in the diagnosis of head injury, various neurological disorders, and differentiation of Alzheimer's Disease from vascular dementia or some other type of progressive dementia.

Dr. Fisher is a well-known speaker and has presented at various workshops, including radio and television, to various professional and lay groups, on such varied topics as ADD, Depression and Anxiety, Comorbid Disorders, Issues of the Aging Population, Alzheimer's Disease, Coping with Angry People, Sibling Rivalry, Nutrition and Comorbid Disorders, and Mothers and Daughters. Dr. Fisher conducts custody evaluations, Neuropsychological evaluations, alcohol assessments, psychological, educational, and achievement evaluation. She is trained in hypnosis and applies this technique to weight loss, smoking, and regressive work for trauma or abuse.

She is a member of American Psychological Association, National Association for Neuropsychologists, American Society of Clinical Hypnosis, and various support groups for both head injury and ADD.

Contents

CHAPTER 1

Understanding Attention Deficit Disorder from a Theoretical Perspective

ADD Is a Lifelong Disorder

Recently, it has come to the attention of the general population that a disorder formerly thought of as only affecting children is now affecting adults. Athletes who had been helped by Ritalin were among the first to point out that this is not merely a disorder affecting children; instead, Attention Deficit Disorder without hyperactivity (ADD) and Attention Deficit Disorder with hyperactivity (ADHD) are problems that affect individuals throughout their lives. Barkley (1990) played an important role in establishing ADD as a disregulation disorder, characterized by inconsistent and variable behavior, due to a biochemical imbalance in the brain. Variable behavior was described by Barkley as a general lack of regulation, whereby moment-to-moment is more compelling. This chemical imbalance was viewed as creating problems with inhibition, and initiating and staying on task, whereby adherence to rules or instructions becomes difficult. When clear external consequences to behavior problems are weak or non-existent, the internal regulating forces do not allow the individual to stay on task.

Barkley was describing ADHD from a substantially different perspective. The original hypothesis of ADD was the diagnosis of ADHD, which was thought to be a disorder of the reticular activating system (RAS) (a multisynaptic system responsible for arousal and alertness in the brain). It is believed that the RAS was immature or underdeveloped and therefore re-

1

sponsive to the stimulant medication, Ritalin. Ritalin appeared to calm the motorically active, ADHD child and rather than operating as a stimulant, operated as a tranquilizing agent instead. The conclusion emerged that this area must be underdeveloped as the opposite occurred of what was expected. As the theory went, once the RAS matured, presumably in adolescence or adulthood, symptoms of the disorder would no longer be seen. Unfortunately, this did not explain the existence of ADD in adults, nor the syndrome of ADHD. Adults are becoming more aware of the symptoms of this disorder and ADD symptomatology explains the unexplainable occurrences in their lives. Medical students were referred for evaluation, due to an inability to either pass their required examinations and/or a lack of success in medical school. A significant number, 78%, were diagnosed with learning disability or ADHD (Banks, Guyer, and Guyer, 1995). This finding points to the versatility and ability of very bright individuals who compensate for symptoms of this disorder and maintain an intact appearance until demand from their environment increases and things become more complex. It is then that problems they have previously managed to hide become obvious.

Neuropsychology as a recently discovered, evolving discipline has provided a viable means of assessing brain functioning. Neuropsychological assessment began to identify and quantify symptoms of ADD in a more-concrete and less-abstract manner. Improvements in neuro-imaging technology contributed to validating and substantiating the results of neuropsychological assessment. Due to this increased technology, it was possible to finally document the presence of ADD within the brain. The result was the hypothesis of a biochemical theory of ADD (Zametkin and Rapoport, 1987), initially citing the frontal area of the brain and hypofrontality to explain commonly observed symptoms of ADHD, a disorder of the frontal-lobe supervisory system and its connections. Symptoms of ADHD were seen to resemble that of a frontal lobe disorder, exhibiting difficulties with planning, organization, sequencing, utilization of feedback and modification of behavior, maintaining and switching of cognitive sets, and flexibility of thinking necessary for problem-solving. Decreased arousal and vigilance resulted in inconsistency, and a high degree of variable behavior. Behavioral symptoms included a loss of motivation and a craving for stimulation.

Currently, ADD is seen as a biochemical disorder involving neurotransmitters, or brain messengers, primarily dopamine and norepinephrine. These neurotransmitters are responsible for arousal and alertness in the brain. The biochemical imbalance results in a lack of the neurotransmitter substance necessary for appropriate arousal and alertness. This lack of arousal and alertness does not allow the brain to function properly in its respective areas nor communicate effectively with other parts of the brain for maximized functioning to occur. Those with the disorder usually present symptoms early in life and continue to present symptoms throughout the lifespan. The disorder is believed to be genetic in origin and statistics have overrepresented the male population three to one. Finally, to rule in ADD as a disorder by itself, brain functioning must be intact. ADD, however, can exist comorbidly with a variety of disorders, often exacerbating symptoms in a cyclical manner.

There is a "wax and wane" of symptoms observed in the behaviors and cognitive skills of the attention-disordered population. Their behavior varies as a result of the natural chemical variability of the neurotransmitter imbalance. In addition, a phenomenon has been observed clinically (which at this point cannot be documented regarding brain functioning), whereby if something is externally stimulating, symptoms of ADD will not be observed. Consequently, ADD symptoms are not seen at the beginning of the task, but in the middle and in the follow-through. ADD symptoms are not observed in a task that the individual enjoys. Thus, the diagnosis of ADD can become difficult and tenuous.

ADD is now thought of as a higher-level thinking disorder, not a behavioral or psychological disorder. The disorder mainly involves the frontal and parietal areas of the brain and their many connections. Blood flow studies, PET scans, MRIs, and EEG studies have contributed to these conclusions. Attention-disordered individuals reveal decreased blood flow, sluggish EEGs, and decreased brain matter. Current research suggests that ADHD and ADD rarely occur alone; often there is an associated condition present. For instance, follow-up research indicates that alcohol and drug use can complicate the presenting picture in one-third of ADHD cases identified in childhood, minor chronic depression can occur in one-fourth of the cases, severe mood swings are also present in one-fourth of the cases, and anxiety problems (nervousness, sleep difficulties, concentration difficulties, and muscular tension) can be present in approximately one-half of the ADHD cases identified in childhood.

There is a general consensus that more work needs to be done in separating and distinguishing the comorbid disorders using differential diagnosis, as well as separating ADD from ADHD. Kwasman, Tinsley, and Lepper (1995) noted wide variations in examining physician's conceptualization and treatment of ADD. The procedure at our clinic has been to first rule in or rule out the attentional disorder and then to address any comorbid disorders. It has become apparent that, due to the disturbance of the biochemical balance involving dopamine and norepinephrine (which are also implicated in a number of emotional and neurological disorders), further disruption results, creating a cascade of other disorders. Thus clinically, ADD does not appear as a singular diagnosis and often the attentional disorder is accompanied by an emotional disturbance and/or a neurologically based disorder. ADD has also been found to be significantly linked to disregulation of the hormonal balance, thyroid disorders, allergies, etc. Generally, ADD individuals (as a population) appear to be specifically vulnerable to other concomitant disturbances.

ADHD versus ADD

Psychologists have thought that persons with ADHD comprised most of the total attention-disordered population. These statistics are expected to change with the advent of improved diagnostic techniques. The disorder that is only recently being documented in the literature and, surprisingly, the more common disorder that we have found in the general population is that of ADD, which appears to operate with a similar neurotransmitter imbalance (notably that of norepinephrine) and involves the parietal area and its connections. As diagnostic techniques improve, the presence of ADD will be correctly distinguished and diagnosed.

ADHD can be likened to a plane being operated without its pilot or control panel. Characteristics are that of inattention, impulsivity, hyperactivity, aggression, poor self-control, disinhibition, easily distressed, overreaction, immaturity, low self-esteem, and rejection by peers. A large percentage of this population is diagnosed learning disabled in reading, writing, math, or language; many underachieve and underproduce; many are immature and demonstrate inappropriate social skills. Many can be classified with oppositional defiant disorder and present symptoms of conduct disorder, seen more often in the male population. This syndrome appears to involve more of the frontal area of the brain and its supervisory system. ADHD children and adults have difficulty with decision-making and planning, error correction and use of feedback, learning of response, faulty judgment, decreased impulse control, and difficulty resisting temptation. All are characteristics and functions of the frontal areas of the brain and its connections.

ADD without hyperactivity has historically been seen by professionals in the field as affecting a significantly smaller percentage of the attention-disordered population. However, it is the presence of ADD without the overt hyperactivity that is the more common disorder to be observed in the mainstream practice of many mental-health practitioners today. Commensurate with the medical model (less severe is more common), the less-severe disorder of ADD is emerging as the disorder seen more often, while the more-severe disorder of ADHD is observed less often. Characteristics of ADD are cognitive sluggishness, daydreams, withdrawal, confusion, fogginess, slowness to respond, lost in their own world, reticent, apprehensive, passive, and non-engaging overall.

These individuals do not call attention to themselves, as do those diagnosed with ADHD, and they tend to be socially neglected (operating on the periphery of the group), not necessarily understanding the world in which they live. There is poor social integration, due to their inability to take in information and comprehend what is occurring around them. Often these individuals have no idea of the conversation and the content in which it is being used. Life basically passes them by. They resemble that dreamy person who appears "out to lunch", and living in Tahiti, having conversations with him/herself. Central cognitive-processing speed is slow and there tends to be a familial history of anxiety. This is vastly different from the ADHD history and its connection to the delinquent, conduct-disordered, alcoholic population. ADD is primarily a true sustained-focus disorder with severe academic underachievement (due to the inability to focus and sustain attention). In addition, there is difficulty with coding, encoding, and retrieval of linguistic information. If the information is not taken in, it cannot be retrieved. These individuals appear to have problems with memory that are truly the consequence of information not being perceived.

This inability to process information received through instructions, directions, and communication in general is one symptom that appears to be highly characteristic of ADD (and sometimes symptomatic of ADHD). Information-processing problems are clinically manifested by an absence of knowledge, "not getting it," and general inability to understand and comprehend, at times, the world that surrounds them. The parietal area of the brain is responsible for the ability to process information received via the senses. The child (and later adult) is unable to process information for utilization. The language problems of the ADD individual tend to relate to spatial problems (inattention to the whole), whereby the individual is unable to discern the whole of the word and compensation is attained via the development of a sight vocabulary. Math skills become deficient, handwriting is very poor, spelling is problematic, time-management issues emerge; there is an inability to anticipate consequences of one's actions, and an overall clumsiness in interacting in one's environment is continually present. This inability to view the whole, whether of a word, situation, conversation, math problem, or movement in space, can impact academic skills to such a significant degree that overall IQ levels drop, grades decline, adolescents quit school and/or do not continue their academic studies. The significant percentage of individuals severely impacted by this specific deficit is both staggering and sobering in understanding the consequences of what we tend to view as a single inability to attend and concentrate.

ADD Has Far-Reaching Consequences

ADD typically impacts the familial and marital systems with the following consequences:

1. Depression can occur regardless of the ADD diagnosis in all family members.
2. Family scapegoating. The ADD child or adult is targeted and held responsible for all mishaps that occur in the household.
3. Hostility toward significant others by the ADD individual, who responds in anger and frustration, whether scapegoated or not.
4. The idea of the child being damaged and abnormal contributes to the family's sense of shame.
5. A parent's confusion about discipline. Parents are unsure of the reason for problematic behavior (can the child change this behavior, or is it due to a more-extensive neurological problem?) and how to treat it. The age-old question arises of whether to punish an individual for an act he/she has no control over. Caretaker of these children remain confused as to what the child can and cannot control.
6. Conflicted marital and familial systems. Conflicts occur over discipline, miscommunication, financial concerns, cohesiveness, and general day-to-day mishaps that characterize the life of the ADD individual.
7. The family's energy is centered around the ADD individual, resulting in a depletion of resources for other family members.
8. Diminished attention and depleted resources lead to the creation of symptoms in other family members in an attempt to resolve their own unmet needs.

9. Impulsivity brings the family into contact with the legal system. Frustration, avoidance and/or impulsive (non-thinking) actions continually lead the individual and the family into situations not within their value system and, on occasion, bizarre events that they thought would never happen to them.

10. Generalized family tension and substance abuse by family members: Family members become angry, unfulfilled emotionally (each for his/her own reason), and may withdraw into separate, individual units. The family, having lost its cohesiveness, becomes tense and a warm, supportive atmosphere no longer exists. Addictions (workaholism, gambling, drug abuse, alcoholism, compulsive overeating, compulsive shopping) provide the means for escape and temporary relief.

Follow-up studies indicate that children diagnosed with ADD also manifested characteristics of ADHD in adulthood. Research presents adults who are seen as restless, exhibiting fidgeting behavior, changing and shifting body position constantly, with fast-paced continual movement, and this appears as the remnant of the motor characteristics of ADHD. What appears as "overactive" behavior can easily be the consequence of a Type A personality, driven-to-succeed individual, and generalized anxiety symptoms. Anxiety can be the underlying reason that individuals shift continuously, or need to hold something or "play" with some object available nearby.

Anxiety is highly prevalent in the ADD-diagnosed individual and readily observable to the naked eye. Individuals are constantly moving hands, legs, and feet in an unconscious reaction to internal anxiety and stress level. Vulnerability to somatic complaints and diseases is substantially elevated. Characteristics such as antisocial behavior, alcoholism, substance abuse, criminal activity, loss of jobs, decreased financial status, auto accidents, traffic violations, divorce and separation, depression, and suicide are commonly observed in both subtypes of this disorder for various reasons.

Generalizations about the ADD Population as a Whole

ADD individuals tend to have children when they are ill prepared to provide and care for them, resulting in adoption and the high preponderance of the adopted population being diagnosed with ADD. Symptoms still evidenced in adulthood are commonly that of poor attention to tasks, distractibility, and disorganization. ADD adults too often lose things, have many unfinished projects or activities, and procrastinate more often than they complete tasks. Many are pegged by family members as "couch potatoes".

These ADD adults fidget, are restless, and have difficulty remaining seated for long periods of time. They are impatient and impulsive, cannot wait in line or at traffic lights, get easily irritated in traffic, readily lose their tempers, and argue with family members and coworkers. They respond poorly to stress and often get upset easily with a minimal amount of it. Reactions to stress are marked by depression, anger, anxiety, or confusion. The subtleties in recognizing, accurately understanding and framing, and coping with emotions associated with interpersonal relationships are often overwhelming for adults with ADD.

The attention-disordered population is excruciatingly aware of its inadequacies, although the source often cannot be identified. They know, perhaps better than anyone, the discrepancy between potential and actual levels of their own performance. Earlier in life, although they understood how to perform a classroom task, they simply could not concentrate long enough to complete the task. Later in life, the scenario may repeat itself in the employment situation. The ADD employee may have an idea that would be of benefit to the company (and her/himself), but somehow becomes distracted from focusing and mobilizing his/her efforts, and again falls short of the conceptualized goal. The idea does not become reality, creativity diminishes, and potential remains unrealized. The ADD individual remains part of the organization, undifferentiated by success.

Adults and children similarly describe themselves as stupid and incompetent. The ADD person is besieged with feelings of grief, loss, anger, confusion, and depression. Significant others cannot understand how in different developmental periods of the lifespan (whereby new tasks and behaviors are an inherent prerequisite), the child, adolescent, or adult, when encountering new tasks to perform, becomes suddenly angry and unreachable, either by withdrawing or lashing out at others. There are no words for the ADD person to adequately express how he/she feels and frequently they are as mystified by their feelings as those around them.

Considerable language problems plague this population and, without words, these emotions and conflicts have little or no chance of being discussed or eventually resolved. Efforts to resolve the conflicts in a therapeutic setting become difficult given the nature of the disorder. Families often change therapists due to ADD individuals becoming frightened or angry, fearful of change and loss, or due to avoidance tactics. Avoidance and procrastination consistently plague the life of the ADD individual, thus reinforcing a sense of failure and devalued self-esteem.

The history of endless failures, projects started and never finished, and being constantly out of communication with parents, siblings, teachers, and employers results in ADD individuals thinking of themselves as "impaired", with accompanying characteristics of being deficient, incompetent, aimless, lazy, and, in a self-fulfilling prophesy, they live up to these negative messages.

The above-mentioned traits are commonly observed with ADD; however, in the case of the ADHD individual, things can be very different. Typically with ADHD individuals, there is less concern (thus less avoidance and less procrastination), because they are not preoccupied with the opinions of others, thus there is no tendency to become depressed or withdraw (rarely does anything bother them); they simply do as they please. This is why individuals interacting with the ADHD child, adolescent, or adult cannot understand why they simply cannot impact these individuals with words, actions, consequences, or anything. ADHD individuals are difficult because there is an absence of connection to draw upon, a low frustration tolerance; when they are ready to leave, they simply leave. The emotional pain is usually not with the ADHD individual, but with those significant to them or who reside with them.

Anger is an emotion that seems to be overused by the ADD population as a whole for a variety of reasons, unresolved grief being the most prevalent and secondarily as an excuse for lack of task completion. Explosive tempers are often ignited by seemingly small incidents or no incident at all, at least in the perception of others. The ADD person can feel less effective (with the knowledge of higher potential) leading to frustration and bruised feelings. The anger seems to come automatically as a defense against the hurt. There is an intensity to the feelings of ADD individuals and they tend to be highly sensitive as a group. Often their reactions do not make sense, their vulnerability is surprising, and their hurt unpredictable. Anger is their protection and in a person with untreated ADD, one is likely to find the sadness of being blamed for not paying attention, and the hurt of being scolded, put down or even physically punished for work not completed. Controlled by an unseen force (biochemical imbalances in the brain), the individual has a sense of helplessness, of not understanding what went wrong or what could have been done to change it. Often, confusion is evident for everyone involved. Husband, wife, child, or teenager diagnosed with ADD responds, "But I was doing the best that I could." They forget birthdays, anniversary dates, special events, or they set off to complete a task only to return home, after the appointed time, having an agenda only partially finished.

Emotions converging in a flood of feelings are very common experiences for the ADD individual. They are not able to adequately screen out emotional stimuli nor incorporate emotional information into the experience itself. Miscommunication is a constant factor. This may occur as a result of a number of interplaying symptoms of the attentional disorder (most notably, the distractibility problem and/or an input or information-processing problem). Typically, only pieces of a given interaction are processed at a given time. Thus, the person misses information, whether parts of a sentence, a whole sentence, a detail, event, time, date, and so on. What is "received" may be substantially different from what was "sent". With only portions of the conversation available, it is very easy to misinterpret, misperceive, and misassume, with the consequence being constant miscommunications and misunderstanding. The ADD individual feels threatened, confused, unaware of what is going on, and may then react impulsively as a result. Thus they find themselves in situations they had no intention of being in and certainly had not foreseen nor anticipated. Criminal and delinquent behavior can often occur in this manner.

ADD individuals can respond with rigidity and inflexibility, lacking any kind of finesse or social understanding, pursuing a course of action without regard to consequences. Their sensitivity and anger can be like emotional blinders, with frustration acting as a trigger to impulsively drive them down a path of self-destruction. To the ADD individual, his/her behavior appears both rational and logical, but to those around them, it seems reckless and without forethought.

The ADD individual who has learned to compensate can lie and manipulate quite well, and can develop such traits as a means of protection and defense against a very confusing and demanding world. Life may become constricted in efforts to control and mitigate symptoms of the disorder. Obsessive compulsive behaviors create a facade to mask inadequacies, mistakes are generally repressed, and the gross errors they cannot cover up are clearly surprising to others and out of context with their appearance. ADD individuals learn to perform, creating a public facade, controlling and repressing emotions to prevent others from noticing the pain and loneliness they experience. The mask is so well affixed that when the slightest bit of intimacy or tenderness is shown, the individual recoils and quickly withdraws. Relationships are avoided, not as a result of being obstinate or self-reliant, but out of shame. Emotional and social competence is often diminished, confirming beliefs that they do not belong and therefore are not allowed to connect with others. Coping mechanisms too often effectively distance the ADD person from relationships early in life and oddly shape the personality. By adulthood, the ADD individual has mastered techniques of evasiveness, double messages, and unresolved grief. They have become emotionally imprisoned by symptoms that began as cognitive deficits. They cannot view the situation from a close perspective to help themselves, and those significant to them have been deliberately kept in confusion.

We have found in our research and study of this population over the last eight years that the emotional symptoms of ADD creates the trauma evidenced, increasing cognitive symptoms beyond that of the attentional disorder. The degree of severity of the disorder, exacerbation of emotional issues, intellectual potential, and drive for success culminate in an intricate interplay of cyclical variables, creating a highly "resistant-to-treatment" situation. The intricate interplay and complexity of the situation determines the necessity for an extremely accurate and specific diagnosis, identifying symptoms, extent and degree of deficits, and underlying comorbid issues. What has been devastating about this disorder is the understanding of its far-reaching consequences and, due to the impact of learning and usage of brain areas for development, the impairment (or type of atrophy) that occurs, due to non-use.

CHAPTER 2

Defining Attention

General Definition of Terms

Attention is defined as the ability to be aware of stimuli. This includes internal stimuli, such as thoughts and memories, and external stimuli, such as sights and sounds (Weber, 1990). Attention is the basis of all mental functions, such as thinking, playing games, coping with household chores and responsibilities, conversation, and so on. Attention is subdivided as either being automatic (applied to tasks performed without being freely conscious of what one is attending to; without a sense of attentional effort), or deliberate (whereby distinct attentional effort is demanded; also labeled concentration). The distinction can easily be applied to everyday life. Initially such routine tasks as learning to ride a bike, to drive a car, to read and write require effortful and deliberate concentration. However, as time passes, such tasks gradually demand less and less attentional effort. Eventually, these tasks are performed automatically and attention can be diverted to other things. Thus automatic attention operates in a very efficient manner as long as there are no changes occurring in the administration of the task. If changes do occur (which is inherent in life), the more purposeful attention and concentration is required and implemented (Schneider and Shiffrin, 1977; Weber, 1990).

Deliberate attention serves to cope with change and to integrate automatically attended skills into the overall situation. As a highly vulnerable, distributed, and parallel processing system, deliberate and effortful attention is necessary for everyday functioning and is easily disrupted by impact to the brain. Deliberate attention can also refer to a controlled and conscious process. Deliberate attention, more specifically defined, delineates focused, selective, divided, sustained, vigilant, intentional, voluntary, and alternating attention. Two basic dimensions can be seen as mediating deliberate and effortful attention: capacity and control. These factors can then be separated into categories of control (being comprised of sensory and responsive selection) and capacity (influenced by variables that affect an individual's attentional state and mediate sustained performance). Factors are not orthogonal and, in fact, share many common neural mechanisms. They are distinct in that they can be individually represented in different task situations and separately influenced by different sets of component processes (Cohen, 1993; Goldman-Rakic and Friedman, 1991; Weber, 1990).

Capacity refers to the amount of information or mental processing a person can attend to within a given time period. Individuals have a limited attentional capacity and are unable to process an infinite amount of information simultaneously. The deliberate form of attending or deliberate processing requires a certain degree of capacity and attending is constrained by the limitations of the individual's specific capacity system. Capacity and speed of processing impact each other in that the less the amount of information that can be attended to within a given time, the slower the processing of that information. Similarly, the faster the processing of the information, the greater the amount that can be attended to within a given time. The key feature of the attentional capacity is that it is limited and such limitation produces the experience of mental effort or concentration and creates the need for selection. The more stimuli we attempt to attend to at a given time, the more sense of effort we tend to experience. Our minds are unable to attend to every sight, sound, smell, thought, memory, and action impinging on us at any given moment. To function effectively, we require a process to selectively focus on some stimuli while neglecting others (Cohen, 1993; Weber, 1990; Schneider and Shiffrin, 1977). This process has been referred to as the ability to "triage", incoming information and attention becomes the mental process permitting the individual to sift through stimuli, directing the attention to the relevant (as opposed to the irrelevant). The idea of "triage" creates a hierarchy of determining what is attended to first. Novel stimuli tends to take precedence, followed by goals or sets, and biological drives and needs specific to the individual (Heilman, Valenstein, and Watson, 1995).

Humans are limited by a maximal rate of information transmission; this limitation is more severe in young children, the developmentally disabled, the very elderly, and those individuals who are demented. The cerebral network becomes the resource allocated to the individual. The extent to which a mental operation interferes with a concurrent unrelated task is the result of how much resource the task engages and where in the network the generated activity for the functions for each task is located. Thus, the more complex the mental operation and the less compatible such mental operations are with one another, the more of the network such operations will occupy (Kinsbourne, 1994).

Factors limiting attentional performance can be either structural or energetic. Structural capacity is limited by the constraints of memory, neural processing speed, the nature of the temporal–spatial representation, and other neural-system characteristics that influence how much information can be processed at one time. These factors combine to affect the global attentional resources of the individual. In addition to these structural factors, there are energetic factors that reflect the short-term capacity of the system: arousal and effort. The concept of arousal has been controversial; however, there is general agreement that it does set the general energetic tone for the system. Effort is another energetic factor that reflects the momentary disposition of the individual toward a task and level of effort is governed by multiple factors including reinforcement and motivational influences. With increasing age, capacity is limited by problems of inhibition and the increased inability to inhibit irrelevant information. The capacity itself or the ability to process information is not limited; however, the ability to inhibit interfering information is impacted by age (Cohen, 1993; Duchek and Balota, 1993).

Control refers to a person's ability to guide the selective process by directing and organizing whatever attentional capacity is available. Normal mental functioning requires an individual to select a limited number of stimuli to be processed at any given moment. The basis for selection needs to be maintained over sufficient time periods to provide coherence to both thought and action. The goal is for the individual to maintain a standard of what is relevant, not be distracted by irrelevant stimuli, and yet continually remain attuned to a wide range of "unattended" stimuli to allow future relevant stimuli to be detected and brought into focus. Shifts of attention for new and different stimuli need to be based on the appropriate relevance of that stimuli to a person's life. If this does not occur, the person would continually respond to irrelevant stimuli and not be efficient in functioning, either by reducing capacity and/or loss of what may have been relevant stimuli (Weber, 1990).

Shifts of attention can be accomplished quickly and efficiently, provided that control of attention exists. The control is usually part of what is referred to as the supervisory attentional system. A control deficit reflects impairment of the executive functioning of the brain (the ability to set appropriate goals, form plans and strategies, and act in accordance with those plans and strategies with appropriate self-monitoring, use of performance feedback, and self-correction). Both capacity and control are *critical* factors. It is the limited nature of capacity that necessitates a selective focus. In the absence of control, attention reverts to an automatic process that does not utilize capacity. Control problems tend to be associated with impairment of the frontal lobes, while capacity problems are associated with diffuse damage to the brain and subcortical structures. Sensory selection refers to the attentional control that initially occurs during relatively early stages of information processing before the development of a response. Component processes of sensory selection involve that of filtering, focusing, and automatic shifting. The earliest form of selection occurs as a result of filtering mechanisms that are attuned to specific neural characteristics. Focusing is accomplished in the higher-order sensory systems and interacts with motivational and response-mediated influences. The neural response of these sensory systems is either enhanced or inhibited by expectancies based on the information that then primes attention. Automatic shifting of attention occurs as a result of focusing in conjunction with the original orienting response, which becomes controlled by habituation and sensitization factors (Cohen, 1993; Shallice, 1994). Madden and Plude (1993) conclude that, with age, the ability to inhibit processing for selective attention also declines.

Attending is influenced by the response demands associated with a situation that then comprises factors relating to response selection. Four component processes appear to be necessary in selective *response selection*: response intention, initiation and inhibition, active switching and executive supervisory control. These component processes are both interdependent and hierarchical. Intentionality and response initiation and inhibition contribute to the individual's ability for active switching and executive control. These processes are mainly under the influence of anterior brain systems located in the premotor and prefrontal cortex. Active attentional switching involves an exploratory search of the environment; an example of this is "looking" and various forms of observing behavior as expressions of active attentional switching (Cohen, 1993).

Neural Overview of Attention

Attention is not seen as a unitary process that can be localized to any one region of the brain. This conclusion is confirmed by a vast amount of research, experimental and clinical findings. The term *attention* is therefore not seen as a unitary function, but rather refers to a class of cognitive and behavioral processes that share one feature, which is the control and selection of stimuli and responses. The neural mechanisms underlying attention vary as a function of the specific characteristics of the behavioral context and the task demands. There are sequential operations that control different stages of selection. Pathways carrying information from primary sensory receptors to primary sensory cortex and to unimodal association cortex areas are arranged as multiple parallel pathways in a top-down approach that also has its own internal hierarchy. Flexibility is ensured via neural connectivity within heteromodal association areas, paralimbic and limbic areas, to allow continual modification to occur. This massive, parallel distributed processing allows for rapid attentional surveying of extensive information to provide cognitive consideration of numerous alternatives and determination of the best fit (Cohen and Sparling-Cohen, 1993; Mesulam, 1995).

Specifically, information received via the sensory systems activates subcortical functioning before any cortical activation or registration of the sensory information at the higher cortical level has occurred. The initial response is thus based on gross informational features (as the cortical areas have not yet been activated) due only to the sensory pathways being activated. As a result, there is little sensory resolution and the detection of an occurrence of a new stimulus is the only information that will provide for more detailed processing. This original response then elicits postural changes in the individual and is associated with an automatic shift of attention to region of space. The individual directs attention spatially to the significant stimulus. The new stimulus additionally triggers reticular activation, which is critical to energizing the system, providing arousal for response preparation, and further stimulating cognitive operation. The occurrence of these events prior to cortical registration suggests that the earliest attentional (spatial) response involves rather automatic activation. The resulting shifts in attentional direction occur as a function of a very gross level of information processing (Cohen, 1993; Mesulam, 1995; Heilman, Valenstein, and Watson, 1995).

Sensory information, upon reaching the sensory cortex, triggers a number of perceptual processes, which then provide for various levels of perceptual resolution of the critical features of the stimuli in question. Stimulus features undergo filtering and analysis during these stages of processing, resulting in a sharpening of the important features of the stimulus and attention to other aspects of information as well. At this point, informational processing is still relatively automatic and not highly modifiable; however, associative information and energetic factors may begin to be influential. After this pre-attentional information processing, information is then integrated within higher cortical systems. Areas of the inferior parietal lobule and temporal lobes appear to be the location of this integration. At this stage, the processing characteristics can be modified and the biases of the system have a direct impact on attentional selection. Thus, information flow has gone through sensory analysis to the processing stage that enables the new information to then be focused and modified in relation to pre-existing biases. Reticular activation elicited at this point produces a general energizing that affects not only sensory processes, but also the response selection systems of the frontal lobes, as well as limbic (emotional behaviors, learning, memory) and hypo-thalamic (internal state) response. Response selection systems can operate to some degree independently of the sensory selection. The frontal lobe has a reciprocal interaction with both the attention systems of the parietal lobe and the limbic system (Cohen, 1993; Mesulam, 1995).

This interaction is critical in the attentional selection as the frontal systems govern the organization of search, as well as the generation of a sequence of attentional responses in complex situations. Although selective attention can be shown to depend mostly on the parietal system, the frontal system still plays a critical role. This allows, in the absence of stimulation, that people can still experience affective, motivational, and other impulses that trigger response intention, preparation, planning, initiation, and control. Based on feedback received from response selection and new sensory input, all of these issues affect the bias for further sensory selection and the direction of sensory attention (Cohen, 1993; Heilman, Valenstein, & Watson, 1995; Mesulam, 1995).

The limbic and paralimbic systems also play significant roles in modulating attentional response. As information is accessed to the limbic system, it is given affective or emotional salience and is then integrated according to the ongoing pressures from the motivational-drive systems of the hypothalamus. Information seems to be filtered or gated within the limbic system (the excitatory and inhibitory influences created by the salience or degree of importance of the new information in relation to prior patterns of connectivity), which creates the bias for learning of certain information. This bias is an important aspect for attention and, as a result of this limbic processing, information is given different weights of importance; thus, the salience greatly influences the allocation of attention or the intensity of focus and may receive more elaborate processing and is subsequently more likely to gain long-term storage (Cohen, 1993; Heilman et al., 1995; Mesulam, 1995).

Information that is well integrated demands less active and controlled attentional allocation. The reticular system, which produces ascending activation, catalyzes the overall system and, to a point, increases attentional capacity, and additional energetic pressures are provided by the hypothalamus (responsible for internal regulation and the site of primitive motivational responses) (Cohen, 1993; Mesulam, 1995). Energetic factors from both the reticular system and the hypothalamus create a pressure to "act" relative to an overall, rather broad goal, and it is only at the level of the limbic system that these pressures are then further specified and modulated based on interaction with pre-existing associative information (Cohen, 1993; Mesulam, 1995).

Neuropsychological research on brain functioning indicates that attentional problems vary as a result of different problems that have occurred within the brain. Lesions in the anterior areas of the brain, such as the prefrontal cortex, are known to cause problems of intention (planning and self-regulation). Unilateral lesions in the sensory association areas are likely to produce problems of attention (neglect in the sensory selection process). The right hemisphere appears to subserve spatial function as a more-dominant force directing attention to both sides of the body and space, while the left hemisphere prepares only the right side of the body and space for action. Lesions in the limbic system are known to affect the attentional capacity by changing memory registration, excitatory–inhibitory behavioral control processes, and the importance assigned or attributed to the signals that are processed. Damage to the lower subcortical centers often tends to disrupt the overall energetic tone and has attentional consequences as well. The neuropsychology of attention is still in its infancy. In process is the development of a unified neuropsychology of attention that requires an integration of information assimilating cognitive, behavioral and neural bases of attention (Cohen, 1993; Heilman, Valenstein, and Watson, 1995; Mesulam, 1995).

Specific Types of Attention

Divided attention refers to an attentional task, whereby the individual must attend to two or more inputs or activities at the same time. This level of attentional capacity is required whenever multiple, simultaneous demands must be managed. Research studies have attempted to determine the impact upon capacity when two or more issues are occurring at the same time. Research is inconclusive; however, what is clear is that attending to two or more tasks will demand more capacity than attending to only one. Control must be involved in divided-attention tasks in order to organize the distribution of attention between two or more sets of stimuli or activities.

Focused or selective attention refers to the selection of some stimuli rather than others as the focus of attention. Selection is the control feature of human cognition when the individual has to attend to only one of two or more inputs. Usually these two or more inputs are concurrent ones and the individual has to attend to one message, but not to the other. Performance under such conditions (such as driving a car while listening to the radio, or holding a conversation during meal preparation) may reflect either rapid and continuous, alternating attention, or dependence on more unconscious automatic-processing components of the attentional network. This level of attention requires the ability to maintain a behavioral or cognitive set in the face of distracting or competing stimuli. Individuals with deficits are easily drawn off-task by extraneous, irrelevant stimuli (which may include external sights and sounds or activities, as well as internal thoughts and concerns). The consequence of directing attention to some information will be at a cost to efficiency in others. Three elementary mental operations appear to be involved in moving attention from one location in space to another: the disengagement of attention from its current focus, moving attention to another location, and engaging attention at that location. Parietal lobe functioning is seen as specifically affecting the "disengage" operation (the ability to disengage attention from its current focus). Mid-brain structures affect the "move" component of the attentional orienting, and prefrontal operations are responsible for the "engage" operation. Selective attention begins early by modifying processing in the cortical areas that encode elementary stimulus features, which precede the fully analyzed patterns, and this is confirmed by studies of electrical and magnetic brain recordings (Nissen, 1986; Mateer, Sohlberg, and Youngman, 1990; Posner, 1989; Hillyard et al., 1995).

Sustained attention refers to an individual's ability to maintain an effective attentional set over an extended period and would be a factor in variability of performance over time. Individuals are required to shift their focus of attention and move between tasks having different cognitive requirements, thus controlling which information will be selectively attended to (Mateer, Sohlberg, and Youngman, 1990). Problems with these types of attentional tasks are evidenced by individuals who are unable to change once a "set" has been established, and thus require extra cueing to initiate new task requirements. Real-life demands for this type of attentional processing are frequent. Sustaining attention and maintaining an accurate level of vigilance would overlap both automatic and deliberate attentional functions. Sustaining attention requires the necessary control to keep a goal in mind and not be distracted by other events, including one's own thoughts.

Sustained attention involves the ability to maintain a consistent behavioral response during continuous and repetitive activity. It incorporates the notion of vigilance. Difficulty with this level of attentional process is observed in the individual who can only focus on one task or maintain response for a brief period of time only or who generally fluctuates drastically in ability to sustain focused attention at all. This skill also takes into account the ability to exercise mental control and working memory with tasks that require the taking in of information and retaining it for use at a later time.

Sustained performance can be considered a consequence of fatiguability and factors that support or do not support vigilance. Fatiguability may be a result of intrinsic biological constraints or the reinforcement and/or motivational factors associated with a situation. Vigilance is also impacted by motivational factors, as well as the frequency of the targets to be detected. Sustained attention is determined on an ongoing basis by sensory selection, response selection and capacity limitations that are always present (Cohen, 1993; Mateer, Sohlberg, and Youngman, 1990).

Intentional attention is associated with voluntary attention and the notion of control. Alternating attention is the ability to move attention appropriately from one selective focus to another, which is an aspect of control that requires capacity. This level of attention also refers to the ability for mental flexibility.

Attentional Functioning Applied to ADD

Brumback (1992) defined ADD as a primary disorder of vigilance, whereby the diminished ability to sustain an alert, awake state resulted in symptoms of poor attention, poor concentration, and problems being "awake". Infants with the primary disorder of vigilance were described as "good sleepers" and easy to care for. Difficulty with attention did not present itself as symptomatic until some type of learning situation became part of the child's life. This disorder of vigilance was found to be a dominantly inherited condition, lifelong in nature, and tends to worsen with age. Adults with the primary disorder may deny sleepiness, but readily admit to boredom in tasks that are repetitious or require continuous mental performance and tend to avoid such activities diligently. Such adults commonly fall asleep when remaining still (as in church), experiencing "naps" that are not refreshing (Brumback, 1992).

Symptoms of ADD occur when the task is not inherently attention attracting (novel, enjoyable, or immediately rewarding) and, at that point, sustained performance requires additional support from incentive (internal) motivators (with its circuitry to be found in the mesolimbic and mesocortical dopaminergic projections, originating in the ventral tegmentum area). Spontaneous exploratory behavior then depends on the integrity of the ventral tegmentum, which can be manipulated by the use of dopamine (DA) agonists and DA blockers. Behavior that is sensation seeking or novelty seeking depends on the reactivity of the mid-brain DA system. When resting, DA transmission is depleted, sensation seeking would then be at a maximum and, under these circumstances, only novel (or rewarded and directly motivating) stimuli would capture one's attention. Stimulus salience has been found to exert control on the attention of ADD children as opposed to normal children. When resting, DA transmission is temporally increased by a DA agonist; the ADD individual finds it possible to persist in tasks that call for incentive (internal) motivation, as well as the ability to work for delayed reward. In the absence of impairment with specific cerebral locus (whereby damage impairs the ability to attend in general, or the ability to selectively attend at different locations, or utilize the selection of different categories of attending), ADD, by virtue of its impact on the DA system, impacts the whole attentional system in a generalized manner (Kinsbourne, 1994).

CHAPTER 3

Manifestations and Consequences of Attentional Deficit

Research in attentional deficit has primarily addressed the head-injured population who frequently experience attentional and memory deficits as hallmark symptoms resulting from mild, moderate, and severe impact to the frontal and temporal lobes. Symptoms noted appear highly similar to those of the ADD population.

Reduced Capacity

The person whose capacity is reduced is unaware of or unable to attend to the substantial amount of information necessary at one time for adaptive, everyday functioning. Consequently, such an individual would require more time to process a given amount of information and be unable to participate in rapid intake and scanning of environmental information. This deficit manifests itself as a described difficulty with concentration, remembering, understanding what others have said, reading speed and comprehension, computational errors, and coping with life's demands at home, school, or work. Although able to perform the same tasks as others, the individual is not able to perform them at the necessary speed or rate. Tasks require more effort, resulting in increased stress and fatigue, and functioning "below normal" levels. ADD individuals evidence overall slow cognitive speed impacting timed assessment, as well as the ability to maintain themselves as integrated parts of a social conversation or setting, business meeting environment and/or classroom or academic system.

Nissen (1986) discusses capacity as the conscious mental effort that is invested in the performance of a task, emphasizing processes requiring attentional or controlled processing (as opposed to automatic), the notion of limited capacity, the result being that the investing of attentional capacity in one task will interfere with the performance of another task that also requires that capacity. The result is a difficulty of performing two tasks at once (unless one is so well practiced that it proceeds automatically) and an overall limited-capacity attentional system. Similarly, the decrement in task performance over long periods of time, which tends to occur with vigilance or continuous performance tasks, is due to the difficulty in maintaining attentional capacity.

The concept of short-term memory is also linked to capacity. The contents of short-term memory are available to general awareness. The capacity of short-term memory provides a working space for active attentional processing. If the primary task becomes more difficult, resulting in an increase of its demand or resources that are shared with the concurrent task, the primary task performance will become more dependent on the shared resource. The consequence will create the necessity of priorities, of the resource allocation available on the primary task performance. The extent to which the two tasks share a common resource determines the degree to which the primary task performance can be preserved at the same level, despite the increased task difficulty, through resource allocation, requiring the sacrificing the secondary task (Näätänen, 1992).

An example of this is passively elicited attention that is initiated by stimuli rather than by the individual will or choice. Stimuli can capture attention by employing novel or salient physical or semantic properties. Certain physical-stimulus events are attention catching with abrupt stimulus onset or change of continuous stimulus. ADD individuals will tend to prioritize attention in a manner not always conducive to task completion and/or long-term process as a consequence of reduced capacity, inappropriate salience, and overresponse to novelty.

Diminished Control

People with control problems may be able to attend fairly well if others are available to aid them in getting started and remind them to stay on-task until it is completed. When individuals with control problems are left to their own initiative, they can easily lose track of what they are saying, doing, or thinking. Consequently, not only is there a problem of sustaining an appropriate focus of attention, there are also problems moving the focus from one task to another in an appropriate flexible though controlled manner that remains somewhat fixed in accordance with set goals of the individual.

Generally, every work setting contains a degree of irrelevant, distracting stimuli and thus requires focused attention. Auditory stimuli have been found to be more of a problem than visual stimuli simply because individuals do not tend to be distracted by stimuli outside of their visual field and, in vision, the act of focusing on specific stimuli automatically precludes interference from the majority of irrelevant stimulation. In contrast to the visual system, however, human voices and mechanical noises are highly distracting. When these sounds are constant, they can become monotonous and the individual can acclimate to them quickly and effectively. People rarely complain of the disturbing effect of the ticking clock or the hum of office machinery; however, friendly and social discussions play havoc with their ability to focus, due to the two-fold impact of pitch and volume, as well as verbal content, both of which serve as distractions. Another factor is that, due to ongoing mental slowness and loss of information, there is a cumulative loss of information and an inability to formulate a mental with which to interpret incoming data set of what is going on in one's environment. As the information system is less effective in filtering, more irrelevant information will tend to dominate thinking, creating more of a problem with focused attention. Thus, a focused-attention problem can also occur as a secondary symptom of impairment in information processing (van Zomeren and Brouwer, 1994).

Mixed Capacity and Control Problems

Individuals can manifest varying mixtures of the two problems of capacity and control. Normal attention function requires the interaction of intact capacity and control. Attention can be flexibly allocated or controlled in different proportions to the parallel tasks. Attention is characterized by resource theories as shareable, flexible, and allocable with different proportions and degrees.

Divided attention tasks occur generally in every occupation, e.g., the office worker completing clerical tasks while answering the phone, interrupted by staff, and having to recall what he/she was doing prior to the interruptions. Thus, the worker must maintain and sustain attention to the task he/she was involved in prior to the interruption, and then focus and attend to the interruption. Other examples are that of an individual in an interview situation, in a courtroom, or teaching a class, whereby he/she needs to recall and sustain attention to the subject material, dividing his/her attention, focusing on the responses of those he/she is interacting with, and thus accounting for a number of variables at one time. Divided attention problems account for overall distractibility, as well as loss of information characterizing the ADD population.

Multiple Resource Failure

Wickens (1984) discusses the idea of multiple resources as more than one commodity in the human processing system that may be assigned resource-like properties of shareability, flexibility, and allocability. The more separate, rather than common, the resources demanded by the two tasks are, the more efficient the time-sharing is. Structured alteration effects or dual task performance occur when a change in task structure affects the amount of overlap in resource demands of the two tasks. If one of the tasks becomes more difficult, i.e., the increasing resource demand involves at least in part resources that are also required in a concurrent task, the latter performance deteriorates. If the increasing resource demand involves resources that are not utilized by the secondary task performance, that performance is not affected (Näätänen, 1992).

The ability to process information is often used as a means of determining if an individual is ready to return to work after sustaining injury to the brain. Information processing and the missing of information depends on a number of functions, such as multiple resource allocation, time-sharing, control, capacity, and so on. This becomes highly problematic in the work setting or in communication in general due to the missing of details, instructions, and directions (notable for ADD), and also impacts the ability to learn new information unless that information is highly stimulating. Efficient time-sharing between two tasks is possible when the two tasks engage different mechanisms and structures. Time-sharing can be said to be perfect when the two tasks can be performed concurrently, as well as separately.

Lack of Alertness

Alertness refers to the general readiness of the individual to act on information. Alertness is characterized as a continuum, with the most severe lack being the comatose state at one end of the spectrum to decreased sustained attentional processes at the other. Individuals with decreased alertness are unable to respond to sensory processing stimuli and changes occurring in their environment throughout a typical day (Nissen, 1986). Sustaining attention is a basic prerequisite necessary for students or any individual involved in the learning of new information. The interaction with others (personally or professionally) in the work setting, driving skill, and competence in any area necessitating sustained focus and attention to task is diminished by an overall lack of alertness that impacts the everyday functioning ability of the ADD individual.

Driving: An Example of the Interplay of a Number of Attentional Factors

Driving skill has been studied in the head-injured population and findings indicate that safe driving demands less in the way of basic ability and fewer resources of the experienced driver as opposed to the beginner. Moderately high correlations were found between driving experience and distance driven, and driving quality and safety. Interestingly, the driving ability of the experienced driver was not predicted in a positive direction based on neuropsychological evaluation, indicating that impairment as observed in a testing situation may not apply to the experienced driver when generalized. In studying driving skill, the variables of speed of information processing and cognitive flexibility were assessed. Reaction time (the speed variable) was not related significantly to expertise in driving. What was suggested from the research was that the ability to switch attention (cognitive flexibility) and the ability to focus attention upon the relevant was significantly related to accident rate. The key issue is that of switching sets and selective attention, and less of an issue for divided and sustained attention. Notable was the finding of a problem with visual distinction in which peripheral information was neglected in the presence of relevant central information. The question arises as to the effect of hemineglect and the impaired ability to disengage attention from the central source of information. Eye disease, information-processing strategy, and general resource limitations can also affect driving skill. Spatial disorientation was used by some researchers to account for accidents and the idea that individuals lose their way while driving. The ability to sustain attention has been viewed as a global indicator of driving skill, especially during long and boring rides, which has been found to be most relevant for epilepsy, and the finding that seizures tend to occur in low event-rate situations (van Zomeren and Brouwer, 1994). Statistics commonly were higher for accident rates for the attention-disordered population similar to that of the head-injured or neurologically impaired (Weiss, 1993; Wender, 1995).

Social Skills Are also Impacted by Interrelationships among a Number of Attentional Factors

Research is minimal relating social skills to injury to the brain;, however, studies indicate that brain-damaged individuals do not notice relevant social cues in terms of facial expression, intonation, and the emotional content of remarks. They miss the subtleties, and thus appear to others to be either uninvolved, shy, self-centered, snobbish, or inappropriate. The impact of social skills has been noted and researched to some degree in evaluating medication efficacy in the ADD population. Expressions of thought and feeling, as well as the ability to communicate, have been noted as common occurrences by both the head-injured and the attention-disordered populations. Research indicates that the head-injured group speaks at a significantly slower rate, with greater monotone, for shorter periods, and is less spontaneous when compared to controls. Social interaction tends to be complex and problematic; information processing is related to poor social skills, not from a speed perspective, but from the need to utilize and have available information regarding a complex interplay of factors. Research indicates that head-injured individuals are not effective in encouraging others to interact with them socially. This relates quite well to the symptoms and observed interactions in the attention-disordered population, in which the delineation of problems with social skills is well researched and noted; both children and adults exhibit problems in interpersonal functioning related to poorly developed social skills ranging from mild to severe. ADHD individuals tend to be rejected due to inappropriate behavior; ADD individuals tend to be neglected because they do not present behavioral problems, and tend to misunderstand and be confused as to what is occurring around them. Problems with speech and language development further exacerbate these communication problems (Flicek, 1992; Giddan, 1991; Landau and Moore, 1991; van Zomeren and Brouwer, 1994).

CHAPTER 4

Anatomical Structures Implicated in the Disorder

Theoretical Basis

Human and animal studies have sought to evolve from a structural perspective of a thorough understanding of the phenomenon of attention that underlies the basic functioning of the human organism and accounts for the impact of neurological dysfunctioning and symptoms observed pursuant to a neurological disorder. Attention is defined as the process allowing for information reduction, whereby individuals are able to process and respond to an infinite amount of information that is present in their environment on a continual basis.

It is obvious that individuals cannot process at one time the vast amount of information present in their environment, and the reduction of information is critical to allow for cognitive processing to occur without overwhelming the individual and creating information overload. Consequently, to allow for information reduction, attention must provide for information selection (meaning that the information must not only be reduced, but also selected to establish a priority of specific information) that is relevant for further processing to occur. As a result, certain stimuli are attended to while others are not, thus allowing for certain information to be selected for the more-advanced processing to occur. Attention can therefore be viewed as the interface between the input of information to the brain via the senses and the higher-order cognition that must occur for the conclusion of behavioral action. An example is attentional neglect, whereby it is not just the registration of the information that is necessary for attention, it is also the cognitive impact that becomes so important in determining what is attended to in the individual's spatial field (P. Cohen et al., 1993; Heilman, Valenstein, and Watson, 1995).

Attention provides for the interaction of incoming information with old learning (or memory components already in existence), i.e., while immediate attention influences the encoding of new information, the existing information (already within the memory systems) influences the characteristics of attention as well, and together this dual impact creates a reciprocal system between attention and memory (Cohen, 1994; Mesulam, 1995).

Attention has been found to be spatially distributed. The spatial characteristics of the stimuli in question can influence the attentional parameters, and attentional selection can then depend on the individual's relationship to the spatial environment. Thus, attention requires several spatially oriented activities to occur almost simultaneously, involving the search of the environment for salient stimuli to be detected, a focus on that stimuli and consequent cognitive processing, all the while rejecting or inhibiting responses to other locations. Humans, as a species, appear capable of diffusing spatial attention to increase the ability of detection from all spatial locations. Presentation in the peripheral visual field, depth, and vertical or horizontal orientation, are all critical factors in determining the parameters of attention (Cohen, 1994; Heilman, Chatterjee, and Doty, 1995).

Attention is also temporally distributed, and this specific variable of attentional processes indicates that attention is a reflection of the selection of information over time. This suggests that attentional control can be governed by the serial processing of human information and that the sequence of incoming information can impact and influence the attentional processes. Failure to maintain an attentional response can occur as the consequence of competing influences that have prevailed; a time factor or temporal element can produce variations in one's attention (J. Cohen, 1994).

There are additional factors of anticipation, preparation for response and the delay of response, which can become additional determinants of attention, stressing the importance of the element impacting as transitional behaviors that occur prior to a response. The relationship between attention and the action to be taken becomes contingent upon the individual's response to time parameters. Anticipation refers to a process of sensitization and general activation that occurs prior to a response demand that is expected to occur at a later time and date. Preparation is the behavioral response to the anticipation of impending demands and is generated to facilitate subsequent performance of action.

Response delay refers to the action of inhibiting immediate responding, despite the presence of anticipatory concerns or other pressures to respond. It is the capacity for response delay that is necessary for sustained attention to occur (J. Cohen, 1994).

Attentional selection and focus of attention are governed by motivational factors, and stimuli can vary in importance and salience (as well as reinforcement strength) for the individual which can comprise many individual differences and idiosyncrasies. Thus, not all stimuli have the same attentional value and some stimuli will have intrinsic qualities that will create process selection and become subject to factors of cue strength. Attention then becomes dependent on and influenced by a whole host of variables that have a bearing on stimulus value, such as novelty, complexity, and strength. The status of the individual (physical and emotional) at any point in time dictates the strength of a particular stimuli and variables present at that time will also impact the strength of that stimuli. Attentional capacity varies as a function of the individual's internal factors. Energetic state, motivational factors, and natural differences differ among individuals and thus influence attentional capacity. Capacity refers to the degree to which the individual is able to divide his/her attention between multiple stimuli, to handle large loads of information, and to sustain attention to task, and thus speaks to the general brain energy available at a given time (J. Cohen, 1994; Mesulam, 1995).

Individuals generally will have a limited capacity for divided attention among multiple sources of information. Demonstrations of parallel distributed processing indicates that individuals have a greater capacity for divided attention, however, than originally thought. Capacity for divided attention is determined by the degree to which the information to be processed or the behavior to be performed is already integrated in long-term memory storage, which would allow for an attentional automaticity to occur in response to well-rehearsed information. There are automatic and controlled attentional operations that are variable, determining the consequence of the effortful demands that a task places upon the individual. Those tasks that can be performed automatically place less attentional effort on the individual and, of course, are more automatic in nature. Attention that is automatic, however, can at some point become more controlled in nature, requiring greater effort if conditions change, such as driving a car and the road detours or weather conditions worsen unexpectedly. The attentional demands created by a task influences the capacity for sustained attention and the subjective experience of effort, and which, after a period of time, sustained effort can produce subjective fatigue. The task that requires greater levels of controlled attention is more likely to produce a conscious awareness, and there continues to be a debate as to whether attention depends on conscious awareness. Individuals are able to attend to a task without being aware of their actions at all times, such as driving a car, and the question is debated as to where one is consciously aware and how to define that phenomenon from attention, and similarly, what do we call attention and what do we call awareness (J. Cohen, 1994; Mesulam, 1995; Weber, 1990).

Attention, generally, is the byproduct of multiple interactive processes and is not a unitary process; it refers to a set of cognitive-behavioral processes involved in the selection of information and in the control of the behavioral response. Attention is determined by numerous multiple factors and by specific subsets of neural systems operating in a parallel distributed network employing a top-down approach. Finally, attentional processes are adaptive and, as such, are sensitive to changes continually occurring within the individual's environment (both external and internal) with attention being enhanced by variations that add excitement and salience to the stimulus set and not enhanced or attenuated (resulting in habituation) as the task becomes more redundant in nature (J. Cohen, 1994; Heilman, Valenstein, and Watson, 1995; Mesulam, 1995).

Summarizing the Neural Mechanisms of the Process of Attention

Attention is not localized to any one site and instead is the result of a network of neural systems involving several major neuroanatomical structures. The neuroanatomical systems involved in attentional control are commensurate with the functional organization of the brain in that the more complex is organized around the basic or less advanced. Thus, higher-order cognitive attentive functions are organized around the basic sensory, motor, and regulatory functions, and it is these higher-order systems associated with the sensory and motor systems that play the fundamental role in the control of attention, presenting a vertical, top-down approach (Mesulam, 1995).

The neuroanatomical systems involved in attentional control are separated into two cortical divisions corresponding to the distinction between the motor and sensory systems. Posterior brain systems are associated with sensory function and are involved in sensory (attention) selection, while anterior systems are associated with motor functions (interior) and are involved in the response preparation and initiation of action. Attention depends on the integration of these two systems. The neural systems are hierarchically arranged in a vertical direction of cortical and subcortical, whereby subcortical systems, such as the reticular system and the hypothalamus, produce active, general-aroused states, directing the individual to respond, and controlling biological functioning, such as the regulation of one's physiological state or appetitive behaviors, such as eating and sleep. At the center of the subcortical system is the limbic system and the basal ganglia modulating impulses from both lower subcortical areas and higher cortical sites. By having both excitatory and inhibitory capabilities, these systems are able to fine-tune the situation and impact less-modulated subcortical impulses (J. Cohen, 1994; Mesulam, 1995; Heilman, Valenstein, and Watson, 1995; Posner, 1995).

These systems appear to be highly flexible in their repertoire of actions, responding to and integrating multimodal sources of information, as well as facilitating the encoding of this information in a highly distributed and diverse cortical system. At the top of the hierarchy, the cortex provides for the multimodal correlation that occurs, whereby new information is associated with what has been previously encoded and learned. Thus, there is an interface between immediate biological pressures that automatically govern behavior and associative processes (incorporating prior learning) that then shape and reshape these pressures in continual concert with the feedback of prior experience. It is this interface and constant interaction that creates attentional control.

The degree to which the cells of particular brain systems exhibit neural plasticity determines their attentional role and cortical regions that have cells with highly crystallized architecture appear to be more "hardwired", resulting in their function being more specific and less subject to variation. Tertiary association cortex areas appear to have less specificity of function and greater neural plasticity, such as the mesocortical areas, as the cingulate gyrus, and the parahippocampal and entorhinal cortex, as they are less differentiated. The limbic system has been found to have a high degree of plasticity. Attention appears to depend on the interaction of the neural systems with less plasticity, which then provide the template to set the experience for the more-plastic neural systems to be modified in accordance with what is needed in terms of behavioral adaptation. The modification of neural cells in accordance with sensory input becomes a means by which attentional enhancement can then occur and also provide appropriate behavioral adaptation.

Processes of habituation, sensitization, and classical conditioning are some of the more-basic behavioral processes that underlie attentional response. Habituation and sensitization are processes that explain the facilitation and continued attenuation of the orienting response to new stimuli and, in more controlled situations, the relationship between the stimulus presentation and these responses can then be specified with some degree of precision (resulting in skilled improvement and automatic attentional processing). Thus, the attentional response to simple stimuli with little informational value and greater predictability due to less variability would provide a starting point from which to build the foundation for classical conditioning, creating a link between attention and memory formations. Habituation and sensitization can be demonstrated with many levels of complexity and these processes become neurally linked with classical conditioning.

Attentional control is then established by the interaction of inhibitory and excitatory processes evident at many different levels of the entire nervous system, from the interactions of large brain systems to events occurring within individual cells. Such arrangements are critical for normal attentional operations to provide the mechanisms that stop, delay, or maintain responding relative to a particular class of stimuli. Several of the relevant inhibitory–excitatory arrangements are the cortical modulation of subcortical impulses, the inhibitory functions of the prefrontal cortex, the reciprocal relationship between amygdaloid and septal influences during limbic system responses of stimuli that is reinforcing, and the lateral inhibition across cells of the visual system that provides the tuning to specific spatial frequencies (J. Cohen, 1994; Mesulam, 1995). The amygdala is seen as playing a critical role in attention, specifically the central nucleus of the amygdala in the regulation of the attentional processing of cues during learning. This area of brain functioning also mediates conditioned fear and anxiety (Davis, 1997). Research provides ramifications for the continual fear and anxiety displayed in the disorder of ADD without hyperactivity and perhaps future studies will pinpoint an anatomical correlation.

The action of the neurotransmitters provides neurochemical mediation to influence the attentional response and modulate the neuronal response. Neurochemical variation is generally slower and produces more gradual change in the attentional tone than that of bioelectrical variation, which provides more direct neuronal activation, and which is likely to produce a more rapid attentional response. It is the neurochemical variation that serves to expand the time horizon of the attentional response and circadian variations in attentional capacity illustrates the presence of these more gradual changes resulting in a number of variations that occur over the course of the day. It is clear that there are both general and specific effects of the neurochemical impact on attention. CNS stimulants are an example of a drug that can produce a generalized increase in vigilance, while other drugs can disrupt the selectivity of attention. Dopaminergic agonists tend to change the ability of the neural systems to gate information, again illustrating the biochemical impact on the attentional processes (J. Cohen, 1994).

Neural processing speed can influence attentional capacity and it has become apparent that a minimal neural processing speed is necessary for incoming information to be able to maintain the integrity of its content. When there is a slowing beyond this level, input losses can occur in terms of the informational content, processing can then become more effortful, and attentional failures can occur as a result. Finally, certain neural cells can have specific or special attentional features and, in addition to the interaction and networking of the brain structures, there are also certain brain sites that provide neurons equipped with specific attentional function. Two areas identified as specific attentional areas are the frontal eye fields and the inferior parietal lobule. These areas seem to be convergence areas with multimodal association cortex capable of processing information on a higher-order level and integrating that information. The frontal eye fields serve to influence sacadic movements and the ability to look and to orient oneself, while the inferior parietal lobule serves to enhance the response to the spatial location prior to an actual stimulus occurring, and this enhancement provides the explanation for the act of attentional focusing (J. Cohen, 1994; Vogt, Finch, and Olson, 1992; Heilman, Valenstein, and Watson, 1995).

The Role of Neuronal Synchronization

Selective routing of sensory information to appropriate motor programs is facilitated by the process of synchronization which integrates the response to specific features and general information of the visual world. The synchronicity of the cell assemblies and their discharges, extending over large cortical areas in the visual and motor cortex play a significant role in visuomotor integration (Roelfsema et al., 1997).

The process of synchronicity allows neurons that exhibit similar selectivity for stimulus features to be linked together and co-activated. Changes occur locally and lead to global changes that influence these networks to operate as a decoding dimension to detect connectivity and to use this as a discriminatory grouping criterion. Co-incident firing by neurons allows for more explicit features, translating firing patterns into a response coded for selectivity. Neurons become simultaneously selective for more than one feature domain. The feature integration theory of attention suggests that the response of selective neurons within restricted regions of the visual cortex corresponds to the focus of attention and is integrated into a coherent perception. The visual field position becomes the determinant of the response. Various feature domains provide the method to link apparently diverse dimensions for perceptual grouping. Neurons exhibit premovement activity that are adapted by the assemblies of synchronous firing neurons that trigger their activity. Synchronizing connections between motor cortical neurons are thought to coordinate and facilitate the selection of the appropriate compatible movement and the cooperative interactions among premovement activity increases the likelihood that appropriate movement components are selected simultaneously. Overall firing rates and synchronous firing rates of neurons via mutual dependence, determine the route along which synchrony may spread and the degree of synchronicity among action potentials in converging afferents influences firing rates (Roelfsema et al., 1997).

Attention as a Process Can Occur in a Step-Wise Fashion

Attention occurs in a specific hierarchical process, commencing with sensory selection determining response selection and control leading to attentional capacity (encompassing structural factors) and, finally, to sustained performance. Sensory selection refers to those attentional processes that operate in association with or soon after the initial sensory registration and perception that a stimulus has taken place. Attention then provides the means by which the individual can select certain stimuli to attend to (over other stimuli), and such selection seems to occur early in the information-processing sequence (prior to the onset of response intention). Sensory selection components are sensory filtering, focusing and selection, and automatic shifting.

Sensory filtering, which occurs quite early in the process, is closely tied with perceptual analysis, and attentional factors seem to influence what information filters through the system (primary sensory cortical systems contain neurons tuned into certain stimulus and spatial features), thus providing a degree of automaticity that can be quite high at this point. Sensory attentional focusing is less closely associated with primary perception and instead is more influenced by the input of other neural systems and sensory enhancement (focusing that occurs in the response of parietal cortical neurons to oncoming stimuli, which is either enhanced or attenuated), based on prior attentional priming. Automatic shifts of attention can occur based on prior learning, habituation, sensitization, and conditioned response. Response selection and control are critical factors underlying the attentional processing and are influenced by four related components: response intention, response initiation and inhibition, active switching, and executive regulation. These components together determine the ability of the individual to become mobilized to attend, to start and stop attentional responses, and to switch between attentional response alternatives. These components, while hierarchical, are also interdependent with one another (J. Cohen, 1994).

Attentional capacity is comprised of two subtypes, energetic and structural capacity, which reflects the idea that attention is influenced by both stable and transient or changeable behavioral and neural characteristics. Stable characteristics are described as being more invariant (specific to the individual species), whereas transient characteristics are more variable (encompassing the individual's status at that moment in time) and including their motivational or biological state. The components of structural capacity are memory capacity, processing speed, temporal-spatial dynamics, and global cognitive resources (which refers to the degree of intellectual capabilities of the individual). Situations beyond the cognitive complexity of the individual are likely to result in attenuation or inattention (J. Cohen, 1994).

Energetic capacity is influenced by several interrelated components of arousal, motivational state, and task-induced effort (which can refer to both the nonspecific arousal and behavior mechanism and the specific motivational and physiological activation of the individual). Arousal and motivation provide a catalyst to create an attentional direction, and it is the reticular activation that then appears to be central to the state of generalized CNS arousal. Motivation then becomes more of a byproduct of the interaction of the biological state of the individual and the reinforcement received or to be received from the environment (whether that is internal or external to the individual). Arousal and motivation can be governed by the nature of the task at hand and situation salience can be modified to influence those motivational factors and thus influence attentional capacity (J. Cohen, 1994; Mesulam, 1995).

Sustained attention as another attentional factor is also a byproduct of the other three factors noted above, and this type of attention can be influenced by variables that affect and impact sensory selection, response selection and control, as well as attentional capacity overall. Sustained attention is seen as a unitary factor to reflect its unique aspects as an attentional process in that sustained attention is more complex and determined by three components: vigilance, fatigue characteristics, and reinforcement contingencies.

Constraints That Can Occur to Impact Attention

The primary factors that can impact and serve to constrain attention are properties of the neural system itself, memory properties of the system or memory dysfunction, spatial representations of attention, the temporal distribution and its impact on the dynamics of attention, the nature of the perceptual representations, and finally, processing speed. These factors cannot only influence and limit what the parameters for attention can be, they also end up setting limits on the individual's attentional capacity as a whole. Variations of these factors would affect the more-transient energetic capacity of the attentional system as well (Cohen, 1993).

Finally, the Flow of Information Through the Attentional System

Evolution has provided the human organism with the ability to take in information from an array of senses, each providing a different "view", and then synergize this information to provide the adaptive ability to deal with minimal or ambiguous environmental cues. Sensory information is originally processed in a modality-specific manner, followed by convergence and integration among the sensory modalities. Attention depends on the ability to take in sensory information, the sensory systems then filter the information in an initial format, signals are analyzed via a system containing sensory comparison processes (utilizing prior learning or existing neuronal templates), a memory system enters, an affective weighing system assigns value or salience to both signals and response tendencies, the arousal system enters, a motivational system creates response pressures based on the individual's drive state, response preparatory and planning systems step in, feedback arrangements occur, and a system is implemented to provide compensatory response adjustments based on noted errors. There is a sequential flow of information; however, parallel processing can occur to account for more complex needs of the individual. The flow of information can become bidirectional as opposed to unidirectional, to account for reciprocity of the systems and continual transactional relationships that occur (J. Cohen, 1994; Heilman et al., 1995; Mesulam, 1995).

Sensory selection and focusing depends on processes that enable particular features or specific stimuli to receive more intensive, cognitive consideration while other stimuli properties or processes are ignored. Once the stimulus is fully registered within the sensory systems, a number of automatic attentional operations can then occur. Filtering describes these automatic processes' ability to sharpen stimulus features, and this early filtering has been referred to as more of an issue of visual perception than attentional phenomenon. It is after the information passes through this early processing stage that attentional focusing can occur and this stage is referenced as focus enhancement for further, more-complex selection and enhancement of the strengths and specific featured components of the stimulus (while other components are attenuated). The final features arising from this process are then subject to a final operation of object recognition and selection. Response selection and control occurs in a similar fashion, moving through parallel and multilayered systems; however, the direction of attention is driven by internal as opposed to external factors and motivation becomes the catalyst for final selection. A decision process occurs based on system biases created by past experiences, the level of arousal at the time, motivation, and factors associated with attentional capacity. The response produces an outcome and feedback determines the motivational system and continues to impact sensory selection and focusing (Cohen, 1993; Stein, Wallace, and Meredith, 1995).

Specific Structures Implicated in ADD

Tucker and Derryberry (1992) investigated the concept of motivated attention, suggesting that the frontal region of the brain appears to play important roles in planning and self-control. They suggested that these roles require close interactions between the cognitive representations of the frontal cortex and more elementary mechanisms of emotional evaluation and motivational control provided by limbic and subcortical structures. The evidence of exaggerated ventral limbic and orbital frontal activity in states of anxiety may reveal the brain mechanisms underlying the elementary processes of vigilant attention and motor readiness. These adaptive influences may be integral to more complex forms of the motivated attention required for effective planning (including such processes as organizing and sequencing actions, evaluating the significance of events, and directing attention toward the future). Thus, the frontal lobes may achieve their executive functions through vertical integration combining the representative capacities of the neocortex with the regulatory influences of the paralimbic cortex and subcortical control system (Mesulam, 1995; Tucker and Derryberry, 1992).

Selective attention was found by Liotti (1995) to involve the circuitry of the thalamus (the pulvinar mechanism specifically), which is controlled directly by axon fibers from the posterior parietal cortex whose cells are driven, in turn, by both bottom-up inputs (originating in the eye) and top-down inputs (arising from the prefrontal cortex). Detailing the structures in further depth, it can be seen how the subcortical and cortical structures interact. Cognitive processes are controlled by their patterns of connections. The dorsolateral frontal cortex receives projections from the sensory and association cortex in both the ipsilateral and contralateral hemispheres. This convergence may allow limited areas of frontal cortex to exert control over widespread sensory and integrative functions of the posterior brain. There may then be a joint activation of the frontal cortex with the associated posterior cortex such that the frontal region tunes the relevant area of posterior or motor cortex to prepare it for the perceptual and motor operation (J. Cohen, 1994; Liotti, 1995; Mesulam, 1995).

Attentional selection operates on a variety of levels within the visual system, attentional orienting operates within relatively late abstract representation, neglect is influenced by retinotopic, body-centered, and environmental reference frames. Attentional behavior in neglect is a disorder of orienting control. Neglect-like object-centered biases (whereby the center is judged to be to the right or left of the vertical midpoint, underestimations of the leftward or rightward extent of the line occur with that portion being less attended) can be evidenced in the neurologically intact brain. Each hemisphere has a contralateral attentional bias which requires that the left and right segments of each visual field must be united into a single form (Reuter-Lorenz, Drain, and Hardy-Morais, 1997). While the encoding and retrieval processes appear lateralized to the left or right hemisphere, respectively, the process linking the object to the location or place is the main responsibility of the right hippocampal region. This demonstrates that when individuals are required to combine information about objects with that of spatial location, the right hemisphere becomes preferentially involved, which is more evident during the retrieval process than the encoding (Owen et al., 1997).

Visual imagery processes include that of a short-term memory system that is stimulus specific, storing the sensory trace, and allowing top-down processes to reactivate it as a quasi-pictorial representation. PET scan and event-related potential studies provide evidence that sustained visual attention is also organized in a top-down manner, with the early sensory input channels being preset and arranged retinotopically. Visual signals arising from specific locations are facilitated at the level of association cortical areas, rather than the primary cortex allowing for attentional control to be exerted for different types of stimuli and tasks. Attention to color provides an example of how selective attention in response to specific features of an object occurs within the same area (involving the processing of features and selective modulation of activity). Neuronal synchronization allows for sensory input to be transformed into motor processes from the primary areas involved in feature selection to the areas involved in response selection and execution. (Clark et al., 1997, Hillyard et al., 1997, Ishai and Sagi, 1997, Roelfsema et al., 1997, Woldorff et al., 1997). The motion singletons differ by presenting a bottom-up control of attention. The purpose, however, is to elicit an automatic attentional response, and in this respect they play a role in the top-down system (Girelli and Luck, 1997).

The auditory system possesses a change detection system allowing for the monitoring of acoustic input and the ability to address deviant signals via a method of attentionally interrupting processing to signal the arrival of deviant stimuli, leading to diminished processing of subsequent stimuli (Schröger, 1996). Subjects were administered an auditory vigilance task while measuring EEG activity as well as blood-flow changes via PET scan. Changes in brain activity confirmed decreased levels of arousal and increased automatic information processing in the performance of very repetitive vigilance tasks. Short-term focusing of attention (60 s) resulted in increased activity of the right ventrolateral frontal cortex in comparison to long-term (>60 s) performance of repetitive attentional tasks resulting in the linear decrease in brain activity within the fronto-parietal cortical network of the right hemisphere. Decreases in both the fronto-parietal network and that of the subcortical structures (thalamus, substantia innominata, and the ponto-mesencephalic tegmentum) occurred simultaneously. The theory of two networks was postulated, one for arousal and alertness involving the subcortical structures [substantia innominata, ponto-mesenephalic tegmentum (midbrain reticular formation) and the anterior cingulate cortex] and the other for auditory attention involving the cortical areas (right inferior parietal cortex, orbitofrontal and dorsolateral frontal cortex, and an FEF-related region, preferentially involving the right hemisphere) (Paus et al., 1997).

The frontal cortex exerts a topographical-specific excitatory control over the reticular nucleus, thus achieving a finely differentiated inhibitory tuning of the posterior cortex. The basal ganglia consists of a set of parallel circuitry connecting widespread cortical areas, subcortical cell groups, and multiple regions of the frontal lobe. Processing along these loops occurs with the development of neural activity in the cortical sensory and association areas.

These cortical processors send transmissions to the cortical regions, as well as excitatory outputs to the subcortical striatum (including the putamen, caudate nucleus, and nucleus accumbens). Upon activation, the striatal neurons carry out aphasic inhibition of the cells in the globas pallidas. Since the pallidal neurons normally function to tonically inhibit cells in the ventral anterior and mediodorsal thalamic nuclei, the net effect of the striatal activation is a disinhibition of the thalamic neurons. The thalamic neurons in turn send excitatory projections back to the cortex leading to increased activity in their frontal targets. Thus, the basal ganglia may apply a form of positive feedback on the cortex. In addition to the converging combinatorial nature of the connections from the cortex to the striatum to the pallidum, it suggests that a process of "focusing activity" is occurring with the frontal targets. This focusing appears to be carried out within multiple and parallel processing loops connecting the basal ganglia and the frontal cortex. Motor and cognitive information appears to be processed within three dorsal loops involving the dorsal caudate nucleus and then projecting to the supplementary motor, frontal eye fields, and dorsolateral prefrontal areas. Motivational information is processed within two ventral loops coursing through the ventromedial caudate and nucleus accumbens and projecting onto the lateral orbital and anterior cingulate regions. Attentional control may emerge from the motor preparation occurring within these loops (Mesulam, 1995; J. Cohen, 1994).

Neurons in the caudate nucleus have been found to be sensitive to the environmental context, but in a manner dependent on forthcoming rather than preceding events. Similar to the expectancy cells of the prefrontal cortex and supplementary motor area, caudate neurons respond in advance of the targets and rewards. The basal ganglia may function as a mechanism for predicting environmental changes and sequencing movements in advance of their initiation. Anticipatory sequencing mechanism could play a central role in learning.

Arousal and attention were found to be intimately linked and mediated by a cortical limbic reticular network (Heilman, Watson, and Valenstein, 1993). Inferior parietal lobe lesions were most often associated with disorders of attention and arousal, and temporoparietal ablations in experimental animal studies indicated attentional disorders. It is from this research that the theory emerged of the involvement of the parietal lobe in attention, and the rate of firing of those neurons designated for attention in the primary sensory cortex appear to be associated with the significance of the stimulus in that the more important stimuli are associated with higher firing rates than unimportant stimuli. Sensory information then projects from the thalamus to the primary sensory cortex and each of the primary sensory cortices (tactile, visual, auditory) project only to their association cortices, whereupon each of these modality-specific association areas then converge on polymodal areas, such as the frontal cortex and both banks of the superior temporal sulcus. These polymodal convergence areas then project to the supramodal inferior parietal lobe. The tempoparietal region not only has strong connections with both the limbic system and the prefrontal cortex, but also contains representations important in determining the meaning of stimuli. The mesencephalic reticular formation (MRF) induces arousal and increased alertness (Heilman, Valenstein, and Watson, 1995).

Weinberg and Harper (1993) define vigilance as steady-state alertness and wakefulness, and propose that the right cerebral hemisphere, predominantly the right inferior parietal lobule and posterior cortices, appear to be specialized for vigilance. The neuroanatomic substrate of lowered vigilance seems to be the loss of modulating influence of the right cerebral hemisphere on the diencephalon and select brain stem nuclei. Filoteo et al. (1994), in researching the Parkinson's population, found that they displayed an abnormal shifting of covert attention, and this was significantly related to the number of perceptual errors they made in identifying target stimuli, suggesting a deficiency in maintaining covert attention, which was postulated to underlie the visuoperceptual impairment observed in patients with this disorder. This research substantiated the involvement of the basal ganglia as playing a key role in maintaining attention. Attentional deficits were examined in temporal lobe epileptic (TLE) patients generalized seizure patients (GSP), and schizophrenics, evidencing impairments for vigilant, self-directed attention for all of the groups. The TLE and schizophrenic groups demonstrated deficits on a task requiring conscious, effortful, preparatory motor set, revealing an inability to profit from predictable repeated presentations. The GSP group evidenced greater attentional errors on the vigilance task, suggesting overall separate cortical- and subcortical-distributed systems involved in the etiologies of these disorders (Goldstein, Rosenbaum, and Taylor, 1997).

The RAS or ARAS System

The RF or reticular formation exerts an excitatory influence on the whole brain by means of a nonspecific projection system, the ascending reticular activating system (ARAS). According to van Zomeren and Brouwer (1994), the ARAS consists of the reticular formation in addition to nonspecific afferents that arise from it to ascend through the intralaminar nuclei of the thalamus, and then these afferents fan out to the various parts of the brain, particularly the cortex. Thus, the ARAS maintains a decisive role in activating the cortex and regulating the status of its activity. The activity of the reticular formation is mainly determined by sensory input, and as its main afferent paths ascend through the brain stem area and approach the thalamus, the branches turn away from the mainstream and enter the RF. The effect of this sensory stimulation is not specific, but instead results in a pooling of excitatory effects, and the ARAS then transmits this pooled excitation through its diffuse projection system to the cortex, thus activating it. Thus, any sensory stimulation will impact the cortex in one of two ways, as a nonspecific part of the whole activating system and as a specific input relayed through thalamic nuclei. Authors note that one cannot look at the action of the RF as a simple energetic model and, instead, although alertness is certainly maintained by stimulation from the outside world, additional factors impact and cause changes in the level of alertness.

There is a distinction made between the upper and lower ARAS at the level of the mesencephalon, which is related to a distinction at the behavioral level, differentiating tonic and phasic changes in alertness. Tonic changes are hypothesized to be mediated by the lower ARAS and phasic changes in alertness mediated by the upper ARAS or the nonspecific thalamic projection system, thus indicating a vertical organization system (van Zomeren and Brouwer, 1994).

The Question of Hemispheric Differences

A right hemisphere asymmetry is noted in the first 3 years as the right hemisphere develops its functions (specifically in the posterior association areas) earlier than the left hemisphere. The asymmetry shifts to the left after 3 years and there is the emergence of hemispheric specialization of functions, the left hemisphere for speech and fine movements and the right for visuospatial processing (Chiron et al., 1997).

Kosslyn et al. (1994) observed hemispheric differences due to attentional effects, and found this as confirmation of observed hemispheric differences in spatial frequency analysis reflecting attentional bias. Attention is adjusted to allow for the hemispheres to monitor outputs from neurons with different size receptive fields. Thus, there is a division of labor with the left hemisphere monitoring high-resolution output and the right hemisphere monitoring low-resolution output, or vice versa. The aspect of encoding is considered to be the most difficult, with the left hemisphere performing the most difficult aspect and the right operating in a complementary fashion. Rafal and Robertson (1995) identified the pattern whereby the left hemisphere is biased to process local information and the right hemisphere tends to process more global information.

Similarly, Goldberg, Podell, and Lovell (1994), in comparing the two hemispheres, found that the right hemisphere is critical for processing novel cognitive situations, while the left hemisphere is a key to the processes mediated by well-routinized representations and strategies. The left frontal systems appear to be critical for the cognitive selection that is determined by the content of the working memory and the context-dependent behavior. The right frontal systems are critical for cognitive selection, driven by the external environment, and critical for dealing with novel-content situations. Finally, the crucial role of the right hemisphere appears to be that of processing cognitively novel situations, and underscores the importance of right frontal systems in task orientation and in the assembly of novel cognitive strategies.

Research has generally concluded that the right hemisphere is more specialized for visuospatial skills and provides information to allow the recognition of relatively unfamiliar faces. The left hemisphere attends to more distinctive features and analysis of the face, resulting in a more durable working memory for faces. It is the right hemisphere that subserves spatial attention for both sides of the body and space, while the left hemisphere only provides information for the right side of space. The right hemisphere prepares both sides for action. The right hemisphere was seen as dominant in oculomotor performance and spatially selective visual attention. It is involved in the purest type of spatial operation and handles fine metric spatial measurement. Left hemisphere was found to play a role in keeping track of decisions and updating decisions with more complex visuospatial tasks and is responsible for categorical spatial relations (Mehta and Newcombe, 1996). Right hemisphere lesions were noted to produce neglect dyslexia in addition to a general visuospatial neglect. Spatial agraphia is a disturbance of graphic expression due to an impairment in visuospatial perception subsequent to right hemisphere lesions (Anderson, 1996; Ardila, Rosselli, Arvizo, and Kuljis, 1997; Lekwuwa and Barnes, 1996; Mehta and Newcombe, 1996). In evaluating stroke patients, Robertson et al. (1997) documented a significant right hemisphere specialization for sustained attention, finding that sustained attention (so critical in the process of learning) was paramount to their recovery of function. The presence of problematic sustained attentional processes at 2 months post-stroke predicted a more detrimental overall functional recovery 2 years later.

Neglect-like symptoms noted are that of a misuse of spaces, stroke and letter omissions, slanting of the lines towards the top or bottom of the paper, underuse of the left side of the paper and tendency to print rather than use cursive. This is the common phenomenon observed in our clinical population of ADD without Hyperactivity with the noted spatial problems that commence as related to ADD and become increasingly severe with time and lack of development. This picture becomes more profound with deficits severe to the degree of brain impairment when there are additional underlying variables of post-traumatic stress disorder, head injury, seizure activation and/or a progressive disorder. Heilman (1997) described all primary emotions as having two or three factors, valence (determination if the stimulus is positive or negative) arousal (satisfaction results in high while sadness results in low arousal), and motor activation (approach or avoidance). The right frontal lobe and its subcortical connections is seen as mediating emotions with negative valence while the left is associated with positive valence. The right parietal lobe mediates arousal response while the left inhibits. The right frontal is important in motor activation, with approach behaviors subserved by the parietal and avoidance by the frontal processes. All of the above form a modulated network associated with connections of the limbic system, basal ganglia, thalamus, and reticular system.

The right hemisphere has the more dominant role for encoding non-linguistic and more affective (prosody) components of language and communications in general. The right hemisphere similarly provides information on the more negative emotional states (vegetative emotional indices) of the individual comprising severe symptoms of depression, while the left hemisphere subserves the more cognitive aspects of the emotional state. The right hemisphere actively anticipates, while the left hemisphere completes the research. Finally, hemispheric patterns in general can additionally be influenced by both gender and strategic information processing (Heilman et al., 1995; Mesulam, 1995; Ross, 1995; Haxby et al., 1995; Prather et al., 1996; Prather, Brownell, and Alexander, 1996).

CHAPTER 5

Pharmacology of Attention

We have considered that the information processing and storing character-istics of the brain depend on chemical communications via synapses within an elaborately complex anatomical organization of neuronal systems. Chemi-cally modulated pathways are in the position to regulate both global behav-ioral states and the emotional motivational salience of events that comprise the mastery of defined emotional disorders.

Specific Actions of the Neurotransmitters

Neurotransmitters act on specialized membrane structures in the postsynaptic neuron called receptors. "Receptor" is a generalized term to denote the mem-brane sites that bind the neurotransmitter molecules. Receptors are composed of proteins that coil in and out of the neuronal membrane and have specialized exterior portions for binding the neurotransmitters. Receptors may be classi-fied by their mode of action on the target neuron as either excitatory or inhibi-tory. There is the fundamental notion that the first messengers or neurotrans-mitters may then cause the release of second or third messengers. Neurotrans-mitters play a key role in transmitting information across cells and can be classified as either excitatory (causing nerve cells to fire) or inhibitory (reduc-ing the responsivity of a nerve cell to incoming stimulation). There is an effect like falling dominos whereby an excitatory neurotransmitter sets off inhibitory properties. Nerve cells have one or more projections — dendrites — whose primary function is to receive information from other cells and pass the infor-mation to the cell body. Bio-elicited changes occur within the nerve membrane

47

that result in information being passed to the nerve terminal situated at the end of the axon. The change in membrane permeability at the nerve terminal triggers the release of the neurotransmitter. One nerve cell may be influenced by reaction to one or more of the neurotransmitters at any given time. The final response of the nerve cell that receives all of this information depends on the balance between the various stimuli that impinge upon it. Neurotransmitters can be released from dendrites, as well as axons. Thus, synapses and/or transfers of information can occur at all of these sites, demonstrating the overall interconnectivity of the brain.

When the transmitter substance is released from a nerve terminal, it diffuses across the synaptic cleft of the postsynaptic membrane, where it then stimulates the receptor site. Any neuron responds to inputs that result from the convergence of several. And because many axons are branched, the target cells may be widely separated and varied in function. Since neurons are linked in an intricate balance, the complexity of transmitter interactions is phenomenal. Neurons can be seen as complex gates that integrate the data they receive and, via their specific collections of transmitter and modulators, move a large repertoire of effects. The majority of neurotransmitters identified can be grouped into four main categories: acetylcholine, monoamines, peptides, and amino acids.

The process of "normal" neuronal function relies greatly on the following:

- Appropriate synthesis and release from the presynaptic neuron
- The successful crossing of the synaptic cleft
- The binding to postsynaptic receptors
- The termination of receptor stimulation by either removal or degradation

Cholinergic neurons (those that release acetylcholine) are distributed throughout a variety of areas in the CNS, including the ventral forebrain, upper brain stem, and striatal interneurons. There are two major classes of cholinergic receptors: nicotinic and muscarinic. Cholinergic systems are hypothesized to play a role in learning/memory process, motor control, stress, affective disorders, and arousal. Monoaminergic systems tend to have long branched ascending and descending axons and are mainly associated with the more diffuse neural pathways. Their cell bodies are typically located in the brain stem area. Noradrenaline, adrenaline, and dopamine are chemically classified as catecholamines while serotonin is classified as an indoleamine (Zasler, 1992).

The Catecholamines and Their Relationship to ADD

The catecholamines are a group of neurotransmitters (including dopamine, norepinephrine, and epinephrine). Their precursor is the amino acid tyrosine, which is enzymatically transformed into the various catecholamines. These chemically defined arousal systems act beyond the receptor at the level of the second messenger systems. The monoaminergic and cholinergic projections activate a variety of receptors, some associated with ion-gated channels and others associated with adenyl cyclase or inositol phosphate. Such interaction seems to underlie the change in neuronal plasticity that occurs as a result of changes in the monoaminergic or cholinergic activity. In this way, activity in these pathways exerts long-term effects that go beyond the immediate course of action (Mesulam, 1995; Robbins and Everitt, 1995).

Dopamine has been found to facilitate learning performance and memory. Typically, its action has been described as connected with appetite and reward-seeking (reinforcing) behaviors. It is involved with the sensory, motor, and neurohormonal activities processing the motivated approach behaviors. It has been associated with fine movement, muscle tone, emotionality, and internal motivation states. Currently in research is the idea that disruption of mesocortical dopaminergic systems results in attentional dysfunction and impedes normal development of corticolimbic circuitry (Randolph, 1995).

Norepinephrine appears to be involved in the regulation of selective attention, as well as attention to significant external stimuli (Cope, 1986). This noradrenergic transmitter is said to produce an alerting, attention-focusing, orienting response. Activities like learning, memory, and awareness are facilitated by norepinephrine. The application of norepinephrine to each of the main sensory areas of the neocortex leads to a general reduction in the spontaneous firing rate, producing a more favorable signal-to-noise ratio. This results in a neuronal response to the sensory stimulus (Robbins and Everitt, 1995). Girardi et al. (1995) suggest that children diagnosed with an attentional disorder demonstrate impairment of sympathetic activation involving the adrenomedullary in addition to the impact of the catecholamines.

Serotonin is found to be an inhibitor of activity and behavior and has been implicated in impulsivity. The amino acid tryptophan is converted by the enzyme tryptophan hydroxylase to 5-hydroxytryptophan, which is then transformed by tryptophan decarboxylase to 5-hydroxytryptamine or serotonin (Shay et al., 1991).

Tyrosine is the amino acid precursor to the catecholamines, dopamine (DA) and norepinephrine (NE). Catabolism of the catecholamines is regulated by two enzymes, monoamine oxidase (MAO) and catechol-O-methyltransferase (COMT). Each of the intermediate compounds formed from the catabolism is then converted to homovanillic acid (HVA). The combined actions of COMT and MAO on NE results in the formation of two principal products, the proportions of each differing in the two major divisions of the nervous system (CNS and ANS). They are vanillylmandelic acid (VMA), the predominant product in the periphery structures and 3-methoxy-4-hydroxylethylene glycol (MHPG), the predominant product in the cortex (Shaywitz et al., 1976).

Animal models have allowed us to hypothesize the behavior of humans and correlate symptoms observed to the clinical condition of ADD. The model that most closely parallels the clinical disorder described initially in 1976 by Shaywitz et al. has since been confirmed by investigators around the world. The model involves the depletion of brain DA and rapid reduction to 10 to 25% as compared to that of controls or normals. Dopamine depletion occurs while NE and serotonin (5-HT) levels remain unaffected. Investigators found that animals with depleted DA were significantly more active than their counterparts. The hyperactivity disappeared with maturity, corresponding to the clinical model whereby hyperactivity tends to be more pronounced until the ages of 10 to 12 years of age and then begins to abate. Associated cognitive difficulties persist corresponding to the avoidance of learning, also evident in the animal experiments. The model also examined the interaction between biological and environmental influences, whereby hyperactivity was significantly reduced by methylphenidate (Ritalin) and avoidance-learning deficits improved by association with normals (Shaywitz et al., 1991).

Wender (1971) suggested that children with ADHD be subdivided into two groups: those with decreased dopamine, and those with decreased NE metabolism. Some factors of ADHD, such as motor overactivity, are pathophysiologically based in abnormalities of NE functions, while problems of vigilance and attention are dopaminergic functions. Levy and Hobbes (1988), using the results that behavioral, but not cognitive impairment occurs with the use of tricyclics, noted that it is only a critical stimulation of the dopaminergic component that causes the improved cognition, with ADHD providing support for the use of the stimulants. Brown and Wynne (1982) proposed a subtype of ADHD, manifested by symptoms of aggression, that is related to the serotonergic pathways.

Investigators believe that ADD is a developmental disorder with characteristic symptoms that change with maturation. Concentrations of NE tend to increase during childhood and adolescence while DA declines. Girls tend to have lower accumulations of DA metabolites and higher accumulations of 5-HT metabolites, representing a more mature or modulated CNS functioning — especially in relation to central inhibitory mechanisms. Thus, there is a marked vulnerability of the whole species toward major neurological and neuropsychiatric disorders (Shaywitz et al., 1991). Zametkin (1992) confirmed that the consistent and well-replicated finding that significant percentages of hyperactive children continue to be symptomatic as adults, indirectly confirmed the hypothesis of the involvement of neurobiology. Using cerebral glucose metabolism and positive emission tomography (PET) scans, hyperactive adults who were the biological parents of ADHD children were examined and found to have abnormal reduced levels of global and regional glucose metabolism. The largest reductions were found to be in the premotor cortex and superior prefrontal cortex. These areas have been associated with the control of attention and motor skills and implicated in attentional disorders. Deficits in these areas produced the motor restlessness associated with hyperactivity in addition to inattentiveness, distractibility, and an inability to inhibit inappropriate responses. Dietary intake of sugar had little impact on cerebral glucose metabolism. Researchers are still not clear what specifically caused these differences, although the overall link between brain chemistry and hyperactivity was clear. Amen (1994, 1995) has done extensive work using SPECT (single/photon emission computed tomography) imaging to validate the significant prefrontal cortex deactivation seen in diagnosed ADHD children and adults in response to an intellectual challenge. Controversy and misconceptions regarding the diagnostic differentiation between ADHD and ADD has related to the intellectual measures used and that neuropsychological measures purporting to measure one variable of brain functioning may in fact be measuring other variables (either in addition to or separate from the variable in question).

Pliszka et al. (1996) presented new information regarding the catecholamine hypothesis of ADHD. They proposed the idea that the central NE system is dysregulated in this disorder and, as a result, does not effectively trigger the cortical posterior attentional system to attend to external stimuli. Effective operations of the anterior attentional system was seen as depending upon dopaminergic input.

Dopamine Intention

Dopamine is a neurotransmitter of itself that has specific projection sites and receptors. It is, however, also an intermediate product in the synthesis of NE. Originating in the brain stem area, this neurotransmitter often overlaps (although patterns of distribution differ) with NE functioning via two systems: the mesostriatal (projections from the substantia nigra and reticular formation to the striatum, comprised of the caudate and putamen, and nucleus accumbens) and mesocortical (projections from the ventral reticular tegmentum of the midbrain to the ventral tegmental area of the cerebral cortex) (Fuster, 1997).

Dopaminergic neurons are suspected to mediate aspects of intention to produce neglect by impacting nigrostriatal, mesolimbic, and mesocortical pathways (Heilman, 1995). There is an abnormally high concentration of DA in the limbic system and its associations. The brain-stem nucleus locus ceruleus has been suggested by Stuss and Gow (1992) as being important in the habituation to irrelevant stimuli. Disorders of attention have been reported after damage to the ventral mesencephalic tegmental area of the frontal dopamine system.

Dopaminergic projections are typically divided into three categories based on length: long, short, or ultra-short. The long tracts emanate from the substantia nigra (nigrostriatal tract) and the ventral tegmentum (mesolimbic/mesocortical tracts). The intermediate length system includes the tubero-infundibular system, the incerto-hypothalamic neurons, and the medullary periventricular group. The ultra-short systems are found in the retina and olfactory bulb. There are several subtypes of dopaminergic receptors known. D1 receptors are believed to be linked to stimulation of the enzyme adenylate cyclase; D2 receptors are not linked to adenylate cyclase. The action of both receptors is necessary for the full expression of dopaminergically mediated motor behaviors, hypothalamic function, and arousal (Zasler, 1992).

The mesolimbic DA system has been implicated in incentive motivational process, whereby evaluative processing is translated into action. Thus, one of the main functions of this system is to achieve the activation of behavior in response to cues that signal the availability of incentives or reinforcers. The role is truly that of activation or energizing of behavior (with a role in response preparation and motor readiness). The effects of elevating DA activity is more behavioral than an improvement in attentional functioning. Attentional task performance does not tend to become impaired as a result of the loss of mesolimbic DA depletion. The DA system also enervates structures such as the caudate nucleus, which does have cognitive functions, including the organization of behavior such as planning, switching response sets, and so on (Robbins and Everitt, 1995). Dopamine functioning correlates with what is observed clinically in ADHD, such as problems of planning and mental flexibility (switching sets and maintaining a set), as well as the behavioral problems and "out of control" reactions so often observed. Hence, the DA system is more associated more with ADHD than ADD.

Mesencephalic DA cells of the ventral tegmental area (VTA) and substantia nigra zona compacta play critical roles in movement, motivation, and mentation. Dopamine released in target areas appears to focus on the processing of inputs and increasing the strength of the behavioral reaction to the stimulus. The appropriate reaction occurs by focusing on the relevant. The firing pattern of mesencephalic DA cells is clearly regulated by both the intrinsic conductance of the cells and the afferent inputs that it receives. Together, this regulation determines the DA release in striatal and limbic target tissues (Seutin, North, and Johnson, 1993).

The presynaptic action of DA on limbic inputs to the nucleus accumbens exerts a focusing or selective effect. The postsynaptic action of DA appears to influence all inputs to the accumbens. It is the presynaptic inhibition action that can selectively reduce certain limbic or cortical inputs while not affecting the transmission of other inputs through the ventral striatum. Transmission of the other inputs may be facilitated by the postsynaptic effects of DA. Thus, DA becomes a focusing mechanism to allow the selected limbic structure to communicate with the motor or extrapyramidal system, and yet it also permits a switching between alternative sources or types of information. This focusing and selecting mechanism of DA is highly advantageous to allow the nucleus accumbens to sift through the multiple limbic inputs, and it is in the accumbens that such input converges. Dopamine permits the expression of a particular behavior associated with a certain pattern of limbic inputs, while suppressing other behaviors that are either inappropriate or conflicting (Mogenson et al., 1993). Stress is found to promote the release of DA within the motor circuit, especially in the areas most closely aligned with the limbic system. The psychostimulants have the capacity to release or to increase the release of DA in the nucleus accumbens (Kalivas, Churchill, and Klitenick, 1993).

Serotonin Impulsivity

5-HT is an indoleamine similar to that of NE and is present in many of the internal organs (gastrointestinal, respiratory, and cardiovascular systems) with cells of origin in the brainstem area. Its pattern of distribution (heavy density in sensory thalamic projection areas) suggests involvement in the processing of sensory information (Fuster, 1997). Serotonin neurons originate in the raphe nuclei of the pons and upper brain stem, and serotonergic pathways involve the hippocampus, hypothalamus, and frontal cortex. Serotonergic axons project into the forebrain, cerebellum, and spinal cord. Functionally, serotonergic systems have been theorized to be involved with arousal, appetite, responses to pain, sleep/wake cycle, regulation, mood and emotion (including aggression), feeding, thermoregulation, ataxia, and sexual behavior (Zasler, 1992). Serotonin is implicated more so in premature or impulsive responding which was the only significant effect of central 5-HT loss. Attentional tasks were not impacted, as was the case for central NE or acetylcholine loss (Robbins and Everitt, 1995).

Serotonin has been consistently implicated in impulsivity and conduct disorder. Low levels of serotonin were found to correlate with impulsivity, oppositional defiant disorder, antisocial behavior, and aggressive behavior according to a review of the research (Halperin et al., 1994; Shapiro and Hynd, 1993; Lahey et al., 1993). Follow-up studies found a constancy related to serotonin in that aggressive behavior continued over time. Research conducted by Halperin et al. (1994) suggests that noncatecholaminergic mechanisms such as serotonin play a role in the evolving of aggressiveness and ADHD as comorbid disorders.

Norepinephrine Attention

Serotonin originates in the brainstem reticular formation, innervating two major pathways, the ventral bundle of axons extending from the pontine and medullary reticular formation cells to the hypothalamus and upper brainstem, and the other has a cortical destination, constituting the locus coeruleus. Traveling a direct hypothalamic route, this second pathway innervates the entire cerebral cortex as well as the spinal cord, cerebellum, and hippocampus (Fuster, 1997). The locus ceruleus in the pons is known to consist entirely of noradrenergic cell bodies, which often send projections to the telencephalon. This contrasts with the noradrenergic projection from the medulla oblongata to (primarily) the diencephalon. Noradrenergic axons enervate multiple structures, both caudally and rostrally, including the forebrain, medulla, spinal cord, and cerebellum. Adrenergic cell bodies are found in the dorsal and lateral tegmentum in the lower brain stem, enervating limbic as well as spinal structures. Noradrenergic and adrenergic systems act at both alpha receptors and beta receptors, and central pathways have been postulated to be involved with sleep/wake cycle regulation, learning and memory, anxiety, behavioral vigilance, and affective disturbance (Zasler, 1992). Specific functions for NE become difficult to determine due to its wide pattern of distribution related to its reticular origin mediating many different functions (Fuster, 1997). Cortical NE has been found to be more important in learning than in performance. NE is implicated in the process of selective attention, while the DA systems contribute to different forms of behavioral activation (Robbins and Everitt, 1995). The levels of concentration of NE are quite high in prefrontal and postcentral somatosensory areas suggesting that there is a more specific role in the processing of somatosensory information (Fuster, 1997).

Norepinephrine is implicated in the ability to pay attention to what is important and only what is important. This correlates with the definition and symptoms of ADD, thus establishing the two different disorders anatomically and biochemically. ADD is characterized by difficulties of attentional focus as opposed to that of the behavioral problems of ADHD. Symptoms of ADD are more responsive to medication targeting NE systems.

Animal research indicates that the postcentral sulcus (somatosensory regions of the neocortex) have much higher tissue concentrations of NE than other cortical regions. There is evidence of asymmetry that may prove to be indicative of laterality in humans. The left pulvinar contains more NE than the right implicating the thalamic NE projection system. The opposite is true for the right ventral posterior thalamic, which involves the mesostriatal DA projections carrying somatosensory afferents to the cortex. Both amine systems are seen as influencing processing in the anterior attentional system associated with executive functioning abilities (Robbins and Everitt, 1995). This neurotransmitter is also implicated in conduct disorder and ADD. Dopamine-beta-hydroxylase (DBH) is one of the enzymes that converts DA to NE. Studies significantly showed that the conduct-disordered, attention-disordered population of boys requires lower levels of DBH necessary for the conversion of DA to NE (Shapiro and Hynd, 1993).

Norepinephrine, Serotonin, and Dopamine Are Interrelated to ADD and Other Disorders

The cortical-striatal-thalamic circuit has been found to correlate with cognitive processing deficits found in schizophrenia (Siegel et al., 1993). Halperin et al. (1994) differentiated aggressive versus nonaggressive attention-disordered children on serotonin levels and found increased aggressiveness with lower serotonin levels. Diminished NE and 5-HT levels were found to be related with increased impulsivity and aggressiveness within the attention-disordered population. Serotonergic neurons have been found to play a role in behavioral inhibition. The involvement of the 5-HT system has been confirmed in impulsive aggression in adults as well (Stein, Hollander, and Liebowitz, 1993). Anger appears to derive from disregulation of NE, DA, and 5-HT. Peptidergic neurons have recently been the focus of intense research regarding their potential role as putative neurotransmitters. The opioid peptides and their precursors have probably received the most attention due to their implication in stress and pain mediation. These neurochemical systems, including that of beta-endorphins, enkephaline, and endorphins, have their cell bodies in deeper, more-primitive regions of the brain, such as the limbic system, reticular formation, medulla, and hypothalamus. Amino acids were found to be the most common of all putative neurotransmitters. Some of the most common are GABA, as well as glutamate and aspartate (Zasler, 1992). Neurometric assessment using a quantitative EEG examination revealed two subtypes, indicating a tegretol-responsive pattern and amantadine-responsive pattern, demonstrating what may be seizure activation or abnormalities associated with the attentional disorders.

Summarizing the Action of Dopamine and Norepinephrine in ADD

The two neurotransmitters most widely implicated in the disorder of ADD are DA and NE. The parallel loops through the basal ganglia are modulated by dopaminergic projection from the ventral tegmental area and the substantia nigra at the midbrain. The ascending dopaminergic fibers contribute to several topographically organized systems projecting to the caudate nucleus, nucleus accumbens, limbic system, and the frontal cortex. The cells of origin in the VTA have been found to respond to environmental cues used for preparation for or initiation of movement. This network represents the extensive convergence of both the exteroceptive and interoceptive information. The hippocampus and limbic system serve as a type of road map, binding the distributed fragments of information into (via the associated cortex) a coherent circuitry (Mesulam, 1995; Tucker and Derryberry, 1992).

Information representing multiple exteroceptive modalities reaches the orbital frontal cortex and the amygdala via the unimodal and polymodal association areas. More direct input also reaches the amygdala via thalamic projections (converging visceral information), which is conveyed by pathways to the amygdala and hypothalamus and also the paralimbic insular cortex (via the thalamus). The insula provides the site of a primary visceral sensory cortex. Such converging inputs place these circuits in a position to evaluate the significance of incoming information. One of the ways significance can be coded is through the gating of the exteroceptive responsivity utilizing the current interoceptive input. Incentive motivation occurs when incoming signals are related to stored representations of pain or reward, with these representations supporting subsequent avoidance or approach behavior. The amygdala conveys information about the conditioned incentive value or salience of stimuli, and problematic functioning would impair the cross-modal integration of the external inputs with its stored interoceptive attributes (Mesulam, 1995).

Problems in the orbital area of the frontal lobe may impair access to a central representation of pain and reward leading to the "experience" but not the "appreciation" of pain. Paralimbic and limbic circuits must first code the adaptive significance of incoming information processing throughout the nervous system. Much of this regulation is carried out via projections to the brain stem centers controlling peripheral somatomotor, neuroendocrine, and autonomic activity. In addition, the limbic circuitry projects extensively to the basal ganglia and cortex, thus providing multiple pathways for modulating activity within the basal ganglia-frontal cortex processing loops. Within the basal ganglia, the amygdala enervates the dorsal (caudate nuclei) and ventral (nucleus accumbens) components of the striatum. Such projections allow the amygdala to temper striatal responsivity to cortical inputs, constraining anticipatory and response processing in terms of the significance of environmental events. The amygdala also influences striatal responsivity via projections to the substantia nigra and ventral tegmental area, the sources of ascending dopaminergic projections to the striatum and frontal cortex (Tucker and Derryberry, 1992).

The amygdala and orbital pathways exert additional effects on the cortex by means of their projections to the nucleus basalis of Meynert and the mediodorsal thalamus. The nucleus basalis, with its widespread excitatory projections to the cortex, constitutes a rostral cholinergic extension of the reticular activating system. The nucleus basalis projects everywhere in the entire center, using a topographical arrangement. Basalis neurons code stimulus significance and their experiential inhibition reduces reward-related discharges into the frontal cortex. Afferents from the orbital cortex and central amygdala appear to govern basalis function and providing feedback control, thus facilitating multiple cortical pathways presenting salience of significant events. The mediodorsal thalamus nucleus also exerts an excitatory influence, which sends an efferent copy to the frontal cortex. This indicates the influence the amygdala is exerting on motor activity. Such a feed-forward mechanism would provide another means for limbic circuitry to contribute to the anticipatory functions of the frontal lobe. In this manner, the limbic and paralimbic circuitry regulates cortical activity via direct projections. Together with orbital projections to thalamic sensory, this circuit relays connectivity and suggests a modulation of early perceptual processing and enhanced attention to objects (Mesulam, 1995).

At subsequent levels within the frontal lobe, the amygdala and orbital cortex project extensively to regions in the lateral prefrontal trend. These ascending influences, along with the lateral system, may provide a route through which multimodal object representations associated with affective significance are formed within the lateral frontal extensions of the ventral limbic system. Sleep loss was found to be related to the disruption of normal frontal limbic RAS connections. Frontal flow typically increases during demanding cognitive tasks, especially those involving vigilance and directed attention, set shifting and decision-making. Such evidence suggests that the level of frontal flow is related to the level of directed mental activity (Tucker and Derryberry, 1992; Goldman-Rakic, 1994).

CHAPTER 6

Information Processing: A Critical Aspect of Attentional Functioning

Defining Information Processing

Information processing is concretely defined as the ability to process information that has been inputted into the brain (or system) to allow that information to be utilized by other modalities and structures within the central nervous system. The idea is that information is processed in a central location, heteromodal association cortex (capable of performing a number of different functions), after initial processing has occurred at modality-specific sensory networks. Information in a parallel, distributed network is then sent to the specific structure (modality) that will utilize the information. On a more-concrete level, when an individual has deficient information processing, he or she will tend to miss little bits of conversation, directions, instructions, communication in general, due to the information not being processed and similarly not being coded for short- and long-term storage and retrieval. Thus, because the information has not been incorporated into this network of processing, it is essentially lost, hence the appearance of a memory problem that is differentiated from a "true memory" problem by the total absence of any knowledge of the information that is lost.

Theoretical Overview

Information processing has been related to processing speed, and although the two can overlap, they are indeed separate entities. Processing speed refers to the speed at which operations can be performed within the brain and tends to operate as a rate-limiting factor for aspects of attentional performance. Thus, there are boundaries on attention that are created by the time required by certain cognitive events (Cohen, 1993).

Broadbent (1958) used the communication system as a metaphor for relationships within the human nervous system and was one of the first to describe mental activities and behavioral responses as components of an information-processing system. According to the description of Broadbent, relationships between structures can be seen as communication systems whereby each of these systems consists of an information source, a transmission channel or channels, and a receiver. The receiver, in turn, may function as a new transmission source. Broadbent referred to filtering as the system that serves to exclude unwanted messages from further analysis, similar to the way one would select one radio channel over another, while excluding other frequencies. The idea being that the individual has a limited capacity to attend to two messages at the same time, particularly if the messages carry vast amounts of technical information that would demand one's full attention. Thus, when the rate of information transmission exceeds the channel capacity of a system, the message will not be transmitted in its entirety. In fact, the messages will then most likely be seriously degraded.

Consequently, if the information presented by the environment exceeds the capacity of the system, then the system is forced to select a limited amount of information to receive and must reject information outside this limited domain or channel. In the human brain, receptors provide vast amounts of information from moment to moment that must be filtered out completely and/or coded from its raw form into a more-succinct form prior to reaching awareness (O'Donnell and Cohen, 1993). Miller (1994) found limitations in the amount of information an individual was able to receive, process, and remember, identifying a capacity problem and the necessity of compensatory techniques to break through the bottleneck.

The question then becomes as to what is the capacity limitation within the central nervous system and the idea is presented that there are many sensations that are received and processed in parallel distributed networks by the nervous system, which are then transmitted across thousands of nerve fibers. As these sensations are organized into perceptions, and these integrated precepts prompt responses, the capacity of the central nervous system would become more and more limited. An example of this is with language, whereby the central limit on processing is quite stringent and typically only one extended message can be comprehended at one time. Further, it does not appear that utilizing different channels or modalities, such as using the right or left ear, visual or auditory, has an impact on the capacity to listen to more than one message at one time. Finally, because of this limit in capacity, the system is forced to exclude unwanted messages in order to attend to the message of interest and thus the evidence of filtering. This filtering is not an "all-or-none" phenomenon and the filtering of unwanted messages does not result in a pure rejection of the information. The filtering system allows some information from an "unattended to" channel to impinge on awareness, although only in a fragmentary way, and instead of the information being lost, it is maintained in this "unattended to" channel. These fragments or bits of rejected messages are limited to a short duration, and there is speculation as to whether a person may be able to develop two higher-order processing systems operating in parallel to encompass relevant and nonrelevant information (O'Donnell and Cohen, 1993).

Broadbent (1958) summarized his conception of the information-processing system as an information flow whereby information enters via the sensory system and is initially processed in parallel networks, and then enters a short-term store or buffer whereby it is then filtered before entry to the limited capacity channel for further transmission into the system. Theories regarding information processing have generally supported the position that individuals are capable of having attentional selections at very early stages of processing. Attentional decisions continue to occur at later stages and are influenced by subsequent response-based factors. Response dispositions are mediated by intrinsic "motivational" and state-dependent factors, which tend to be moderated by both intrinsic and extrinsic cues from the internal and external environment.

Effort is another important issue in considering attentional factors. Attentional efforts reflect the allocation of cognitive and behavioral resources, and response demands create a pressure for attentional processing. Overall, attentional effort is a consequence of the demands for response preparation of selection and production and of the limited capacity of the system as a whole. Attentional capacity, effort, and fatigue are intricately related to one another and together they influence vigilance, as well as the ability to sustain attention on complex tasks (Cohen and Sparling-Cohen, 1993). Information processing is seen as dependent on cognitive maturation over and above basic processing skills. Attempts have been made to identify information-processing skills that allow the individual to efficiently allocate resources. Identified skills comprising attentional factors are the ability to acquire external information, handle temporary information, and verbal processing.

Research confirmed the necessity of the above skills and the idea that all attentional resources need to be coordinated to meet task demands and that although the initial adaptation was difficult, individuals were able to exert the required effort to complete complex task performance. The idea was postulated that information processing needs to remain constant and it is the continual shift from one input channel to another that excludes the use of cognitive strategies and skills to acquire information in an efficient manner (Nettelbeck and Wilson, 1994; Schweitzer, 1994). Cerella and Hale (1994), in their extensive survey of research in information processing, concluded that if viewed from a developmental framework information processing may be seen as a large number of small steps that are homogeneous and interconnectable similar to that of neural networks, changing neural elements interact with constant components to alter functioning over the lifetime of the individual affecting other aspects of cognition in a reciprocal manner.

Current Research Applying the Concept of Information Processing

Recent research is beginning to address the problem of information processing as applied to specific issues of functioning. Younger children (ages 6-1/2 to 8 years) were found to have some difficulty with decoding facial emotional stimuli; however, more significant differences were found for the ADHD population when examining variables of complex auditory processing, affective (emotional) processing, and extended use of working memory (Shapiro et al., 1993). Crick and Dodge (1994) found that problems with information processing and the tendency to miscue or misunderstand led to social problems in children. As a result, there were evidenced tendencies towards hostile attributional biases (as well as disturbances in), intention cue-detection accuracy, response access patterns, and evaluation of response outcomes, resulting in causal factors leading to decreased sense of self-competence and social status. Dodge (1986) proposed a model of social information processing to explain children's social behavior. It was proposed that children, when faced with a social situation cue, then proceed to engage in four mental steps prior to enacting competent social behaviors. The steps involve that of encoding the situational cues representations, interpretation of those cues, a mental search for positive possible responses to the situation, and finally, the selection of a response. During the initial steps of encoding an interpretation of the social cues, it was proposed that children focus in on and encode particular cues in the situation, and then, on the basis of these cues, proceed to construct an interpretation of the situation. During the latter steps it was proposed that children accessed possible responses to the situation from long-term memory storage, evaluated those responses, and then selected the most favorable one to act on. Crick and Dodge (1994) proposed a reformulated social-information processing model of children's social adjustment to include the following steps:

1. Encoding of external and internal cues
2. Interpretation and mental representation of those cues
3. Clarification or selection of a goal
4. Response access or construction
5. Response decision
6. Behavioral enactment

It is during Steps 1 and 2 that the encoding and interpretation of social cues that children selectively attend to occurs. There are particular situations and internal cues that are processed and they then proceed to encode those cues and interpret them. The interpretation may consist of one or more independent processes including the following:

▪ A filtered, personalized mental representation of the situational cues as a result of long-term storage
▪ A causal analysis of the events that have occurred in the situation
▪ Emotional inferences about the perspectives of others in the situation, which would include attributions regarding intent
▪ An assessment of whether the goal has been obtained
▪ An evaluation of the accuracy of the outcome expectations
▪ Self-efficacy predictions based on past performance, inferences regarding the meaning of the past and present exchanges for the self (meaning self-evaluation) and for peers (evaluation of others)

All of the above-mentioned interpretational processes are guided or influenced by basic information stored in memory and results in further impact upon memory systems as a result of changes or revisions to the basic information after interpretation has occurred (Crick and Dodge, 1994).

Upon interpreting the situation, during Step 3, children then select a goal or desired outcome for the situation or continue with a pre-existing goal. Goals are seen as focused arousal states that function as orientation toward producing (or the desire to produce) particular outcomes, and it is proposed that children bring goal orientations or tendencies to the social situation, but also revise those exiting goals and construct new goals in response to immediate social stimuli in their environment. At the Step 4 interval, children access from memory possible responses to the situation, and if the situation is novel, they may then construct new behaviors in response to the immediate social cues. By Step 5, children then evaluate the previously accessed or constructed responses and select the most positively evaluated response for action. A number of factors have been proposed to be involved in the children's evaluation of responses, including the outcomes they expect to accrue after using each response outcome in terms of outcome expectations, and the degree of confidence they have in their ability to enact each response (self-efficacy), and finally, their evaluation of the appropriateness of each response in terms of response evaluation. By Step 6, the response that has been chosen is moved into action (Crick and Dodge, 1994).

Processing of social information would appear to impact social adjustment and the ways in which peers respond to a child, whether that be aversion, avoidance, neglect, or affection. This influences the ways in which the child thinks about him- or herself and those responses received from others are important factors in determining the child's social self-perception and confidence. The child's perceptions about acceptance from others then influences their behavior towards peers and the process continues in a cyclical manner. Children who have social problems have been traditionally found to misattribute feelings (thinking that others think something that they do not, which is usually negative) believe they have the situation analyzed, and disallow new information. Attentional problems can clearly impact social information processing not only in the ability to process the information received, but in problems of being distractible and thus missing the subtle nonverbal cues that help to correctly assess a social situation and determine appropriate behavior. Neglect has been well documented as contributing to the lack of facial recognition and in all probability contributes to social misreading of facial expression, contributing to problematic social functioning in the ADD population.

The social abnormalities characteristic of autism and Asberger's syndrome (characterized as a social isolation disorder) has been linked to a deficient attentional system; the impaired ability to selectively attend to critical aspects of one's perceptual world to appropriately discriminate stimuli and to shift focus of attention as needed to accommodate rapid and unpredictable task demands. Deficits are seen as inherent in the supramodal, attentional base for the integration of sensory experiences, consistent with the theory of information processing. Deficits then produce an incoherent integration of external and internal sources necessary for the accurate representation of reality (Smith and Bryson, 1994). Perry and Braff (1994) administered measures of information processing and thought disorder to adults diagnosed with schizophrenia. He found a significant correlation between thought disorder and problems of information processing.

Kujala et al. (1994) attempted to evaluate the type of slowing of information processing associated with multiple sclerosis and how this possible slowness is related to the cognitive deterioration observed in this disorder. Patients diagnosed with multiple sclerosis were compared with control subjects. Subjects were identified as having mild cognitive deterioration, and preserved cognitive capacities. Using computerized testing, separate stages of information processing were assessed, automatic and controlled processing and motor programming. Results indicated that patients with mild cognitive deterioration were slower than patients with preserved capacities or the controlled population in every stage of processes measured. The preserved patient evidenced signs of mild slowing in automatic visual processing and results indicate that with multiple sclerosis there is a widespread information-processing slowness associated with multiple sclerosis-related cognitive deterioration. Authors hypothesized that information-processing slowness in MS may be due to diffuse demyelination changes, which would disrupt some of the essential components in the information-processing network.

Raymond et al. (1996) discuss visual information processing, identifying numerous processes involved in disorders of higher-level, more-complex visual processing, resulting in impairment in the identification of the spatial properties of objects and the mental manipulation of those properties. Disturbances due to deficits of visual information can produce the following symptoms:

1. Impaired visual analysis and synthesis-separation of foreground from background
2. Impaired judgment and assessment of objects in relation to self in space
3. Problems with direction and distance, the spatial positions of objects and depth perception
4. Prosopagnosia or impaired facial recognition
5. Visual object agnosia, failed recognition of objects despite intact vision
6. Body image disturbances

Visual processing is viewed as the culmination of functioning from critical brain areas. This confirms the idea that information processing is a concept encompassing all of the sensory modalities, integrating and interacting at the most complex level of brain functioning.

The auditory system, similar to that of the visual system, relies on supplemental areas and bilateral neuronal activity for internal auditory imagery to occur. Using cerebral blood flow as a measurement, research identified that the process of perceiving and imagining songs is dependent on functions subserved by the frontal and parietal areas (judgment of pitch, perception, and imagery), supplementary motor area, and secondary auditory cortical areas (superior temporal gyrus). Inferior frontal polar cortex and right thalamus are hypothesized to be associated with retrieval and/or generation of auditory information from memory (Zatorre et al., 1996).

The processing of numbers involves a similarly complex cascade of interactions among a number of areas: posterior activation provides early visual processing; posterior occipito-temporal activation provides comprehension (verbal lateralized to left hemisphere and bilateral for arabic); bilateral temporo-parietal to address hard length; right lateralized parieto-occipito-temporal activation for distance; motoric areas for response, and medial superior prefrontal activation for error detection. The right hemisphere was found to possess abilities to identify digits and its relationship to other numbers (Dehaene, 1996). Superior information processing of numbers by Asian children suggests the impact of multicultural factors (Mardell-Czudmowski, 1995).

Problems of information processing have been defined as a central auditory processing disorder and associated with ADHD. Riccio et al. (1994) addressed the question and the diagnosis of CAPD and ADHD as representing a singular disorder and found that the two actually are distinct and different disorders, although there is considerable overlap. They questioned the considerable overlap of attentional disorders and language problems. Moss and Sheiffele (1994) examined the problem of under-diagnosis of ADD and its overlap with a central auditory processing (CAP) problem, suggesting the need to differentiate separate symptomatology for both diagnoses and for treatment ramifications.

A processing deficit approach has been used as a means of identifying learning disabilities and the idea that adequate processing skills of chronological awareness, pseudoword decoding, abstract and nonsense word memory, confrontation and rapid naming are predictors of reading success. Schuerholz et al. (1995) found that linguistic processing deficits, specifically that of phoneme segmentation and rapid naming, is an approach to identify children at risk for learning disabilities. There was a significantly higher percentage of deficits in phonemic awareness for those diagnosed with reading disabilities and associated with comorbid elevated attentional ratings.

August and Garfinkel (1989) identified a cognitive version of ADHD related to severe academic underachievement and including information-processing deficits related to inadequate encoding and retrieval of linguistic information. Evoked potential studies confirmed abnormalities characterizing the comorbidity of ADHD, poor reading ability, and decreased ability to allocate the attentional resources to complete the task. There is a question of the involvement of more posterior regions subserving the information-processing deficits related to dyslexia (Duncan et al., 1994). We have found consistent language problems associated with the attentional disorders, which probably represents the longest lasting and most devastating of the symptomatology associated with ADD. The dual deficits of spatial issues characterizing ADD in addition to information-processing problems and the missing of information results in considerable speech and language difficulties. ADHD-diagnosed individuals experience learning problems in addition to missing information to experience the language deficits, although the etiologies appear to be quite different.

Summarizing the Attentional Information-Processing System

Generally, information is received via the unimodal sensory systems and this activates subcortical functioning before any cortical activation has occurred and/or registration of the sensory information. There is only the detection of an occurrence of a new stimulus that is transformed for more-detailed processing. This response creates an automatic shift of attention to the specific region of space. Reticular activation critical for energizing the system and for preparation for action enters the formula. These resulting shifts in attentional direction here at this point continue to involve automatic activation remaining at very gross levels of information processing. Upon reaching the sensory cortex, sensory information is coded for specific critical features.

Filtering and analysis processing results in a sharpening of the important features of the stimulus and attention to other aspects of the information. Informational processing remains relatively automatic and not highly modifiable; however, associative information and energetic factors then become influential. Subsequent to this pre-attentional information processing, information is then integrated within higher cortical systems integrated by areas of the inferior parietal and temporal lobes. At this stage, the processing characteristics can now be modified and the biases of the intrinsic system begin to have a direct impact on attentional selection.

Information flow moves through sensory analysis to the processing stage, enabling the new information to be focused and modified in relation to pre-existing salient and relevant biases. Reticular activation continues to provide a general energization that affects not only sensory processes, but also the response selection systems of the frontal lobes, as well as limbic and hypothalamic response. Response selection systems appear to operate independently of this sensory selection. The frontal lobe has a reciprocal interaction with both the attention systems of the parietal lobe and the limbic system. The frontal systems govern the organization of search as well as the generation of sequences of attentional responses, and continue to play a minor role in selective attention. Thus, in the absence of direct stimulation via frontal processes, the individual is still able to experience affective, motivational, and other impulses that trigger response intention, preparation, planning, initiation, and control. Based on feedback received from response selection and new sensory input, all of these issues continue to affect the bias for sensory selection and the direction of sensory attention in a reciprocal manner.

CHAPTER 7

Frontal Lobe System

Functional Analysis

The frontal lobe system is seen as being heterogeneous and complex, subserving cognitive and emotional thought processes. There is such variability in the morphology and individual differences in the position, size, and shape of the inherent structural areas of the frontal lobe that the various classical maps of the area are substantially different. Rajkowska and Goldman-Rakic (1995) suggest that such variation provides an explanation for the individual differences in the visuospatial and cognitive capacities for which this area is responsible. Current research supports separate regions for cognition and emotion and a separate region for interrelated processing between the two, rather than overlapping neural substrates (Grattan et al., 1994). The supervisory system of the frontal lobe is necessitated in five different types of everyday life situations:

1. Situations that involve planning or decision-making
2. Situations that involve the need for error correction and/or trouble-shooting
3. Situations where responses are not well learned or contain novel sequences of actions
4. Situations that are judged to be dangerous or technically difficult
5. Situations that require the overcoming of a strong habitual response or resisting of temptation

The idea is that the individual with problems or deficits related to frontal lobe functioning is impaired in his/her ability to develop an appropriate strategy to deal with any problem situation where no routine procedure is available to implement (Shallice and Burgess, 1991).

Frontal lobes have been implicated in the following actions:

1. The frontal lobes decide what is worth attending to and what is worth doing in terms of an action response. Frontal systems play a special role in regulating both attentional and intentional functions. The inability to prioritize attention and intention factors produces distractibility, poor sustained attention and mental effort, rambling speech, aimless behavior, preoccupation with irrelevant or trivial matters, perseveration, confabulation, confusion when confronted with choices, and failure to apprehend the significance of events in the environment.

2. The frontal lobes provide the continuity and coherence for assessing behavior across time (temporal sequences). This allows for such complex functioning as planning, providing overall coherence and predictability to behaviors. Deficits in the ability to prioritize and temporally integrate may lead to problems with planning and executing a sequence of behaviors necessary to meet a goal. This results in the tendency to be driven by the irrelevant and to become directionally lost. There is an inability to conceptualize oneself in the future, to grasp the relationship between long-term plans and the sequential steps required to meet them, as well as an inability to decide which actions fit most appropriately to attain a given goal.

3. The frontal lobes modulate affective (emotional) and interpersonal (social) behavior to allow internal drive states to be met within the confines of the individual's external and internal environments. The frontal cortex serves as a bidirectional function in constant communication with the internal milieu of the hypothalamus. The limbic system energizes the cortex to direct action in efforts to satisfy basic human drives, and the frontal cortex then modulates those drives to meet the contingencies of an extremely complex and highly technological society (integrating the individual's internal and external environment). Deficits in affective modulation can result in emotional liability, emotional flatness and indifference, belligerence and aggression, childishness, euphoria, and abnormal jocularity.

4. The frontal lobes monitor, evaluate, and adjust. This is the critical role for the supervisory system, operating as overseer, adjuster, and corrector. If dysfunctional, there is an inability to benefit and learn from

experience, resulting in an overall rigidity. Things can best be described as knowing what one needs to do, but not being able to do it. Such behavior can easily be misinterpreted as resistant or lacking in motivation (Hart and Jacobs, 1993).

Structural Circuitry

The frontal lobes are considered as the cortical suprastructure of this attentional system. The prefrontal region, specifically the orbitofrontal and dorsolateral areas, is the primary functioning area, and is distinctly different. Five parallel anatomical circuits link regions of the frontal cortex with the striatum, globus pallidus, substantia nigra, and the thalamus. Circuits originating in the supplementary motor area, frontal eye fields, dorsolateral prefrontal region, lateral orbitofrontal area, and anterior cingulate cortex comprise open loop structures that provide input to and/or receive output from specific circuits that share overall functions, cytoarchitectural features and phylogenetic histories. These circuits mediate motor and oculomotor function, in addition to executive functions, socially responsive behavior, and motivation. Neuropsychiatric disorders of the frontal-subcortical circuits include impaired executive function, disinhibition and apathy, and mood disorders of depression, mania and liability. Neurotransmitters, modulators, receptor subtypes, and secondary messengers within the circuits serve to provide the chemoarchitecture that underlies these loops. Disruption of these circuits results in various disorders ranging from the cognitive to the psychiatric.

Five circuits are identified and named according to their function and/or cortical site of origin. The primary motor circuit originates in the supplementary motor area and the oculomotor circuit originates in the frontal eye fields, with both circuits dedicated to motor function. The dorsolateral prefrontal, lateral orbitofrontal, and anterior cingulate circuits are designed to subserve executive functions, cognitive functions of a higher nature, personality, and motivation. Each of the five circuits has the same basic member structures, including the frontal lobe, striatum, globus pallidum, substantia nigra, and the thalamus. Each circuit uses the same neurotransmitters at each anatomic site. Anatomic positions of the circuits are specifically preserved in each circuit structure. The dorsolateral prefrontal region projects to the dorsolateral region of the caudate nucleus. The lateral orbitofrontal region projects to the ventral caudate area and the anterior cingulate cortex projects to the medial striatal nucleus accumbens region. There is a reduction of activation of the circuits at the subcortical level as compared with the cortical regions.

The basic anatomic organization shared by all of the circuits has its origin in the frontal lobes with excitatory glutaminergic fibers that then terminate in the striatum (caudate, putamen, and ventral striatum) (Mega and Cummings, 1994).

These striatal cells then project inhibitory (GABA) fibers to neurons in the globus pallidus interna/substantia nigra pars reticulata as a direct loop connection and neurons in the globus pallidus externa as an indirect loop connection. In the indirect loop connection, it is the external globus pallidus that projects to the subthalamic nucleus via the inhibitory GABA fibers and the subthalamic nucleus then connects with the globus pallidus interna/substantia nigra pars reticulate through these excitatory glutaminergic fibers. The direct pathway or connection utilizes substance P with its GABA projection to the pallidum and expresses dopamine D1 receptors, whereas the indirect loop connection combines enkephalin with GABA and receives its dopaminergic influence via the D2 receptors. The globus pallidus interna/substantia nigra pars reticulata then projects inhibitory GABA fibers to specific targets in the thalamus to complete the circuit by sending a final excitatory connection to the site of the circuit's origin in the frontal lobe (Mega and Cummings, 1994).

Each circuit comprises a closed loop, which has specified neurons that remain anatomically separate from the parallel chains of neurons comprising the other circuits. There are, however, unspecified (open) elements in each circuit that receive inputs from regions outside of the loops that serve to modulate the circuit's activity. The circuits also project to areas outside of the closed loop and the "open" afferent and efferent components of the circuits are regions that share functions with each specific circuit.

Circuits mediating limbic function then have connections to the other limbic areas of the brain and those involved with executive functions have connections and interact with brain regions closely involved with cognition. As a result, the circuits integrate information from anatomically different (but functionally related) and interrelated brain regions. This supports the idea that there are circuit behaviors specific to each within each of the circuits mediating a defined set of related behaviors. The dorsolateral prefrontal subcortical circuit mediates executive functions, the lateral orbitofrontal-subcortical circuit mediates socially appropriate restraint and empathy and the anterior cingulate–subcortical circuit mediates motivation. The numerous structures and the various neurotransmitters, receptors, and modulators involved in these circuits provide an explanation for the occurrence of lesions in different brain areas that have similar behavioral effects and that a variety of pharmacologic interventions tend to have similar effects on behavioral disturbances (Mega and Cummings, 1994).

Dorsolateral Prefrontal Circuit

The dorsolateral prefrontal–subcortical circuit originates in Broadman areas 9 and 10 commencing on the lateral surface of the anterior frontal lobe. Neurons in these regions project to the dorsolateral head of the caudate nucleus and fibers from the caudate nucleus project to the lateral aspect of the mediodorsal globus pallidus interna and rostrolateral substantia nigra pars reticulata via the direct pathway or loop. The indirect pathway or loop sends fibers to the dorsal globus pallidus externa, which then projects to the lateral subthalamic nucleus and fibers from the lateral subthalamic nucleus then terminate in the globus pallidus interna and substantia nigra pars reticulata. Output that occurs from these two pathways (direct and indirect) then terminate in the parvocellular portions of the ventral anterior (direct pathway) and mediodorsal thalamus (indirect pathway). The mediodorsal thalamus closes the circuit by projecting back to the circuit's origin, areas 9 and 10 of the dorsolateral prefrontal–subcortical circuit (Mega and Cummings, 1994).

The dorsolateral prefrontal circuit is responsible for executive functioning, which includes the ability to organize a behavioral response to solve a complex problem (learning new information, using creativity or mental flexibility, and memory search), activation of remote memories, self-direction, goal-directed behavior, planning, temporal coding of external and internal events, judgment, insight, shifting and maintaining a set, and using verbal skills for internal speech necessary to guide behavior. Damage to the dorsolateral areas can be characterized by a pseudodepressed state and will produce a range of symptoms across such areas as slowness, perseveration, and general lack of initiation (Knight, 1991; Mega and Cummings, 1994).

Lateral Orbitofrontal Circuit

The lateral orbitofrontal circuit originates in Broadman areas 10 and 11 and sends projections to the ventromedial caudate. The ventromedial caudate projects directly to the most medial portion of the mediodorsal globus pallidusinterna and to the rostromedial substantia nigra pars reticulata. The ventromedial caudate also sends an indirect loop through the dorsal globus pallidus externa to the lateral subthalamic nucleus, which then projects to the globus pallidus interna and substantia pars reticulata. Neurons are sent from the globus pallidus and substantia nigra to the medial section of the magnocellular division of the ventral anterior thalamus as well as an inferomedial section of the magnocellular division of the mediodorsal thalamus. The circuit then closes with projections from the thalamic region to the lateral orbitofrontal cortex (Mega and Cummings, 1994).

The orbitofrontal circuit mediates emotional control and appropriate emotional responses for empathy, socially appropriate behavior, impulse control, social integration, and judgment. Personality change is the hallmark of dysfunction in the orbitofrontal areas and damage to this area tends to result in prominent emotional disturbance: problems that can center around disinhibition and lack of control resulting in anger; inappropriate laughing, crying, or sexuality; general disinhibition, and hyperactivity and/or mania. The individual is aware of the behavior, however, he/she is unable to control it. Irritability, liability, tactlessness, and fatuous euphoria are often descriptions of individuals with damage to this area. Individuals do not respond appropriately to social cues, show undue familiarity, and are unable to empathize with the feelings of others. There are rapid shifts from one mood to another, resulting in covert emotional liability. Another aspect of dysfunction in this area is that of obsessive compulsive behaviors, which can be observed in overall increased behavioral control, resulting in overconcern about social behaviors, disease contamination, and an excessive investment in social appropriateness, and which appears to be the result of increased metabolic activity in the orbitofrontal area and increased caudate metabolism (Duffy and Campbell, 1994; Knight, 1991; Mega and Cummings, 1994).

Anterior Cingulate Circuit

The origin of the anterior cingulate–subcortical circuit are the neurons of the anterior cingulate gyrus originating in Broadman area 24. Input is provided to the ventral striatum (which includes the ventromedial caudate, ventral putamen, nucleus accumbens, and olfactory tubercle). These structures comprise the limbic striatum and projections from the ventral striatum enervate the rostromedial globus pallidus interna and ventral pallidum (the region of the globus pallidus inferior to the anterior commissure), as well as the rostrodorsal substantia nigra. There is the possibility of an indirect loop projecting from the ventral striatum to the rostral pole of the globus pallidus externa. The external pallidum connects to the medial subthalamic nucleus, which returns projections to the ventral pallidum, which provides some input to the magnocellular mediodorsal thalamus. The anterior cingulate circuit closes with projections from the dorsal portion of the magnocellular mediodorsal thalamus to the anterior cingulate gyrus (Mega and Cummings, 1994).

The anterior cingulate–subcortical circuit impacts motivated behavior; impairment in this area produces a state of overall amotivation and lack of movement and/or deficits of motor movement (particularly that of skilled movement). Apathy signifies damage to the structures of this circuit. Individuals are profoundly apathetic, rarely moving, incontinent, eating and drinking only when fed. Displaying a total absence of emotion, these individuals evidence complete indifference to their surroundings and circumstances (Knight, 1991; Mega and Cummings, 1994).

Degos et al. (1993), in evaluating ischemic lesions in the left anterior cingulate gyrus and in the head of the right caudate nucleus, reported clinical symptoms, that included complex disorders, such as distractibility, docility, emotional unconcern, manual grasping, comprehension and utilization behavior, perseveration, and anterograde amnesia.

Specific Functional Deficits

Distractibility can be a prominent feature of prefrontal lesions and has been effectively revealed by animal studies, as well as human studies. Distractibility has been hypothesized as an inability to inhibit attending and responding to irrelevant events in both the internal and external environment. Studies have shown that it is the prefrontal cortex that provides inhibitory response and modality-specific suppression of the sensory transmission through the thalamic relay nuclei for divided attention processes. It is through this inhibitory pathway that a gating mechanism operates to gate transmission to primary sensory regions. This prefrontal thalamic gating mechanism provides a powerful neurophysiologic system for early filtering of sensory inputs capable of intra- and intermodality suppression of irrelevant stimuli, allowing relevant stimuli to be effectively processed (Knight, 1991).

Sustained attention appears to be due to the combination of the enhancement of neural activity to the attended channel and active suppression of neural processing to the nonattended channel. The ability to inhibit irrelevant signals subserves the phenomenon of this gating process. As seen from the perspective of frontal functions, sustained attention may be impacted by a variety of deficits in executive processes.

Weintraum and Mesulam (1985) refer to an "attentional matrix" that corresponds to the function of the ascending reticular pathways and the frontal lobes. The elements of this attentional matrix consist of concentration, vigilance, perseverance, and response inhibition. Mental control, another term for the attentional matrix, involves:

1. Arousal and alertness
2. Vigilance
3. Ability to initiate set shifting
4. The ability to inhibit inappropriate set shifting (response inhibition)
5. Speed of cognitive processing

Using this concept of mental control, attentional deficits can be defined as perseveration, impulsiveness, distractibility, impersistence, slowness in processing, and confusion.

The brain structures involved in this system can be considered as part of a frontal diencephalic brain stem system (Auerbach, 1986). The mesencephalic reticular activating core has long been considered a critical component of arousal and alertness. The brain stem reticular formation receives collaterals from a large number of ascending and descending pathways and then provides major ascending cholinergic and monoaminergic pathways to thalamic and neocortical targets. The thalamus acts as a major relay between cortex and reticular formation. The reticular nucleus of the thalamus can be thought of as an attentional valve for thalamocortical transmission mediating the inhibitory influences of the frontal lobes and the excitatory impact of the reticular formation (Auerbach, 1986).

Clinical attentional disorders are generally described as impairments in the direction or regulation of concentration and effort to specific demands of the environment over a defined period of time. Developmental abnormalities were identified in the frontal striatal circuits of children diagnosed with ADHD, using qualitative measurement of caudate volume and asymmetry. Smaller total brain volumes and absence of normal caudate volume asymmetry (right greater than left) was noted (Castellanos et al., 1994).

The brain stem reticular activating system has been hypothesized as responsible for overall arousal and alertness and, if problematic, can result in "drifting attention". If the individual is alert and cooperative, but easily distracted, classified "wandering attention", this tends to be more related to the thalamic projection system. Finally, disturbance of the frontal thalamic gating system, controlling the ascending reticular activating system, somatosensory fibers, and the descending frontal cortex tracts would produce disturbance in planning, selection, and monitoring of performance. Disorders of directed attention may occur with relatively focal frontal areas producing symptoms of inflexibility and perseveration, impulsivity, distractibility, and rapid alteration of attention (Stuss and Benson, 1986).

Impulse and Behavioral Control

Copeland (1991) discusses the impact of central nervous system underarousal on the reticular activating system, RAS. The RAS is viewed as a monitor or gatekeeper allowing selected stimuli to be relayed to the appropriate cortical areas. An underaroused RAS may (in its sluggishness) transmit messages inefficiently and ineffectively. When the RAS is deficient, too many stimuli enter consciousness, resulting in poor attention, concentration, impulse control, distractibility, poor organization, low frustration, and other symptoms associated with ADD. Once thought to play an important role in ADD, the effects of this system are secondary to that of the frontal lobe and its connections. The basal ganglia utilizing the neurotransmitter, dopamine, was viewed as responsible for modulating movement and integration of sensory information; when not operating effectively, it produced a loss of the support role between the various systems and the assurance that they were communicating effectively. The limbic system, although not fully connected with the reticular system until adolescence, was found to be particularly delayed in ADD, thus lacking the inhibitory system impulse control, maturity, and judgment (Copeland, 1992).

Executive functions comprise those mental capacities necessary to formulate goals, plan to achieve them, and carry out the plans effectively, and are at the heart of all socially useful, personally enhancing, constructive and creative activities. With executive functioning intact, an individual can suffer dysfunctioning and impairment in any of the other areas of the brain and still be able to function within his/her environment. Impairment or loss of executive functions severely compromises an individual's life and deters the ability to survive independently and productively (Lezak, 1982).

Intention, Planning, and Goal-Oriented Behavior

The system of executive functions can break down at any stage in the sequence of events that make up a planned or intentional action. The capacity to formulate a goal or to have an intention is involved with motivation and with awareness of self and how one's surroundings affect the individual. The ability to create motivation to attain a goal from past experience, appreciation of needs or imagination and hope require self-awareness on a number of different levels (including the awareness of internal status and an experiential sense of self). People who lack the capacity to formulate goals may be unable to initiate activities beyond basic instinctual responses to internal or external stimuli. Individuals who may be capable of complex activities may not consider doing anything due to a lack of the capacity to formulate a goal (Lezak, 1982).

Several capacities are necessary for planning, primarily, the capacity for sustained attention. Planning also requires the ability to think of alternatives, make choices, and evolve a conceptual framework aimed toward the specific activity. Defective planning can occur when individuals are able to formulate goals, but lose track of their intentions. They make plans, arrive at plans, but such plans are unrealistic and impossible to attain. In addition, the individual may experience difficulty creating a conceptual structure and providing a blueprint and subsequent time schedule to carry out such a plan. Impulsivity also interferes with planning. Thus, an individual may be well energized and motivated, yet still unable to succeed at a goal, due to defective planning skills. These individuals eventually become very frustrated and may become involved in some form of acting-out behavior. The translation of an intention or plan into a self-serving, productive activity requires the capacities to initiate, maintain, switch and stop sequences of complex behavior in an orderly and integrated manner. Disorders in the programming of activity can interfere with an individual's ability to carry out reasonable plans, regardless of motivation, knowledge, and skills. Programming disorders can appear as perseveration. The effectiveness of behavior depends on the individual's ability to monitor, self-correct, and regulate the delivery. Erratic performance becomes the hallmark of impaired executive functions (Lezak, 1982). Individuals do not perceive their mistakes and thus cannot correct them. The ability to self-monitor is critical to improve on performance and utilize feedback from one's environment.

Inhibitory Influences

Inhibitory influences are seen as crucial and necessary for allowing the brain to coordinate reflexive responses with goal-directed behavior. Inhibitory processes, operating in attentional selection, inhibit both primitive reflexes while tonically inhibiting sensory processes at the level of the thalamus, to influence all subsequent perception and action. Selective attention involves the ability of the individual to maintain goal-directed behavior by gating the flow of perceptual information into the response systems, while continuing to emphasize goal-relevant information. This involves the action of the prefrontal lobes in gating the flow of activation from posterior perceptual systems to frontal motor planning and execution systems. Attentional gating requires that internal goals comprising target specifications remain constant while they are matched against high-level perceptual representations. Matched representations are facilitated while nonmatching representations are inhibited. This precise mechanisms allows for efficient selection over the intricate and continuous range of the processing substrate providing for the automatic control of inhibition so that the strength of the inhibition continually adapts to the strength of the "to be ignored" input. This self-regulating feedback mechanism allows for nontarget stimuli to have an activation level that is equalized below that of target stimuli and above that of resting levels. Rebound behavior utilizing opponent mechanisms allows for rapid attentional switching, providing inhibition of return to allow for continual self-regulating inhibitory feedback (Rafal and Henik, 1994).

Frontal Processes Are Seen as Reflective of Overall Brain Functioning

Reitan and Wolfson (1994, 1995) question the historic claim that the frontal lobes are actually the seat of analytical reasoning, executive functioning, and abstract reasoning. Research has not supported the hypothesis that there is more specific and severe impairment found in individuals with frontal lesions than in those with nonfrontal lesions (Reitan, 1994). Unsupported by research is the hypothesis that the anterior frontal areas are related to the general indicators of neuropsychological impairment and the more posterior areas located in both right and left cerebral hemispheres are the ones that subserved the more specific functions (depending upon the hemisphere involved). Since the frontal lobe constitutes such a large anatomical area, there is a large undesignated area, largely in the anterior portion, that has not been defined as involved in any specific behavioral function, and it becomes tempting for theorists to assign the higher level of brain functioning, such as reasoning, planning, logical analysis, and executive functions involving the final output of the brain with respect to organized and effective responses, to this anterior frontal portion. Reitan and Wolfson found that patients with frontal lesions show more indications of general impairment rather than specific deficits. They propose the idea that other cortical areas share essentially all of the higher level cognitive functions of the frontal areas of brain functioning.

Walsh (1994) refers to the frontal lobes as capable of numerous functions involving higher-level thinking processes, including planning and problem solving, error utilization, cognitive flexibility, visual search and analysis of complex material, and abstract thinking. The term *frontal lobe syndrome* is seen as very general, covering the disruption of a vast geographical area, including areas that are both functionally and structurally distinct. The frontal system is seen as a superordinate functional system utilizing the temporal structures to allow the individual to deal with four major characteristics of behavior (adaptive function, changing demands, novelty, and complex integration over time) and, to be successful, the system must be able to anticipate and plan future outcomes, while retaining the basic schema or plan (with the specific elements to be executed) until the goal is attained, while simultaneously being able to avert interfering influences that threaten to disrupt this process.

Seger (1994) provides evidence that identifies the importance of the basal ganglia, association cortex, and frontal cortex in implicit learning (learning of complex information in an incidental manner without awareness of what has been learned), in addition to some involvement of the hippocampus. The basal ganglia appear to be involved in the area of response programming, the association areas appear to be involved in the perceptual aspects of implicit learning, and the frontal lobes appear to be involved in the evaluation of implicit knowledge in making conceptual fluency judgments. Implicit learning is seen as a complex process that depends on attention and working memory processes, and the quality and quantity of learning that depends on which of these processes are used during learning. Implicit learning is then stored as abstract information and interacts with explicit learning and other cognitive processes in complex ways.

Moscovitch (1994) found that the strategic retrieval processes mediated by the frontal lobes system placed greater demands on cognitive resources than the relatively automatic associative retrieval processes mediated by the temporal lobes. The frontal component was seen as a central system structure operating strategically on both the output and input of the memory structure. Prefrontal cortex is beginning to be seen as underlying functions that are less hardwired in nature (with greater plasticity) operating in the position of director, orchestrating, and integrating other cortical areas with appropriate behavioral responses (Mesulam, 1995). Diminished attentional resources due to head injury reduce the capacity for allocation (Schmitter and Edgecombe, 1996).

Goldman-Rakic (1994), in his research with diagnosed schizophrenics, maintains that the cortical feedback pathways are specifically important for bringing representational data into line with reality via the anatomical structures. Prefrontal projections to the parietal and temporal association areas may be able to gate sensory (real-world) information that these areas received from the thalamus and secondary sensory areas. An impairment in this process could lead to an altered consciousness of sensory experience. Impairment in some of the feed forward projections to and from the prefrontal cortex may lead to certain negative symptoms seen in schizophrenia, such as lack of initiative, poverty of speed, and lack of goal-directed behavior. In diagnosed schizophrenias, the disruption of cognitive ability may either directly or indirectly involve the cortico–cortical and cortico–subcortical pathways that establish the inner models of reality and adjust them to environmental demands. The prefrontal cortex is thus seen as a component of a larger network of cortical areas. Frontal processes are viewed as providing a nonspatial form of attentional control over divided or focused attention processes (Godefry, Lhullier, and Rousseaux, 1996). The thalamus has been implicated as inherent in the regulation of cognitive and sensory input, abnormalities in sensory gating contribute to being overwhelmed by sensory information.

Giedd and associates (1994), using quantitative neuroanatomic imaging, assessed structural brain abnormalities relevant to frontal lobe circuitry in children with diagnosed ADHD. The midsagittal cross-sectional area of the corpus callosum was divided into seven sections and measured from magnetic resonance images of boys and compared with matched controls. Two anterior regions, the rostrum and the rostral body, were found to have significantly smaller areas in the ADHD group, and these findings correlated in the expected direction with teacher and parent ratings of hyperactivity-impulsivity dimensions. Findings supported the theory of abnormal frontal lobe development and function in ADHD. The rostral body corresponds to the premotor and supplementary motor areas of the cortex and would explain the defective response inhibition seen as the core deficit in ADHD. The rostrum contains projections from the caudate orbital prefrontal region and other studies have implicated these areas in ADHD. Findings support the assertion that the primary deficit in ADHD is that of response inhibition and attention rather than attentional problems. Authors conclude that it is doubtful that a single area would be found to account for the variety of symptoms found in this disorder; however, there are subtle differences between the brain morphology of ADHD individuals and normal comparison subjects. Recently, and contrary to prior findings, Hall et al. (1996) noted significantly larger areas of volume for ADHD on the corpus callosum, hypothesizing overactive and excessive transmission. The perisylvian gyral region was also noted as significantly different for ADHD and LD (Hynd et al., 1996).

CHAPTER 8

Parietal Lobe Functioning

Importance of the Parietal Area
and Its Relationship to ADD

The parietal lobe provides the primary reception area for somatic sensation and is rich in noradrenergic transmission. The parietal cortex contributes to sensorimotor transformations located at the crossroads of four sensory systems — visual, auditory, vestibular, and somatosensory — projecting to several frontal and premotor areas (Pouget and Sejnowski, 1997). It is heteromodal or association cortex, posterior to the post central gyrus, which is thought to deal with the combination of discrete elements into meaningful wholes, also providing a central processing area responsible for higher-order information processing, subserving functioning of the parallel distributed attentional networks. It is critical in the function of this area of the parietal lobe, which is responsible for intersensory or cross-modal association and integration. The role of spatial representations is to code the sensory inputs and arrange signals in such a manner that subsequent computation for the generation of motor commands can be achieved. Basis function neurons (approximation of single parietal neurons) reduce nonlinear transformations involved in sensorimotor coordination to linear mappings. They have the advantage of not having to depend upon any coordinate system or reference frame; thus the position of an object can be represented in multiple reference frames simultaneously (Pouget and Sejnowski, 1997). The common "spatial" finding related with ADD is that it reveals the consistently confirmed clinical pattern of problematic reading, writing, math, and spelling skills, which is typically found correlated with a "neglect of the page" or hemineglect. It is this unilateral neglect that emphasizes a lack of activation of the parietal area of the brain and implicates its association with the attentional disorders. The presence of this hemineglect correlates with what would be evidenced in damage to parietal areas of the brain and has been documented in our research as correlating with ADD. On a consistent basis, to a greater or lesser degree, evidence of a hemineglect is observed across several different measures and correlated with symptomatology suggestive of the impact of this deficit on functioning specifically: difficulty with spatial issues, or an inattention to the whole, resulting in significant academic problems, specifically in the language areas, as well as social miscuing.

This *inattention to the whole* or *inability to view the whole* has emerged in our research over the last 10 years of administering our attentional battery as a common phenomenon characteristic of the ADD without hyperactivity population and correlated it with the impact to posterior attentional symptoms and with the predominance of the neurotransmitter, norepinephrine being less available. Above-noted symptoms impact the academic-skill development to a varying degree, as well as social functioning, and overall thinking abilities. The ADD individual is not as adept at sizing up the social situation, interpreting the nonverbal social cues in a wholistic manner, and grasping the gestalt of the situation and the manner in which specific social interactions comprise the whole. Characteristics of being unable to anticipate the consequences of one's behavior, saying or doing the wrong thing at the wrong time, appearing less emphathetic due to an inability to perceive the ramifications of the whole situation, as well as diminished problem-solving abilities due to not thinking of another possible solution or not viewing the whole picture, are common issues which occur and disrupt the individual's life. Attributes previously described as ADHD issues of poor social control, poor problem solving, and inability to learn from one's mistakes, can be applied to the without-hyperactivity population when considering the impact of this pervasive inattention to the whole.

Individuals have been noted to have difficulties with time management, the space of time (being unable to anticipate how long tasks will take), and the ability to correlate tasks with the appropriate space of time available to complete the tasks. There are issues of directionality, of becoming disoriented and lost, and a lack of understanding of the differentiation and ability to utilize directionalities. Right-left confusion is rather common phenomenon plaguing this population, as well as difficulties with dancing and the use of the proper right foot versus left. Having to move through the whole alphabet to get to a letter, not being able to repeat numbers backward as accurately as forward, using piece by piece analysis rather than the gestalt to problem solve, are further issues.

Finally, reading and math difficulties emerge as the most disturbing of the problems. Lack of development in either of these areas, particularly that of reading, has been highly predictive of academic difficulties and the tendency to avoid any unnecessary educational pursuits. Tendencies to misread words which leads to comprehension problems, missing words on the page, misinterpreting a sentence (as a result of learning contextually to read), getting multiple-choice questions wrong (due to reading the question incorrectly), and difficulty with the types of evaluations that utilize computer scoring, are common roadblocks to learning and academic achievement. These are often subject to misinterpretation by professionals and wrongful diagnosis of learning disabilities.

Figures 8.1 through 8.16* are various renderings of the Bender-Gestalt designs. The individual is asked to copy these designs, drawing all nine designs on the one sheet of paper. Time taken to complete this measure is noted in the figure captions. Generally, within the normal population, all nine designs are completed within 2 minutes. Drawings are assessed relative to the individual's own performance. Due to the necessity of capturing the gestalt and inability to complete the design utilizing logical skills, the same two designs emerge as being difficult on a continual basis, across gender, age, and neurological insult. The remainder of the profile may be almost perfect in renderings of these designs in contrast to those designs necessitating the view of the whole. The pattern remains similar in this respect despite the individual being male or female child, adolescent, or adult, young or aged, and/or having seizure activity or impact to brain functioning. Impact to brain functioning becomes highly notable in the distortions evidenced in renderings, whether damage is subsequent to a progressive disorder, trauma, or other type of neurological insult. Obsessive-compulsive behavior is noted in the counting of the dots and time taken to complete the task (usual time is that of 2 min although no exact time period is specified to the individual) (Figures 8.8 and 8.9). Perseveration also provides evidence of impact to brain functioning. Findings of distortions and perseveration provide initial indices of impact to brain functioning, targeting this already weakened area, and generally occurring with seizure activation arising either by itself or related to some other type of neurological disorder. The presence of disorders such as drug or environmental

---

*All figures were recreated by Matthew T. Rivard.

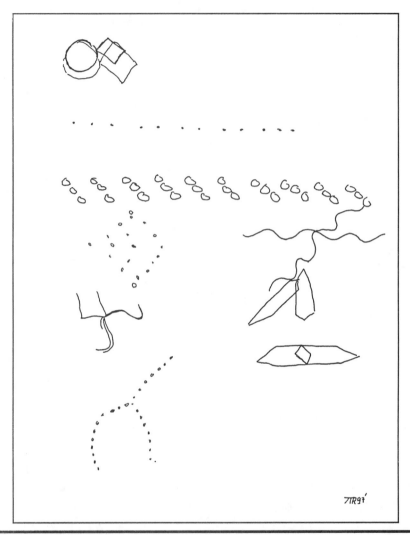

Figure 8.1 Female, aged 13 years, diagnosed ADD without hyperactivity, no brain pathology. Time taken to complete was 6.33 minutes.

toxicity, dementia (especially Alzheimer's disease), sleep apnea, and/or injury to the brain are confirmed with further neurological and neuropsychological evaluation and investigation (see Figures 8.10 through 8.13).

Figures 8.14 through 8.16 indicate the beneficial effects of targeting a specific area of brain functioning for remediation, in this example, the parietal/spatial areas have been directly trained with the use of a variety of materials,

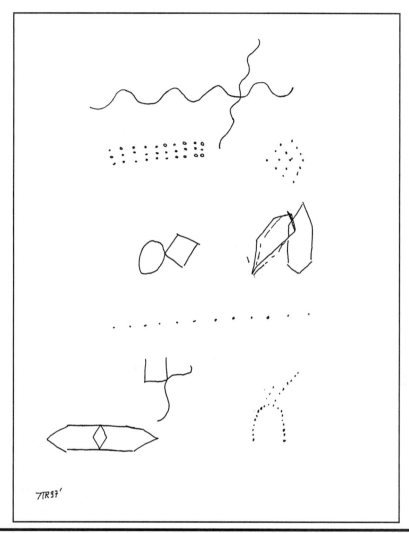

Figure 8.2 Male, aged 14 years, diagnosed ADD without hyperactivity, no brain pathology. Time taken to complete was 3.52 minutes.

including computer software that forces use of the spatial modality. Drawings reveal the progress of this child, diagnosed ADD without hyperactivity, over a period of 3 years. Progress is confirmed by her improved reading and overall academic skill level. At the time of the original assessment, she was having difficulty with her letters and elementary stages of reading. She is of above-average intelligence. There remains some question of brain pathology and she

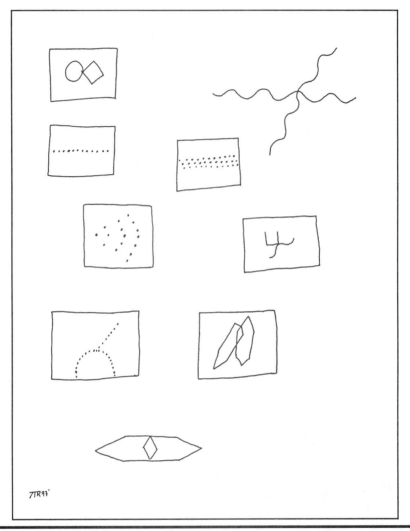

Figure 8.3   Male, aged 24 years, diagnosed ADD without hyperactivity, no brain pathology. This man is a graphic artist who drew all of these reproductions. Time taken to complete was 6.73 minutes.

is being closely observed with regard to any development of seizure activation while on the stimulant medication.

Hemispatial neglect is viewed as a very complex and multifaceted disorder composed of independent processes. Disturbances to the areas of temporal-parietal, dorsolateral, frontal and deep frontal structures are equally likely

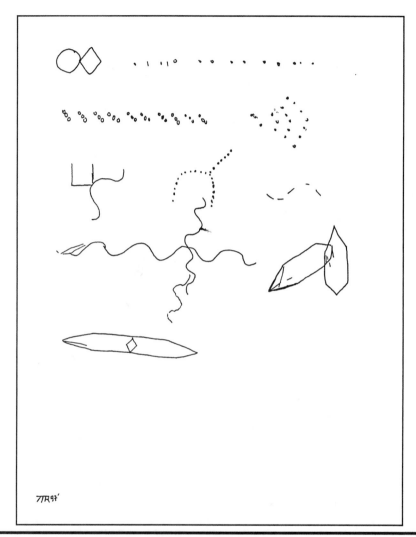

Figure 8.4   Female, aged 12 years, diagnosed ADD without hyperactivity, no brain pathology. Time taken to complete was 6.48 minutes.

to be implicated. Word reading was found to represent an aspect of visuospatial neglect and the failure to read to the left side of a word or sentence, often making substitutions to form alternative words or sentences of equal length. Generally associated with right hemisphere lesions creating an attentional deficit and decreased spatial resolution with the difficulty being the inability of specify or maintain the absolute location of letters within a multi-item

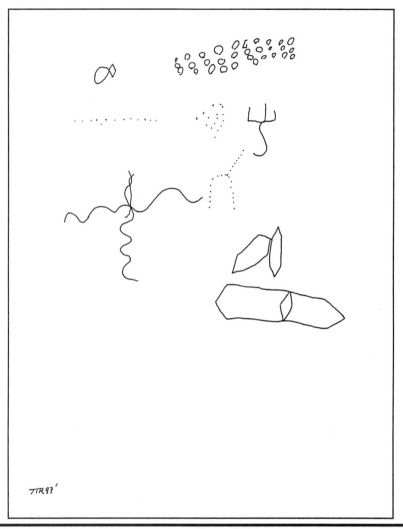

Figure 8.5   Male, aged 7 years, diagnosed ADD without hyperactivity, no brain pathology. Time taken to complete was 9.28 minutes.

array. Right hemisphere lesions produced a neglect dyslexia in addition to a more general visuospatial neglect. Serious phonological weaknesses have been cited in children who still managed to develop adequate reading and spelling skills (Anderson, 1996; Marshall and Halligan, 1996; McGlinchey et al., 1996; Saffran and Coslet, 1996; Snowling and Hulme, 1996). Syntatic features of words are accessed independently of phonological content and

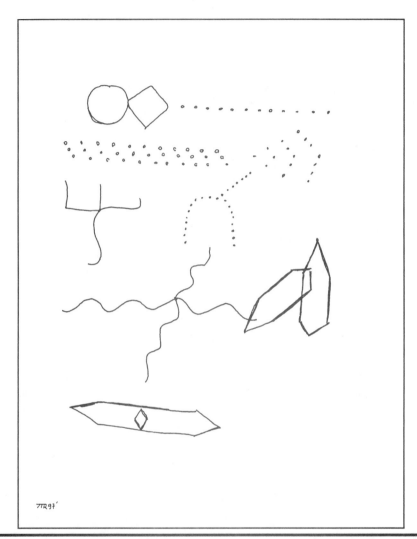

Figure 8.6   Male, aged 19 years, diagnosed ADD without hyperactivity, no brain pathology. This man is an artist and drawings provide a very close rendition to the ideal placement of the figures although three figures remain somewhat incorrect. Time taken to complete was 7.32 minutes.

subserved by distinct neural structures (Miozzo and Caramazza, 1997). Thus, ADD individuals become contextual readers, learning to read via a whole language approach, rather than phonetic. The problem occurs with the misreading of intonation, substitutions of words and the failure to develop reading skills due to the overall difficulty of phonetic learning.

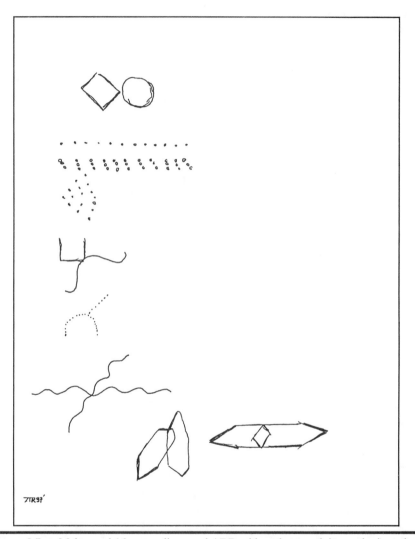

Figure 8.7   Male, aged 16 years, diagnosed ADD without hyperactivity, no brain pathology. This is the usual pattern seen with this population, notice the placement of the designs on the page and clearcut failure to use the right hemispace. Time taken to complete was 4.23 minutes.

Kinsbourne (1994) summarized research findings relating attentional problems to neglect and indicated that it has been more frequent and more often associated with damage to the right hemisphere causative lesions hypothesized to involve specifically the inferior parietal lobule and, when subcortical, the thalamus or the basal ganglia. Theoretically, there is the idea

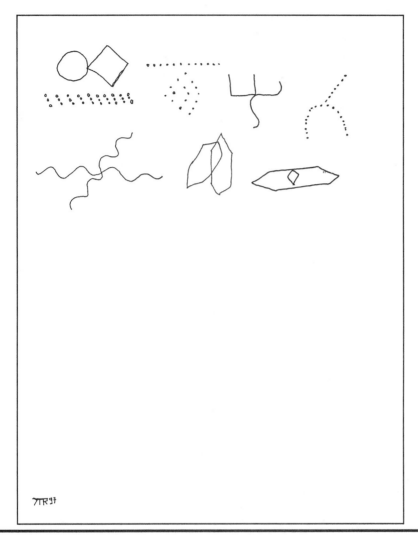

Figure 8.8   Male, aged 13 years, diagnosed ADD without hyperactivity, no brain pathology. This is another common pattern evidenced with this population, especially characteristic of those individuals who have compulsive tendencies, they reduce the size of the drawings to make it easier to draw them perfectly and/or to make their mistakes less noticeable. Time taken to complete was 4.59 minutes.

that there is an attentional bias in the sweep of the inner "eye" that scans the passively represented input for attentional purposes, and while the input itself or the image is fully represented, the inner monitor sweeps only to one

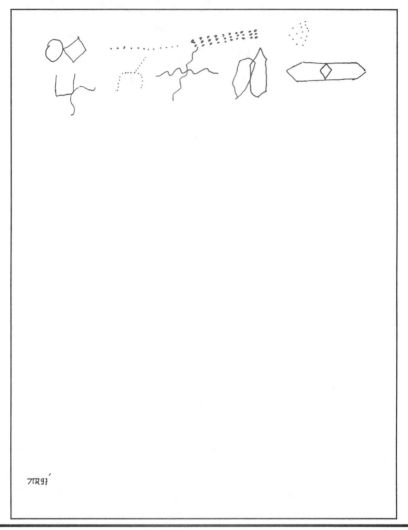

Figure 8.9   Male, aged 16 years, diagnosed ADD without hyperactivity and Obsessive Compulsive Disorder, further evaluation was in process to determine evidence of Tourett's Syndrome. Notice the shakiness of the lines, very minute small hand tremors are evident when there is a question of seizure activation. (However this shakiness can also be observed in a hypoglycemic reaction.) Time taken to complete was 3.34 minutes.

side, similar to the idea of receptor orientation to external objects being laterally biased. Visuospatial impairment in Parkinson's disease is viewed as the consequence of dysfunction of the dorsolateral prefrontal and posterior

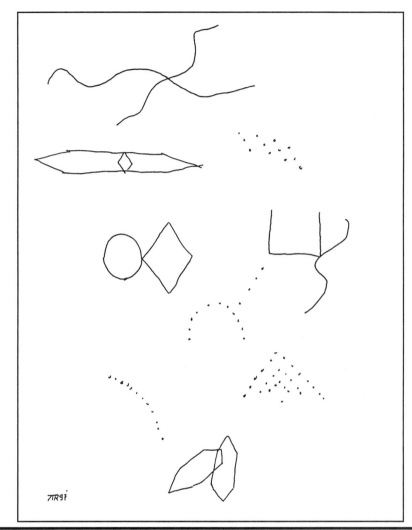

Figure 8.10   Male, aged 9 years, diagnosed ADD without hyperactivity. The distortions of some of the designs is quite noticeable. Further neurological evaluation provided evidence of a longstanding seizure disorder. This child is unable to read a single word due to a deteriorated spatial condition and significant memory impairment. Lacking any of the compensatory mechanisms with which to develop reading despite consistent tutorial work he remains unable to read due to the lack of ability to memorize words and/or learn phonetically. In addition he possesses minimal motivation, is highly labile, and is self-derogatory in his thinking due to personality changes subsequent to seizure activation. Time taken to complete was 4.37 minutes.

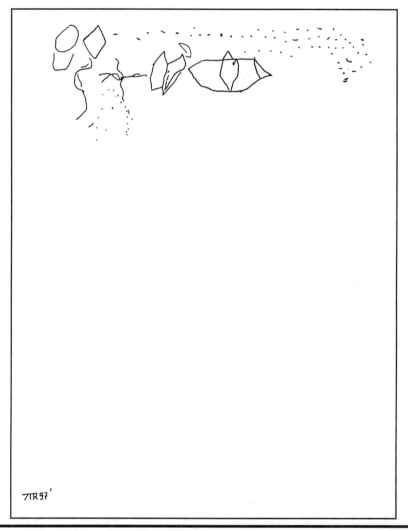

Figure 8.11   Female, aged 6 years, diagnosed ADD without hyperactivity, there is a question of brain pathology. She talked throughout the completion of these designs, "dot, dot, dot", "circle, circle, circle…". The distortions are quite evident as well as the failure of the gestalt on some of the designs that is not age appropriate. Time taken to complete was 4.00 minutes.

cortices comprising the basal ganglia-thalamocortical circuit (Cronin-Golomb and Braun, 1997). Functional MRI imaging analysis during a shifting task identified visuospatial attention regions in the parietal and frontal cortices,

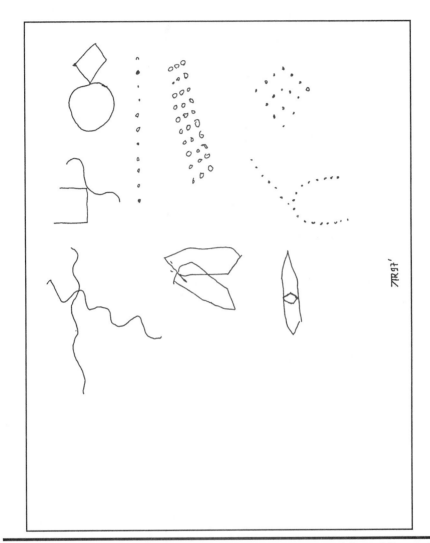

Figure 8.12 Male, aged 35 years, diagnosed ADD without hyperactivity and Traumatic Brain Injury as a result of a motor accident whereby he was a pedestrian. Neuropsychological evaluation revealed significant parietal impairment of basic sensory areas in addition to the more complex problem solving of the tactual modality. He drew these designs without turning the cards or the paper which is indicative of the spatial distortions and deterioration to this area of functioning subsequent to seizure activity. He was on anticonvulsants at the time of evaluation. Memory processes are significantly impaired and there is evidence of frontal lobe pathology, executive dysfunctioning. Time taken to complete was 5.02 minutes.

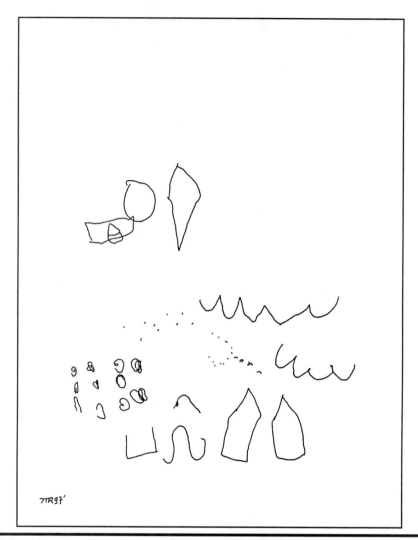

Figure 8.13 Female, aged 5 years, diagnosed ADD without hyperactivity, distortions and lack of the gestalt is highly evident. She displayed symptoms of idiopathic seizure activity with behavioral outbursts, blank staring spells, continual restless movement and thrashing of legs at night, emotional liability, and noise and light sensitivity. Time taken to complete was 2.00 minutes.

presenting bilaterally in the post-central and intraparietal sulcus and middle frontal gyrus (Corbetta et al., 1997).

Given the idea that selective attending is implemented by enhancing the activation of the particular representation, neglect would occur when the two

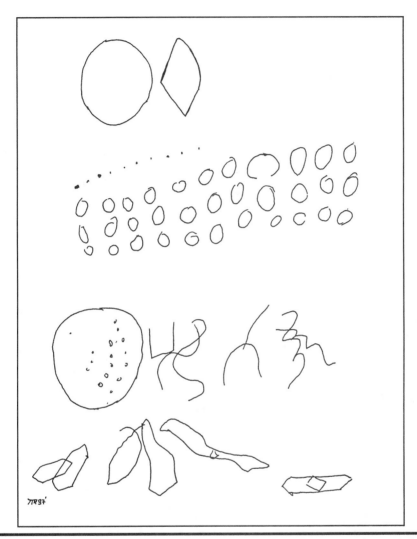

Figure 8.14 First evaluation, aged 5 years 6 months. Time taken to complete was 6.12 minutes.

half-brains activate the cell assemblies that represent stimuli disposed along the lateral plane in a complementary fashion. Each hemisphere would then contribute activation to that portion of the representation that is excited by contralateral segments of the stimulus. With graduated change in this continual interaction, the normal individual would be able to attend selectively to either side or any intermediate part of the representation at will. When neglect occurs, however, the component of the cell assembly that represents the

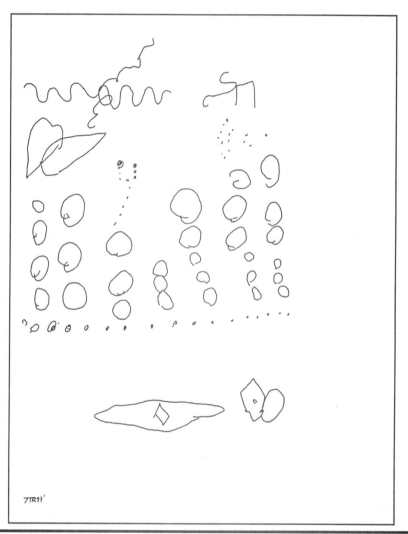

Figure 8.15 Second evaluation, aged 6.5 years. Time taken to complete was 6.13 minutes.

contralesional section of the stimulus is underactivated and, as a result, contralesional contents are not experienced, nor do they excite reaction. Chatterjee et al. (1996) conclude that damage to either hemisphere can result in abnormal deviations in orienting attention within a region of space. The right hemisphere was seen as subserving attentional abilities across regions of space.

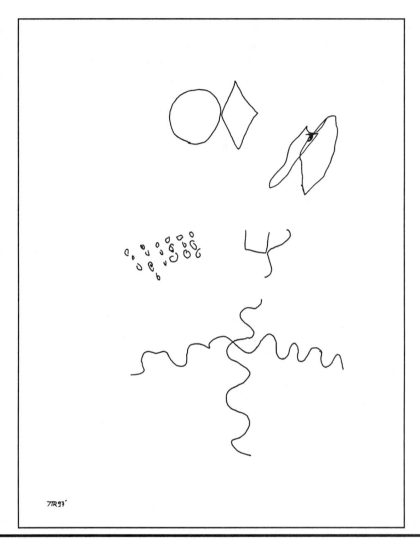

Figure 8.16 Third evaluation, aged 8 years. She was not asked to draw all of the designs.

In addressing visuospatial attention, the posterior attentional system was found to be well preserved and less impaired in the healthy aged population in comparison to selective-attention processes involving the anterior attentional system. Alzheimer's patients as well as older adults experience changes and breakdowns in functioning in the posterior attentional system (associated with the early filtering of information); however, the anterior attentional system (and top-down control of processes) associated with the control or selection of a response for action, was found to be considerably more impaired. Authors proposed confirmation of the right hemisphere as aging more rapidly than the left and the idea of diminished interhemispheric transfer of information as an age-related decline in functioning (Faust and Balota, 1997). Làdavas et al. (1997) presented evidence that neglect patients with parietal lesions do not evidence a lack of oculomotor control, uncontrollable leftward eye movements and left attentional shift that the neglect patients who have sustained frontoparietal lesions do. The presence of separate systems responsible for attentional and gaze orienting is suggested to be mediated by corresponding roles of the frontal and parietal lobes in the selective turning of the eyes towards the stimulus location (overt orienting) and the shifting of attention to the visual object (covert orienting). Knight (1997) reports similar findings using event-related potentials indicating a pattern of results confirming the presence of an association cortex, interhemispheric network involving the prefrontal and posterior cortex for early visual processing activated during orientation to novel events.

This can be applied to the biochemical theory of ADD in that the underactivation, rather than lesions, would create the lack of excitation or inability to view the whole that are so commonly seen in the ADD population.

The reason that the parietal arc and its subservient process appear responsible is that this inattention, neglect, and/or inability to conceptualize the whole of some object, event, or idea transcends basic sensory modalities, reflecting more complex functioning of the spatial area and its connections. Common complaints provide testimony to the uniformity of this deficit:

1. Individuals cannot compute numbers in their head or view numbers to repeat a sequence backwards.
2. They cannot draw a straight line.
3. Social situations are often inappropriately sized up. The individual is in the wrong place at the wrong time, says the wrong thing, cannot anticipate or predict consequences related to sequential events (which is not related to sequencing deficits).
4. Individuals miss items that are in front of them.
5. ADD individuals with this imperception of the whole are clumsy, bumping into things, and cannot gauge their size in relationship to sizes around them. The management problems occur due to their inability to estimate the span of time necessary to complete tasks.
6. They have right left confusion.

7. One must go through the whole alphabet to arrive at the intended letter (e.g., A-B-C-D-E-F-G- to get to the H).
8. Time management problems occurred due to the inability to estimate the space of time necessary to complete tasks.
9. There is difficulty in anticipating consequences in the environment, based upon their behavior as an antecedent causal factor.
10. There exists an inability to size up the whole picture of things, appearing myopic in seeing all of the parts of a situation, thus impacting decision-making skills.
11. Movement in space and direction becomes problematic, there is a tendency to move to the opposite direction in response to verbal or visual request, such as a dance routine and confusion with turns and directionality, especially as that direction is continually changing.
12. They have significant handwriting problems, reading, spelling, and mathematical difficulties as it becomes more spatial in origin.
13. Individuals appear lacking empathy due to a difficulty perceiving the whole or gestalt of a situation to fully interpret the meaning of the individual's feelings.
14. There is an inability to connect several facts and ideas together to view a situation from a whole perspective.
15. At times, a disorientation or loss of directionality exists.
16. Stuttering, due to an inability to organize language internally and/or attempting to say something too quickly without the ability to integrate and modulate the speech pattern exists.

Anatomical Basis of Attention

Cortical areas in the temporoparietal-occipital junction, as well as subcortical structures and structures involving the limbic areas, were found to be important in mediating arousal and attention. Researchers have concurred that inattention or sensory neglect can be defined as an attentional arousal disorder, the consequence of a dysfunction involving the corticolimbic reticular formation network (Heilman and Valenstein, 1972; Watson et al., 1981; Mesulam, 1981). Heilman, Watson, and Valenstein (1993) cite references from animal research suggesting that this neglect may be connected to the striatal dopamine depletion and restoration of dopamine or dopaminergic activity has been found to reinstate ability and lead to recovery of function regarding neglect issues.

Corballis (1994) indicated that there is no general agreement as to the specific brain mechanisms underlying hemineglect, and theorists have postulated that it may be attentional and/or related to the failure to disengage attention from the side of space ipsilateral to the lesioned area. Damage to the posterior parietal lobe has been suggested as responsible for perceptual hemineglect. Finally, conscious awareness of visual input appears to depend on the geniculo-striatal pathway leading to the inferior occipital regions, and hemineglect may be the consequence of damage to this localizational system in the parietal lobe. The processing and analysis of spatial frequency information using cerebral blood-flow studies was found to primarily activate occupied and parietal regions (Gulyas and Roland, 1995). Significant impairment on tactile perception tasks subsequent to Parkinson's disease presents evidence of abnormal frontostriatal functioning as accountable for somatosensory abnormalities impacting the decision-making process for correct analysis of incoming sensory input (Sathian et al., 1997).

Various research studies have implicated the mesencephalic reticular activating system (MRF), cingulate cortex, and nucleus reticularis of the thalamus as having a major influence affecting the cortical processing of sensory stimuli. Rapid MRF stimulation or behavioral arousal inhibits the nucleus reticularis and is thereby associated with enhanced or activated thalamic transmission to the cerebral cortex. Lesions of the thalamic relay nuclei or primary sensory cortex induce a sensory defect, as opposed to neglect. Primary cortical sensory areas project to unimodal association cortex, and association cortex synthesizes multiple features of a complex stimulus within a single sensory modality. Thus, lesions of the unimodal association cortex may result in perceptual deficits limited to a single modality. Unimodal association areas converge on polymodal association areas. In the animal, this is represented as prefrontal cortex and includes both banks of the superior temporal sulcus or STS, whereas in the human this area is defined as the inferior parietal lobule (IPL) and unimodal association areas may converge on this area after synapsing at the prefrontal and temporal sulcus areas. Polymodal convergence areas can subserve cross-modal associations and polymodal synthesis and analysis. Polymodal synthesis can detect novelty and significance and, in contrast to the unimodal association cortex (that only projects to specific parts of the thalamic nuclei) thereby gating sensory input in only one modality, these multimodal areas are convergence zones for a more-general inhibitory effect, and then provide further continued arousal after further cortical analysis has occurred. These convergence areas may also project directly to the reticular formation to induce a general state of arousal because of diffuse multisynaptic connections to the cortex or increase thalamic transmission via connections with the nucleus reticularis, or both (Heilman and Valenstein, 1993).

Spatial bias in normal subjects are separate and task specific. Task specificity determines the predominance of one system over another (sensory attentional versus motor intentional) isolating a primary and secondary system with commensurate influence (Schwartz et al., 1997). PET scan activity confirmed the presence of a general neural system with right hemisphere dominance, underlying visuospatial attention, consisting of the cortical areas of the anterior cingulate gyrus, intraparietal sulcus, medial and lateral premotor cortices. The superior temporal sulcus (STS) region, while activated by the majority of subjects in response to the visuospatial shifts of attention, did not meet the criteria of significance. The subcortical structures were difficult to pinpoint anatomically and the only structure to emerge with significance was that of the pulvinar nucleus of the thalamus (the limited size of the array of the PET detectors may have created problems of detection and influenced the lack of significance (Nobre et al., 1997).

Disturbed visuospatial attentional processes in Alzheimer's disease are subject to bilateral impact of the parietal regions, disturbing spatial and object components of attentional shifting by affecting the jointly operating system of the right and left, superior and inferior lobes. The right superior parietal lobe subserves the spatial orienting of attention while the left inferior parietal lobe is involved in the maintenance of attentional selection, creating separate yet parallel representations of the relationships occurring between the parts of a single object and between the separate objects themselves (Buck et al., 1997).

Specific Manifestations of Spatial Orientation Disorders

Disorders of spatial orientation can occur whereby the individual cannot appreciate spatial relationships between and within objects in extrapersonal space. Spatial disorientation encompasses a number of different disorders and principal categories are those disorders in which (Walsh, 1974):

1. Impaired judgment of the location or orientation of stimuli, both with respect to each other and to the person
2. Impaired memory for location

3. Topographical disorientation and loss of topographical memory
4. Route finding difficulties
5. Constructional apraxia
6. Spatial dyslexia and dyscalculia

Disorders of location and orientation are noted by Benton (1969) as the difficulty with the perceived spatial relation between two or more stimuli, which could be termed a difficulty with relative localization. Tests of more-complex spatial relations bring out difficulties not seen in simpler tests. *Impaired memory for location* may be part of a general amnesic disorder or may be seen in association with other spatial difficulties.

Topographical disorientation and loss of topographical memory encompasses several different types of difficulties:

▪ The inability to recall the spatial arrangement of familiar surroundings, such as the way a room is arranged
▪ The inability to recall and describe well-known geographical relationships with which the person was familiar prior to injury to the brain

Welsh (1974) notes that in the research these areas are beginning to receive attention. Different studies point to the impairment of both personal and extrapersonal space as due to legions of the posterior part of the left hemisphere of the parietal area. Anterior lesions were found to impair personal (but not extrapersonal) orientation. Studies indicate that parietal patients have difficulty with reversible mental spatial operations, while other patients do not. Soeldner and Fedio (1972), in comparing left frontal and right parietal patients found that the frontal and parietal regions mediate qualitatively different spatial abilities. Spatial orientation to external objects was found to be mediated by the parietal regions, particularly the right hemisphere and spatial discrimination, whereas orientation involving the individual's own self was mediated particularly by the frontal region, left hemisphere. Benton and colleagues (1974) attempted to more systematically study this hypothesis first generated by Teuber. Geographical orientation was assessed in patients with unilateral cerebral disease utilizing two different tasks requiring localization of states and cities and a verbal test of the directional relations between places. Findings identified clear differentiation between the two groups, suggesting neglect of the visual field contralateral to the side of the lesion in some of the patients, and demonstrated that there is an interaction of deficits involved in producing this type of impaired performance on complex tasks. The relationship between the locus of the lesion and the topographical loss is less clear than with a number of the other spatial disorders. Research indicates that the most frequent reports are after posterior lesions, whether they are right, left, or bilateral (Welsh, 1974). McGlone, Losier, and Black (1997) found no gender differences for post-stroke patients. Greater severity and incidence of neglect was more notable subsequent to right hemisphere lesions. It was only when comparing ipsilesional versus contralesional reaction times on a visual search task that gender differences emerged with significantly more women (76%) than men (62%) evidencing neglect with the etiology of right hemisphere lesions.

Route-finding difficulties are addressed by Welsh (1974), who indicated research conclusions of only occasionally reported cases, whereby the principal deficit lies in the patient's inability to find his/her way around in surroundings that have been familiar for a long period of time. They may be able to provide adequate verbal descriptions of familiar routes; however, they are unable to execute them either by drawing or taking such routes in real-life situations, and thus become lost en route. In defining *topographical agnosia,* Welsh (1974) notes the importance of separating out the issue of the inability to recognize objects that serve as landmarks along a route from the individual, being able to follow signs to a goal, learning their way about and, instead of learning discrete movements, learning orchestrated sequences of movements and meanings. Thus, the individual learns not just a movement pattern, but significant relations and a behavior route. Aspects of route memory was found to be susceptible to aging effects as older adults performed worse than younger subjects and experienced difficulty memorizing, navigating, or retracing the route. They intended to make more errors, presenting impairments in the selection or effective utilization of critical visual cues, consequently making more errors, despite an intact ability to encode and recognize landmarks (Wilkniss et al., 1997).

Specific cases for *topographical amnesia* are rare, whereby this forms the sole complaint. The amnesia may include long-stored topographical information, as well as material more recently acquired. Welsh (1974) cites research whereby patients are described with a very short forgetting period for spatial information. It is important to differentiate between spatial information that can be gained from a single viewpoint (visuospatial perception) and the topographical schema of large-scale space, which is usually acquired by personal locomotor experience.

Early investigators found that with *constructional apraxia,* the failure of individuals in such tasks as drawing and route-finding reflected a visuospatial disturbance; however, it also became apparent that those with severe difficulties with drawing did not always necessitate a spatial deficit. To this end, constructional apraxia has been said to be an impairment with combinatory or organizing activity in which details need to be perceived and combined in a relationship made up of component parts to a whole entity, thus the Gestalt of the design needs to be intact to be correctly drawn. Researchers have argued whether constructional apraxia represents a single entity and different varieties have been suggested. Factors to consider are the inability to analyze the model visually, a disruption of the spatial schemata, or the inability to initiate, monitor, or execute a plan for the solution of the task, whether it be drawing or a combination of blocks, as seen on the Weschler subtests. Welsh (1974) concludes that the research generally shows more impairment to the right hemisphere than to the left, while posterior lesions for either hemisphere produced more consistent disturbances than anterior lesions. Problems observed clinically with drawing of Gestalt of the design may relate to an attentional disorder and inattention to the whole.

Spatial dyslexia can be distinguishable from dyslexia in that the individual can recognize letters and words, but not be able to read due to difficulty in putting letters and words together as a whole entity. Part of this difficulty may be attributable to a difficulty with the continuous scanning movements necessary for reading. The disorganization of the directional control of the eye movements can vary from individual to individual and, in those severely disabled, the fixations appear to be made at random. Thus, the fixation may jump from one part of a line to another, and from one line to another, and so on down the page. As a result, the individual would be unable to make sense of printed material as it is listed on a page, those less severely affected are able to compensate due to missing only a few words and consequently they are able to piece together the whole due to having more information (rather than less), when compared with those who are severely affected. Thus, reading difficulties can depend on unilateral spatial neglect, and spatial dyslexia is seen more frequently with right hemisphere lesions (Worthington, 1996). Benton (1969) indicated that observations are of individuals initially fixating on a point that is some distance to the right of the beginning of the line, and they then read to the end of the line to return to a point on the next line, which is again somewhat to the right of the beginning of the line, and the result is that as time goes on, they become increasingly confused. Alzheimer patients were found to exhibit reading difficulties due to a loss of location and impairment was greatest when the words were less distinguishable from one another (upper vs. lower case letters) and in the presence of other words (as opposed to viewing words in isolation). Reading text becomes more difficult and contextual errors occur when the mechanism designed to enhance processing of one letter string over another fails to do so. Location information was seen as a significant factor in reading impairment in this population relative to visuoperceptual disturbances (Saffran and Coslett, 1996).

Knivsberg (1997) noted that phonological deficits comprise the underlying problem in the majority of reading disturbances. Characteristic symptoms of difficulties with word decoding, particularly nonwords (inability to string letters in a meaningless manner), reflect phonological difficulties. In evaluating children with dyslexia, abnormalities emerged in urine samples and serum analyses which may be related to underlying peptidase deficiencies for the proteins gluten and casein, similar to abnormalities related to syndromes such as Tourette's, Autism, ADD, Schizophrenia, and Depression. Fiez (1997) proposes the idea that the left inferior prefrontal gyrus is seen as being complementary for both semantic and phonological processing.

The connectionist model of reading, that real words and pseudowords are processed within a common neural network, was confirmed by evaluation of normal adult male subjects. Phonological (pseudowords) and orthographic (real words) pronunciation activated left superior temporal gyrus, significantly greater activation was noted for phonological pronunciation. Phonological decision making resulted in intense and widespread activation for the left inferior frontal cortex and occurred to a much lesser degree of orthographic decision making (Rumsey et al., 1997). The orthographic method of reading resulted in the ability to incorporate the lexical representation of the printed word without the use of phonological mediation. This was rendered an implicit visual operation requiring visual feature analysis and visual coding ability to provide a direct route for word meanings to exist, almost as if they were entries in a mental dictionary which could then be accessed directly (Rumsey et al., 1997). PET scan studies were used to analyze speech and language production occurring with developmental stuttering, determining that stuttering symptoms were associated with anterior forebrain regions located almost exclusively in the left hemisphere. As speech became more fluent, the anterior and posterior perisylvian areas of the right hemisphere became activated, suggesting the positive intervention of right hemisphere processes in the mediation of stuttering (Braum et al., 1997).

Phonological dyslexia is defined as the ability to read at a normal rate; however substitutions are made. These substitutions increased in diagnosed dyslexic children when they read faster and also tended to sound out words to a lesser degree. When attention is diffused and distributed over the entire word, it is recognized more quickly (Hendriks and Kolk, 1997). Spelling involves both orthographic and phonological processes and is not solely phonologically mediated (Coltheart and Coltheart, 1997).

Delayed phonological development was seen as a causal factor for reading and spelling deficits. These deficits were determined to be the result of delayed development of mappings from orthography to phonology and unreliable mappings between individual graphemes and phonemes (Snowling and Hulme, 1996). Longer words were more prone to errors (Worthington, 1996). Performance improved on a visuospatial task utilizing left hemisphere input in the fact of severe right hemisphere deficits. The idea is proposed that attentional vectors of the cerebral hemispheres can be modulated by both perceptual task demands and motor response demands (Marshall and Halligan, 1996).

Evans and Seymour (1997) reported the development of an extensive word recognition vocabulary using almost exclusively logographic (whole word) processes due to extremely poor phonological development subsequent to genetic abnormalities associated with the 48, XXXY syndrome.

The ability to develop proficient reading and spelling skills despite serious phonological difficulties (limited knowledge of grapheme and phoneme correlations) an inefficient decoding strategy, was evidenced in a child of average intelligence, as measured over a period of 3 years, who learned to read via the development of mappings between orthography and rudimentary phonological representations. Difficulty with phonological processing increased with time and maturity despite the continued occurrence of compensatory processes. This child was not viewed as dyslexic, learning occurred in an atypical manner (left to right decoding strategy was not utilized) and instead semantic content and partial decoding (corresponding to words already present in her vocabulary) using the spoken word to form a fully adequate orthographic system was implemented for intact reading and spelling (Stothard, Snowling, and Hulme, 1997). Language was acquired as late as 9 years of age using only right-hemisphere processes and it was postulated that language can fully develop provided that it is acquired or re-acquired before the onset of puberty and hormonal changes which bring a close to the period of cerebral plasticity (Vargha-Khadem et al., 1997).

Holmes and Standish (1997) in studying a young woman with above-average reading comprehension noted that she had compensated for impaired phonological processing capacity with the development of superior orthographic processing ability. She was identified at above-average efficiency in her ability to choose correct spellings and lexical status of both short words and nonwords. She excelled at orthographic processing in silent reading and demonstrated an exceptional efficiency in lexical decisions for short word and nonword sequences. Their research demonstrated that remediation for problematic phonological processing and memory can occur with programs directed towards training in orthographic segmentation and discrimination skills.

Spatial Dyscalculia (Acalculia)

The role of the left hemisphere has been addressed in the research and general findings report left-hemisphere lesions with dyscalculia. Hécaen (1962) was one of the first to report a predominance of right hemisphere lesions with a type of mathematical difficulty involving spatial problems. Adults who had suffered unilateral lesions were administered a test of computation and numerical series completion. The left-hemisphere group, as expected, performed worse than the right hemisphere on the computation measure, however the two groups were equally impaired, to a severe degree, on the numerical series completion. Findings suggested the necessary interaction of input from both hemispheres to perform tasks requiring arithmetic reasoning. Abstraction of numerical relations was found to rely upon right-hemisphere functions as a result of the role of spatial skills. The spatial processing of the right hemisphere contributes to an initial overall appreciation of the series progression, while left-hemisphere processes allows for the generation and evaluation of formulas, use of computational rules, and calculation process (Langdon and Warrington, 1997). The left parietal lobe was implicated in the performance of simple multiplication problems and the ability to retrieve arithmetic facts from memory (Whalen et al., 1997).

Mathematical problems are fairly common in the ADD population, specifically those diagnosed with ADD without hyperactivity. These problems appear to be well correlated with spatial issues, an inattention to the whole, and inability to grasp the mathematical concepts, complete equations, and comprehend geometric issues. Children generally do not experience considerable difficulties in math until later grades (junior high and high school) for this reason.

DeLuca et al. (1997) used fluorodeoxyglucose PET and proton magnetic resonance spectroscopy (MRS) to document hypometabolism in right parietal and bilateral superior temporal cortices in two male children ages 11 and

12 years, who demonstrated a right hemisphere learning disability on neuropsychological evaluation, evidencing symptoms of poor arithmetic skills, visual spatial difficulties, diminished deductive reasoning skills, and intact reading, spelling and rote verbal skills. Other measurements of neuronal status were within normal limits.

Unilateral Spatial Neglect

Unilateral spatial neglect can result primarily in syndromes of both motor-spatial and personal neglect. Premotor and perceptual factors are seen as related to unilateral neglect (Sterzi et al., 1996). Central processes and messages from peripheral processes move across a neural network of generally segregated pathways towards response system outlets (Berti, LaDavas, and Corte, 1996). Robertson et al. (1997) presents the idea that spatial knowledge must be accurate and specific to allow for the correct perception of features for attentional selection and subsequent rapid search for these features in a multi-item display. Impact to parietal cortices disrupts the accurate rendering of spatial representations fundamental for spatial awareness and, ultimately, for object perception.

Heilman et al. (1972) postulated an attention arousal hypothesis to explain the mechanism of neglect. Authors argued that the sensory and perceptual hypothesis that preceded their work could not explain in a sufficient fashion all of the cases of neglect, especially since the neglect was often produced by lesions external to the traditional sensory pathways. Finally, neglect was often found to be multimodal, and thus could not be explained by a problem in a specific sensory modality.

Heilman is one of the leading authors on neglect and defined it as the failure to report, respond, or orient to novel or meaningful stimuli presented to the side opposite a lesion. Neglect occurs in the absence of sensory or motor defects and has been predominantly associated with parietal lesions, although it can also be found with lesions of the frontal lobe as well. According to Heilman, neglect may be spatial or personal, an individual may be inattentive to stimuli in space or to themselves. They may fail to act in a portion of space, in a spatial direction, or on a portion of their own body. Although there is a continuum of individual differences, major behavioral manifestations are that of inattention or sensory neglect, extinction to simultaneous stimuli, motor neglect, spatial neglect, personal neglect, allesthesia, allokinesia, and anosognosia, which is total denial of an illness or lost limb (Heilman, 1993).

Parietal lesions are seen as unbalancing the interplay that exists between orienting and attentional maintenance mechanisms to produce "disengagement" deficits. Disengagement is the process that occurs due to the interactions between mechanisms whose role it is to maintain attention and to reorient attention to other objects (Humphreys, Boucart, Dator, and Riddoch, 1996). Walker, Findlay, Young, and Lincoln (1996) view neglect as a disorder of spatial awareness and do not subscribe to the disengagement hypothesis and instead attribute symptoms to cortical and subcortical areas who each have their own neural representation and present faulty programming of the motor outputs under visual guidance. The problem then becomes one of orienting attention within an object-based frame of reference. Deficits on tasks which were dependent upon spatial information were found to be due to the disruption of a spatial map, representing visual information accumulated across saccades in an egocentric coordinate system. Impairment of judgment of the location of visually and auditorially presented target was found with visual attention remaining preserved. Disturbance in the processing and/or use of spatial information is seen as common manifestations of damage to the parietal area. Impairments may take various forms ranging from deficient performance on a spatial problem solving task to clear disabilities as a result of a lack of responsiveness to stimuli on one side of space (Hemispatial neglect) to an inability to reach accurately to visual targets (ataxia). There are two types of spatial dysfunction identified, one involves the restrictions on attentional capacity, the failure to allocate attention to one side of space. The second addresses the loss of an underlying capacity for spatial representation, evidenced as a visual disorientation (Start, Coslett, and Safran, 1996).

Sensory neglect or inattention refers to a deficit in awareness of contralateral stimuli and has been identified in both the human and animal populations with lesions in locations other than the primary sensory areas or sensory projection systems. The distribution of attentional deficits may vary from individual to individual and may also vary depending on the method of evaluation utilized. Individuals may fail to attend to visual, auditory, or tactile stimuli, and their inattention may be to stimuli in space or to stimuli on their own person. The situation becomes even more complex, in that the distribution of attention in space can depend not only on the position of the stimulus in the visual field, but also on the relative position of the stimulus to the individual's space or body position. The visual field and the spatial fields (as defined by head and or body position) are only congruent with one another when the individual is looking straight ahead. Thus, movement, whether of the eyes or of the body, will result in noncongruent fields. Individuals with unilateral visual inattention will find deficits vary with direction of gaze (Heilman, 1993). There is evidence for the interaction between linguistic knowledge and cognitive mechanisms underlying visual attention (Coring, Kritchevsky, and Bellugi, 1996). The evaluative coding principle recognizes the persistence or significance of the encoded attribute in the cerebral cortex. Information has value when endowed with the factor of persistence that modifies subsequent treatment (Koechlin and Burnod, 1996).

Action Intentional Disorders (Motor Neglect)

Sensory loss and inattention may account for the unawareness of stimuli. There are those who fail to respond even though they are aware of the stimulus. These disorders are termed by Heilman and his associates as action-intentional disorders characterized by akinesia, motor extinction, hypokinesia, and motor impersistence.

Akinesia is the failure to initiate movements and is most often associated with dysfunction of movement when the motor system or any disorder involving the motor neurons is not involved and cannot account for the failure to initiate. Thus, it is a problem of the systems necessary to initiate the action or movement. According to Heilman, akinesia can involve different body parts, such as the eyes, the head, a limb, or the whole body, and it can vary, depending on where in space the body part is moved and in what direction. In *directional akinesia,* there is a reluctance to move in a direction that is contralateral to the lesion and directional akinesia may be associated with a directional motor bias and the tendency to deviate to the side of the lesion. The failure to move in response to a stimulus, despite the presence of spontaneous movements that are accurate and good motor strength, is often attributed, according to Heilman and associates, to an elemental sensory defect or to sensory inattention (Heilman, 1993).

Motor extinction occurs when the individual can report stimulation of both sides of the body, but will only move the ipsilateral limb (Heilman, 1993). *Hypokinesia* impacts individuals with more mild deficits and reveals itself in a slow response, slow to initiate, and initiation that occurs after an abnormally long delay. Hypokinesia can be observed in both the limbs and the eyes, and can be hemispatial, resulting in some movements being slower than others. *Motor impersistence* is the inability to sustain the act and appears to be the intentional equivalent of the distractibility symptom of an attentional disorder. Motor impersistence can be demonstrated when utilizing a variety of body parts and individuals may experience difficulty with maintaining overall motor activation.

Allesthesia and *allokinesia* are defined as deficits that do not allow the individual to determine where touch occurred (Heilman et al., 1985, 1993, 1995). *Spatial dysgraphia,* a writing disorder, was identified in a patient with cerebellar damage. The cerebellar system is proposed as having a modulatory effect on structures involved in the planning of the motor response and in the actual performance involved in this writing disorder, normally evidenced with only right hemisphere lesions (Silveri et al., 1997).

Spatial Neglect

The process of neglect occurs when different aspects of spatial cognition are disrupted, and is not attributable to a single etiological deficit (Coslett, 1997). The overall definition as provided by Heilman (1993) is that the individual fails to act in body-centered space or on the side of the stimuli contralateral to the area damaged. Individuals can demonstrate both body- and object-centered spatial neglect. Individuals with neglect may fail to read part of a word or a portion of a sentence and may only write on one side of the page. There is horizontal neglect, neglect of vertical and radial space that has been identified. Neglect may be viewer, body, object, or environmentally centered. When an individual neglects the left-sided stimuli in the upright position, then lies on the right side and neglects stimuli to the left side of the body, he/she may have body-centered neglect. If the individual neglects stimuli in the left side of the environment, he/she may have environmentally centered neglect. Individuals can neglect stimuli to the left of the body and on the left side of the environment having both body- and environmentally centered neglect (Heilman, 1993). Spatial attention was found to operate in isolation from preattention processes, these processes interact, however not in a mutually dependent manner, and may actually mutually constrain one another in the selection process (Vecera and Behrmann, 1997).

Personal neglect can occur with the individual who fails to recognize his/her contralesional extremity as their own and may complain of someone else's leg or arm being in bed with them. Frequently, these individuals will fail to dress or groom the abnormal side, and this can also appear as dressing apraxia and/or a profound visuospatial disorder. When referencing unilateral spatial neglect, it is indicated that there is a clear tendency to neglect one half of the extrapersonal space in such tasks, and drawing, reading, dressing, etc.

to a greater or lesser degree. Thus, individuals may be found to neglect food, collide with walls, and so on. A spatial component was determined as involved in a condition of *amusia* (lack of musical appreciation) subsequent to a right hemisphere infarction between the middle and posterior cerebral artery areas, demonstrating the involvement of areas beyond that of the primary auditory cortex (Griffiths et al., 1997).

Significance of the Inferior Parietal Lobe

The idea is that the "what" and "where" describing the stimulus in question occurs in the inferior parietal lobe (IPL) and lesions in that region produce unawareness or neglect due to receiving not only polymodal sensory input, but also because it is the convergence site for the perceptual cognitive systems that deal with both the "what" and the "where" aspects of environmental awareness. Anatomic and electrophysiological data substantiate this hypothesis in animals and it is in process of being validated in humans. As a convergence area, information is received from the cingulate gyrus and the dorsal lateral frontal lobe. Lesions in both areas have been shown to produce neglect. The dorsal lateral prefrontal region appears to be important in the mediation of goal-directed behavior and provides the convergence region of the IPL with information that is related to long-term goals (as opposed to immediate drives and biological needs), while the cingulate gyrus provides information about biological needs and drives as part of the limbic system structure (thus supplying the "what" and "where") cognitive and motivational information to arrive at attentional computations (Heilman, 1994, 1995).

Heilman hypothesizes that the IPL has reciprocal connections with the ventral temporal "what" region and the parietal "where" region based on the animal models. This area is found to be important in the cortical control of arousal and the supermodal synthesis that leads to neuronal activation in the ventral temporal "what" and dorsal area "where" systems. Thus, if this area is dysfunctional, it not only can fail to make attentional computations, but also cannot arouse or activate (directly or indirectly) those areas that determine both the location of objects and their identity. This failure of activation accounts for the individual not being aware that there is a stimulus in the space opposite the side of the lesion. Heilman has demonstrated a hemispatial anteriograde memory deficit associated with neglect, confirming that lesions in this area may be associated with the inability to activate old memories or form new memories of objects that are located in the hemispheric space contralateral to the lesion. This area has been found to have connections with the hippocampal region (important not only in memory, but also in retroactivation of sensory association areas) and this accounts for the failure of retroactivation and imagery memory deficits (Heilman, 1994).

Individuals with neglect fail to fully explore their environment, especially the neglected portion of space that may be related to connections of the IPL, with the frontal arcuate gyrus region found to be important in the initiation of purposeful saccades to important visual targets, and thus this region is important for the initiation of voluntary arm movements to important visual stimuli. Legions of this region, as well as that of the basal ganglia and thalamus, are part of the intentional functional network that may then induce motor intentional neglect. When, in animal models, sites of the prearcuate region and correlate IPL are lesioned, a hypoarousal is noted. Although neglect may be in association with both right and left hemispheres, it has been found to be more severe with right-hemisphere lesions (due to the right-hemisphere dominance for spatial functioning) (Heilman, 1994).

Finally, recent research further indicates that the IPL is not simply a sensory-association region and that it acts in parallel with the retinostriate system, and thus functions as an interface between attention to, reception of, and response to significant events that occur in extrapersonal space. The light-sensitive neurons of the IPL provide for the continual updating of the neural image of extrapersonal space and allow for the attraction of attention toward events in one's peripheral vision. Neurons in this region are movement independent, and thus not only subserve attention to extrapersonal space, but also process information to determine its emotional or motivational significance.

IPL and the Attentional Model

Heilman and associates propose the model that unilateral inattention will follow unilateral MRF lesions due to the loss of inhibition of the ipsilateral nucleus reticularis by the mesencephalic reticular activating system, which decreases thalamic transmission of sensory input to the cortex and/or because the MRF does not prepare the cortex for sensory processing and/or both conditions occur. Unilateral lesions of the primary or association cortices result in contralateral unimodal sensory loss or the inability to synthesize contralateral unimodal sensory input. Corticothalamic collaterals from the association cortex to the nucleus reticularis (NR) serve unimodal habituation and attention processes. Unilateral lesions of multimodal sensory convergence areas of the IPL that project to the MRF and the NR induce contralateral inattention as the individual cannot be aroused to process multimodal contralateral stimuli. Thus, a lesion in the IPL area, due to its reciprocal connections with polymodal areas such as the prefrontal and temporal sulcus areas and the limbic system, can impair the person's ability to determine the significance of a stimulus from their environment. The right hemisphere is more involved in parallel processing, while the left is more specialized, consequently the impact is greater for right-hemisphere lesions (Heilman, 1993).

The IPL seems to be responsible for selective spatial attention, independent of behavior and any IPL neuron that is enhanced to one type of behavior will also be enhanced to others (Heilman, 1993). In summation, the presented construct of attention is that the brain is bombarded with stimuli, both external and internal, and it is the job of the structures within the attentional system to decrease the amount of input by attaching significance to it. It is the IPL that makes the decisions of both "where" and "what" and determines the attentional decisions by being a convergence area. The reticular activating system provides overall activation, but it is the IPL that decides and allows the response to occur by activating the necessary systems. A lesion anywhere in this circuit can impair processes and produce inattention.

Consequences of IPL Dysfunction

Welsh (1974) details disorders of intersensory association or cross-modal integration. Damage to this area (the conjunction of the temporal, parietal, and occipital lobes) is believed to produce the most marked losses of cognitive function. The left inferior parietal region has been related to a "quasi-spatial" deficit, first termed by Luria. This quasi-spatial deficit may impact the ability to perform mathematical operations with increasing difficulty, requiring the individual to employ some degree of "spatial" or "carry-over" element. Lesions of the IPL may also impact logical relations of syntax.

According to Welsh (1974), the impact of spatial components on such relationships as those involved in the *learning of language* can be greatly affected by the sequence of words, by the introduction of relational terms such as prepositions of space or time, or by more-complex syntactical structures or sentences. In other words, the spatial issues can impact the learning of language, even the learning of words and how they fit into sentences, and are used as a whole for adept verbal communication. Identical words can take on completely different meanings just by the way they are used in a sentence or by how they change the whole of the sentence, such as "my sister's husband" or "my husband's sister" or "they overdid it" or "they did it over." The idea is that the spatial element can have a huge impact on one's ability to communicate. The problem is clearly related to the IPL area, whereupon the individual can understand the specific components, but not the whole, and not be able to apply such components into an integrated whole.

Walsh and Perrett (1974), in discussing the value of *social attention,* noted that visual gaze forms the basis for the vast majority of the different communicative nonverbal signals that happen as part of the social interplay between individuals and, further, how essential it is for the individual to comprehend the spatial reference of that gaze and to understand the subtleties present to benefit from any visual or auditory communication. The STPA region (superior temporal polysensory area), which is usually thought of as a component of the temporal processing stream, appears to have an additional role decoding the direction of another individual's attention and gaze, requiring this region to access information from both major streams of cortical processing that flow dorsally (parietal) and ventrally (temporal) from the primary visual cortex. They conclude that the visual pattern of a face and eyes, which are analyzed with the ventral visual pathways, also appears to provide a strong control over dorsal parietal mechanisms for direction of attention and gaze. Anatomical studies support the STPA region as providing considerable output projection to the parietal cortex. Connections from the STPA to the parietal cortex may form a conduit through which the STPA cell sensitivity to the direction of another individual's attention exerts an influence over the spatial attention of the observer.

Platz (1996) identified preserved tactile feature analysis and ability for cross modal matching of features while tactile identification of the specific entity was impaired. The interactive mode of function of the disturbed network system was seen as responsible for feature analysis. There is evidence of a lateralized organization of the network responsible for tactile object agnosia. The ability to appreciate the significance or nature of an object from tough is the ability to formulate meaningful conceptualizations based upon learned unimodal feature entity relationships. In tactile agnosia the ability to combine features to form entities is defective and represents that perception and knowledge are mediated by distributed neural ensembles that encodes both features and specifications for binding features into entities with local and multimodal convergence zones.

CHAPTER 9

Genetic Influences on ADD/Comorbidity Factors

Wender (1978, 1995) suggests that brain catecholamines are influential in the genesis of ADHD. The demonstration of a heritability pattern for ADHD is often the first clue to detecting the biochemical disturbance. Investigation of parents with ADHD and adoption studies provide the links between ADHD and genetics. Findings are consistent in pointing to a depletion of dopamine (DA) and norepinephrine (NE), but not 5-HT, and that motor regulatory systems involving subcortical and frontal systems are abnormal in the ADHD population. A neural model to explain the characteristics of ADHD (inattention, impulsivity, and hyperactivity) can be seen in reviewing brain–behavior relationships, particularly those structures subserving attention and motor control (Hynd et al., 1991; Shaywitz et al., 1991; Voeller, 1991).

Family Studies

Family studies suggest a genetic link of problem behavior indicating a general hyperactive conduct disorder entity rather than hyperactivity syndrome (Pauls, 1991). Data suggest a genetic factor in the relationship between childhood hyperactivity and later alcoholism, sociopathy, and hysteria (Ferguson and Rapoport, 1983). Data collected from a 10-year followup study provided confirmation of the high degree of inheritability in addition to the impact of environmental factors of this disorder. Families of ADHD children were found to have more difficulties than that of controls (Hechtman, 1996). Gillis et al. (1992) examined the genetic etiology of ADHD using identical and fraternal twins, whereby at least one member had a reading disability. Analysis supported the concept of ADHD as highly heritable. Biederman et al. (1986) conducted a pilot study to investigate ADHD as a familial disorder and results indicated positive findings. Based on these results, they proceeded with a study that was more in-depth to explore the genetic and psychosocial risk (Biederman et al., 1990, 1994). Findings reflected ADHD as a highly familial disorder. There is a statistically and clinically increased risk for ADHD to occur in children if present in either of the biological parents, regardless of social class or family disruption. Genetic factors and sibling interaction (competitiveness) emerged as an interactine in twin studies (Thapar, Hervas, and McGuttin, 1995).

ADHD was found to be highly familial for both genders. These findings support the continuity of ADHD from childhood to adolescence to adulthood. ADHD diagnosed in adulthood was found to have stronger genetic link factors than the pediatric diagnosis (842 of adults diagnosed with the disorder also had children meeting the diagnostic criteria). Methodological limitations are that diagnosis depended on meeting criteria detailed in the DSM-III-R and was reliant on only self-reported symptomatology.

The parents of ADHD children were more likely to be separated or divorced as compared to controls. There was a weak trend in the entire sample for separation or divorce to predict an increased risk for ADHD among relatives. The notion of "nature vs. nurture" emerges and the idea that adverse psychological conditions may account for a nonfamilial form of ADHD. In some families, parental ADHD may have been a cause for the turmoil that led to separation. Follow-up studies and longitudinal research consistently indicated that childhood ADHD persists into adulthood in 30 to 50% of the cases. Thus, there may be the issue that external environmental influences also have an impact on the ADHD child, and it is proposed that there is a continuing and reciprocal relationship between the genetic predisposition, resultant family interactions and the exacerbation of symptoms developmentally through the life span. ADHD children with familial pathology of the disorder were found to have the greatest impairment on neuropsychological evaluations measuring sustained attention, response inhibition, selective attention, and visual scanning, verbal learning and memory, motor speed, and handedness, as well as being more at risk for psychiatric comorbidity (Seidman et al., 1995; Bernier and Siegel, 1994; Biederman et al., 1990, 1994).

Beiderman et al. (1991) evaluated the familial association between ADD and anxiety disorders. His team of researchers found the following specific trends:

1. The overall risk for anxiety disorders among the relatives of patients with ADD was significantly higher than the risk among relatives of normal comparison subjects.
2. The risk for anxiety disorders was greater among the relatives of ADD with anxiety disorder than those without.
3. Families of both ADD and ADHD with anxiety had significantly higher risks for anxiety disorders than did relatives of normal children.
4. There was a tendency for ADD and anxiety to converge within families and thus the risk for anxiety disorders was two times higher in relatives of ADD with anxiety disorder than ADD without anxiety disorder individuals.
5. There is a comorbidity factor in those families with ADD than without ADD for anxiety disorders.

Beiderman et al. (1992) completed a study with a large population of ADHD children, finding over half with comorbid disorders that included depression, anxiety, and conduct disorder. These results extended previous findings implicating family genetic influences in ADHD. Beiderman's work provides a mean for subgrouping the population based on comorbid disorders. Relatives of ADHD when compared with normals had a markedly higher risk for ADHD, antisocial disorders, major depressive disorder, substance dependence and anxiety disorders. Analysis suggests that familial transmission of ADHD could be due to an autosomal gene, promoting the idea of genetic vulnerability. ADHD and bipolar disorder were found to be linked, possibly representing a separate and distinct entity (Wozniak et al., 1995).

A second study conducted by Beiderman and his group (1992) indicated that the familial transmission of ADHD can be attributed to the effects of a single major gene. Research proposed the idea of a genetic and nongenetic ADHD. Adoption studies indicate that the biological families of ADHD children exhibit a significantly higher rate of childhood ADHD among first- and second-degree relatives than do their adoptive families (Alberts-Corush et al., 1986). A biological parent adjudged to be delinquent or to have an adult criminal conviction predicted increased ADHD in adopted-out sons, as well as increased adult antisocial personality (Cadoret and Stewart, 1991).

ADHD and Parental Psychopathology

Schachar and Wachsmuth (1990) examined the relationship between hyperactivity and parental psychopathology and found that children with a diagnosis of ADHD show higher rates of parental psychopathology. In addition, results revealed rates of parental childhood history of hyperactivity significantly higher than for normals or the emotionally disturbed population, but closely resembling the conduct-disordered population. When hyperactivity was accompanied by the presence of conduct disorder, the rate of parental psychopathology was significantly increased. Thus, the family history profile of ADHD with or without conduct disorders (CD) is characterized by significantly elevated rates of childhood hyperactivity in either parent. ADHD in the absence of CD is not associated with high rates of parental psychopathology. Marshall et al. (1990) measured parent and child attitudes and interactional behavior with the presence or absence of associated aggressive symptomatology in families with an ADHD child. The study supported the idea that aggressiveness and a negative family climate may be separate factors in determining the long-term cause of ADHD in children.

Phares and Compas (1992) reviewed research regarding relatives between paternal factors and child and adolescent psychopathology. They found that fathers of ADHD differ from normal controls on a variety of characteristics, such as attention span, behavioral interactions, perceptions of parenting behavior, and parental self-esteem, as well as expectations for future compliant child behavior. There are consistent differences between fathers of ADHD children and normals on measures of attention and reaction time and ADHD fathers had lower expectations for future compliant behavior. Fathers did not differ on measures of paternal psychopathology. Mothers of ADHD children did report significantly more symptoms of depression than mothers of normal children. It was found that with ADHD children's life satisfaction in the family was most strongly predicted by paternal support, followed by paternal discipline, paternal indulgence, and maternal support. Finally, fathers of ADHD children reveal almost no differences from mothers of ADHD children and what is significant is that there appears to be more similarities between the two groups (Alberts-Corush et al., 1986; Phares and Compas, 1992).

Murphy (1991), however, found no significant differences between biological parents of ADD children and normals on selected tests, thus failing to support the notion of parents exhibiting similar deficits to their children. The author concludes that tests may not have been sensitized enough to discriminate the presence of the disorder. Goldhammer (1991) found a co-occurrence rate of 49.41% for ADHD and dyslexia. The ADHD with dyslexia group was found to be more impaired in reading skills and more likely to repeat a grade. There was a moderate relationship between the severity of ADHD and dyslexia and both were found to have significant inherited components.

A study appeared in the *New EnglandJournal of Medicine* by Hauser et al. (1993), revealing a new genetic link finding a strong association between ADHD and generalized resistance to thyroid hormone, which previous studies have shown is firmly linked to mutations in the genetic coding from the thyroid hormone receptor. This remains inconclusive, however, and subject to considerable controversy.

Biological Factors

Review of the literature to determine the biological validation of ADHD indicated that pre- and perinatal measures support only some complex multivariate notion of "risk" in association with diverse pathology rather than a specific behavioral profile of ADHD. Association between neurological soft signs and ADHD is weakened, nonspecific, and does not support validation of the syndrome. The relationship between congenital developmental deviation, physical anomalies, and problem behaviors did not validate a hyperactivity syndrome. It did validate a spectrum of behavior labeled "oppositional-defiant disorder" or "difficult temperament".

Accumulated data support the theory of CNS underarousal for a subgroup of hyperactive children, especially if they are engaged in tasks required to attend to external signal stimuli. There is a general correlation between hypoarousal and impulsive deviant behavior. Toxic substances do not directly correlate with the syndrome of hyperactivity. Evidence is inconsistent regarding specific food allergies and the ingestion of toxic substances. High lead levels in the body have been related as a causative factor in hyperactivity, but still needs further research as to application to the general population. Fetal alcohol syndrome has been associated with a subgroup of hyperactive children, but represents basic behavior and learning problems as a consequence of general CNS disturbance. The authors conclude that there may be a final common path of biological disturbance (catecholamine depletion, receptor hyposensitivity) resulting from exposure to toxins, fetal brain damage, genetic transmission, and even early social deprivation. The weak association and lack of specificity relating biological factors to hyperactivity may reflect that it is not an etiologically and biologically unitary disorder.

There is considerable debate over the question of a targeted gene as responsible for dyslexia, and the association between a reading disorder, immune disorder, and motor preference. Research has not confirmed this association. There remains a question of immune system deficiency that results in other comorbid pathology. It has been well documented that ADHD co-exists to a significant degree with additional pathology with the predisposition of being neuropsychiatric in nature (associated with brain abnormalities) that is beyond what would be expected for simple interactive effects and predisposition. The diagnosis is emerging as a significant predictor of other comorbid pathology (Warren et al., 1995; Cardon et al., 1995; Milberger et al., 1995; Biederman et al., 1995).

CHAPTER 10

Cognitive Differences Between ADHD and ADD Nosological Issues

Attention problems may also be secondary to other medical problems, such as hypothyroidism, hyperthyroidism, pituitary problems, narcolepsy, hypoglycemia, and seizure disorders. Bipolar disorder, depression, and other emotional symptoms may mimic ADHD or ADD. Medications taken for allergies or seizure disorder may result in attentional problems. Environmental toxins may produce attentional symptoms in addition to head injury or general CNS dysfunctioning due to some other sort of trauma to the brain. Finally, stress may operate as a causal factor or enhancer of those already present with some sort of CNS dysfunctioning (be that ADD or brain injury). Considering all of these factors, diagnosis is subject to:

1. Ruling in or ruling out an attentional disorder
2. Distinguishing ADD with hyperactivity from ADD without hyperactivity.
3. Addressing other possible neurological or emotional variables that would present similar behavior.

DSM-III, DSM-III-R, and DSM-IV Findings

Historically, children were labeled "hyperkinetic reaction of childhood" or "minimal brain dysfunction". The diagnostic nomenclature of the American Psychiatric Association (DSM-III) separated various symptoms formally grouped under "hyperkinesis" into "attention deficit disorder" with (ADHD) or without hyperactivity (ADD) and two distinct behavior disorders, Oppositional Disorder and Conduct Disorder. DSM-III taxonomy represented the shift from the assumption of underlying brain damage toward the establishment of specific behavioral criteria for diagnosis (Ferguson and Rapoport, 1987).

Following its introduction of ADD in 1980, the subtyping of attention deficits was criticized as being empirically unfounded and led to its removal in the DSM-III-R, established in 1987. This test classification substituted two disorders, attention deficit hyperactivity disorder (ADHD) and undifferentiated attention deficit disorder (UADD) for the previous ADD categories (Goodyear and Hynd, 1992). The third revision estimated the occurrence of the disorder as present in as many as 3% of the total population of children; Barkley (1995) estimated 3 to 5% of school age children, comprising 30 to 40% of total referrals to child guidance clinics.

The problem with this classification is the "polythetic" approach to the diagnosis of ADHD that requires the presence of at least 8 to 14 symptoms associated with ADHD's essential features. With this approach, the diagnosis of ADHD could be made without the requirement that symptoms from each of the essential features be present. The effect of this is that any combination of symptoms of inattention and/or impulsiveness and/or hyperactivity can result in an ADHD diagnosis. Thus, it is possible to make the diagnosis of ADHD without considering any of the attentional items (Goodyear and Hynd, 1992). The idea was to have ADHD represent predominant features of inattention and impulsivity, while UADD required only the diagnosis of inattention.

Healey and associates (1993) investigated the DSM-III-R dimensions identifying ADHD and data from the study provided further validity to the distinction between inattention and hyperactivity symptoms, while finding that items related to impulsivity did not significantly load for either of these two dimensions. The majority of impulsivity items were more associated and highly correlated with the hyperactivity dimension than with inattention. Further, the hyperactivity-impulsivity factor scores were related to test performance of response inhibition problems, while the inattention-disorganization factor scores were related to problems of attention and visual search. A two-factor model was supported; however, there was not enough validity for impulsivity to be represented as a third independent factor or dimension. Dykman and Ackerman (1993), after a thorough review of the research, identified three subtypes of ADD: ADD, ADHD, and ADD with hyperactivity and aggression.

The DSM-IV introduced a three-factor system:

1. ADHD primarily inattentive subtype (ADHD-I)
2. ADHD primarily hyperactive-impulsive subtype (ADHD-HI)
3. ADHD combined subtype (ADHD-C)

The primarily inattentive subtype is a variant of ADD, while the combined subtype represents the latest version of ADHD. Understanding and diagnosing the newest subtype, ADHD primarily hyperactive-impulsive, which requires at least six hyperactive-impulsivity symptoms, but fewer than six inattention symptoms, becomes a difficult task. McBurnett (1995) addresses this issue, and indicates that those children who would qualify for this subtype will be early first grade or younger who have essentially the same disorder as children diagnosed with ADHD-C. He hypothesized that this group would evidence inattention symptoms as they progress in school and eventually ADHD-HI will become ADHD-C. Further, he indicates that these children will probably have less problems of aggression or oppositional behavior.

The DSM-IV field trials were conducted by Lahey et al. (1994) to determine the optimal diagnostic thresholds using children aged 4 to 17 years. In that study of 380 children referred to clinics, 152 were diagnosed with ADHD-C, 74 with ADHD-I, 50 with ADHD-HI, and the other 104 children comprised either no or other diagnosis group. Findings supported the distinct categories of the DSM-IV and that ADHD-HI is distinctly different from ADHD when using symptoms of the DSM-III. Children meeting the criteria of ADHD-HI had fewer symptoms of inattention than the combined subtype; however, they also had fewer symptoms of the hyperactivity-impulsivity dimension, thus suggesting that this would be a less severe form of ADHD.

Clinicians who determined the diagnosis of ADHD-HI also found that the children would meet the criteria for ADHD (87.5%) and also diagnosed these children as having the same level of overall impairment. The ADHD-HI group was found to contain 20% girls, which is midway between the percentages for ADHD-C (12%) and ADHD-I (27%). Children who were diagnosed with the ADHD-HI (76% were between the ages of 4 and 6 years) were found to be of younger ages than those diagnosed with ADHD. Interestingly, the average age of the ADHD-HI diagnosis was 5.7 years, while the average age for the ADHD-HI diagnosis was 8.5 years and average age for the ADHD-C was 9.9 years, thus substantiating that ADHD-C may well be the later version of ADHD-HI. Further, children with ADHD-HI had fewer symptoms of ODD and CD than did those children diagnosed with ADHD-C. ADHD-HI did not differ from ADHD-I with regard to comorbid disorders, even after controlling for age differences, suggesting that ADHD-HI may be a less severe form of the classic ADHD. Children with ADHD-HI had the same degree of academic difficulties as the control group, which was less than that found for either ADHD-C or ADHD-I, again after controlling for age and comorbid differences. Children with ADHD-HI had the same frequency of accidental physical injuries as ADHD-C, which was higher than that of controls. Finally, children with ADHD-HI and ADHD-I were similar in impairment of peer functioning and social skills and both groups were less impaired than ADHD-C even after controlling for comorbid behavior problems and age. Authors concluded that the subtyping represented a correct decision and identifying symptoms correctly distinguished between the groups. de Quiros et al. (1994) continued their study in the presence of three clinical variants: inattention, impulsivity, and hyperactivity as representing distinctly different disorders and question if all disorders should be seen along the singular continuum of ADHD. Similar questions point to the need to consider the interaction of comorbid disorders and multicultural issues for accurate diagnosis, in addition to assessment behaviorally and neuropsychologically to arrive at a specific problem-focused treatment plan (Sabatino and Vance, 1994; Wright and Beale, 1996; March, Wells, and Conners, 1995; M. L. Cohen, 1996).

Barkley (1995) questions some specific issues regarding DSM-IV diagnosis, such as the clarity of the predominantly inattentive type as a subtype of ADHD, the appropriateness of items for different developmental periods, adjustment of criteria based on gender, and the problematic requirement of substantiation from two of three environments. Given the heterogeneity of ADHD and various anomalies associated with this rather diverse behavioral and cognitive picture, Barkley (1997) has attempted to arrive at a more unified theory by viewing this disorder as primarily representing a deficit in behavioral inhibition. The idea is postulated that a deficient response inhibition (resulting in increased impulsivity) results in secondary impairments specifically targeting four neuropsychological abilities (working memory, internalization of speech or self-talk, self-regulated affect and reconstitution, behavioral analysis and synthesis) that are dependent, to some degree, upon inhibition processes for effective execution. These abilities are viewed as being dependent upon self-regulation and the ability to have control over one's behavior with internally represented information, as allowing for the targeting of behavior and persistence of that behavior towards future goals, as well as the ability to re-engage goal-oriented behavior if interrupted. Research appears to support the components of behavioral inhibition, working memory, poor self-regulation of motivation, sequencing and motor control (reconstitution and internalization have not been as well researched) providing confirmation of this proposed theory.

Bilateral orbitofrontal hypoperfusion was evidenced on the Brain 99mTc-HPAO SPECT which specifically targets nonconvulsive epilepsy, in a child presenting symptoms of ADHD. His father, who presented similar symptoms, revealed left orbitofrontal hypoperfusion. Both father and son were diagnosed with orbitofrontal epilepsy. Although outwardly displaying symptoms of ADHD characterized by inattentiveness, impulsivity, poor concentration and motor restlessness, they had additional symptoms highly characteristic of seizure disorder, that of nonresponsive starting, complex automatic behavior, amnesic periods and atonic drop-attacks (in the son) and responded quite well to medical management with antiseizure medication (Powell et al., 1977).

Clinically, we do not subscribe to the theory of a combined subtype, seeing the two subtypes of ADD as having different anatomical correlates and different neurotransmitter systems. When criteria meet a combination subtype, it is usually the overfocused subtype of ADD, displaying behavioral symptoms of ADHD. In using the DSM-IV criteria, the group to emerge with the greatest difficulty, behaviorally is the combined subtype (hyperactive, impulsive and inattentive) evidencing more symptoms of conduct disorder and oppositional behavior and displaying social problems (Eiraldi et al., 1997, Gaub and Carlson, 1997).

Clinical and Research Differences Between ADHD and ADD

Brown (1994) discusses undifferentiated ADD and finds that it includes many of the following symptoms:

1. Often easily distracted by extraneous stimuli
2. Often difficulty following through on instructions from others
3. Difficulty sustaining attention
4. Often does not seem to listen to what is being said

5. Tendency to lose things necessary for tasks or activities
6. Often fails to give close attention to detail
7. Difficulty organizing goal-directed activities
8. Often shifts from one incompleted activity to another

Brown (1993) further indicates that many of those with ADD report chronic problems with getting tasks completed and getting "cranked up" to complete them. If they do complete a task, it will tend to have been an urgent one due to a crisis situation. There is difficulty activating oneself to complete tasks and sustaining energy in task completion. Often those with ADD complain of feeling drowsy even if they have had a good night's sleep, and report fighting off drowsiness while studying, listening to lectures, or attending meetings. Chronic problems in activating and sustaining arousal can make life difficult and things are especially problematic for the highly intelligent individuals. They are seen by others as very bright, and thus it becomes all the more frustrating when behaviors such as those mentioned prevent achievement and the attainment of potential. The wide gap between potential and actual achievement makes these individuals very vulnerable to demoralization and resignation to failure.

Lahey and Carlson (1991) in reviewing the research on ADHD and ADD found that children with ADHD are often characterized by serious conduct problems, while children with ADD are more likely to display symptoms of anxiety, depression, and shyness. Goodyear and Hynd (1992) presented a review of the literature comparing ADHD and ADD/WO for behavioral and neuropsychological differentiation. Studies suggest that girls are less likely to be referred than boys with ADD and there is a risk of under-identifying girls with ADD who are impulsive. The average age for ADHD sample populations is 9.4, 9.8 years for ADD samples. Authors concluded that ADD are referred and identified later than ADHD individuals, who are more noticeable and create more stress for both parents and teachers. The vast majority of studies are based on clinical samples. IQ differences between ADHD and ADD are insignificant.

Conduct disorder more frequently occurs among ADHD than ADD children. ADHD was associated with parental ADD and hyperactivity in maternal substance abuse, while ADD was associated with maternal anxiety disorders and learning disabilities in siblings. ADHD children who are identified somewhat earlier may have input difficulties related to behavioral problems associated with activity level and/or impulsivity, whereas ADD children identified later manifested output difficulties associated with neurocognitive processes associated with dysfunction of automatized information processing and slow cognitive speed. A conceptualization of ADD emerges that involves neuro-cognitive deficits of poor long-term retrieval of verbal information, lack of automaticity with number facts, and slow writing speed. ADHD and comorbid conduct disorder are also associated with lower socio-economic status and poor academic achievement.

Borchending et al. (1988) compared ADHD with normals and found that they differed not in automatic processing capabilities, but with effortful processing tasks involving learning. The combination of ADHD and LD resulted in demonstrated information processing difficulties, resulting in a substantial loss of information. It is only the combination of ADHD and LD that result in such a significant loss of information. The transfer of information is implicated as more critical than processing the type of memory process, and results suggest the idea of an application deficit rather than an ability deficit (Kataria et al., 1992). Schachar and Logan (1990) found that ADHD boys had longer reaction times to performance of a secondary task, indicating problems in the area of shifting capacity from one process to another. The problematic issue was not that of capacity in general, but it was the necessary shift that caused poor performance. Levy and Hobbes (1989) investigated male ADHD children for reading and phonetic spelling ability and found that a vigilance factor was significantly related to the diagnosis of moderate and severe ADHD and the vigilance factor correlated with a phonetic spelling ability.

The social information-processing abilities of hyperactive children were evaluated and confirmed that hyperactive boys that were rejected had distinct difficulties with social information processing than those hyperactive boys who were not rejected. There were deficiencies in being able to socially reason (take another person's perspective), to attend to and encode social cues, to attend to changing social cues, and to amend the social interactive style as task demands shift, in addition to a tendency toward negative attributional bias. Social rejection was the consequence of deficient overall social skills leading to inappropriate, disturbed interpersonal interactions and overall reaction (Moore, Hughes, and Robinson, 1992; Frederick and Olmi, 1994). Negative child characteristics and mothers with diminished social resources contributed to an increased risk of child abuse (Ammerman and Patz, 1996). ADHD symptoms were found to be less apparent when the child was engaged in an externally stimulating activity such as television or playing video games, although their behavior was still not within normal limits and symptoms of restlessness, inattentiveness, and being overly talkative, continued to be observed during these extrinsically stimulating activities (Tannock, 1997).

Diagnosed ADHD teens involved in substance abuse were found to have lower self-esteem and to be involved in substance abuse as a means of self-medication (Horner and Scheibe, 1997). ADHD was found to be a highly significant predictor of cigarette smoking as well as early initiation of smoking, and smoking was highly correlated to co-morbid disorders of depression and anxiety (Hughes, 1997; Milberger et al., 1997). In examining ADHD adults, Murphy and Barkley (1996) noted a significant degree of oppositional behavior, conduct disorder, and substance abuse (greater illegal usage) as well as psychological maladjustment, more driving risks and changes in employment. Driving licenses had been suspended, job performance was poor with firings, marriages were multiple, there was a history of poor educational performance with disciplinary action and the noticeable absence of anxiety or depression. ADHD adults did not appear as emotionally intense nor responsive to reinforcement, positive or negative (Braaten and Rosén, 1997). Large populations of adolescents were examined for driving offenses and the relationship to inattentive and hyperactive behaviors. Findings indicated that ADHD symptoms and symptoms of conduct disorder were more significantly correlated (Nada-Raja et al., 1997).

Predictors of ADHD persisting into adulthood were that of genetic factors (ADHD) in the family, psychosocial adversity, comorbid conduct disorder, depression and anxiety. Follow-up assessment after a 4-year interval confirmed the likelihood that symptoms will remain in evidence (Biederman et al., 1996). Variables of the parent's love for their spouse, similar child-rearing viewpoints, traditional role identification, and paternal ADHD interacted with the factor of father involvement to predict parental practices of less effective discipline, diminished love for wives, and high degree of identification with traditional roles (Arnold, O'Leary, and Edwards, 1997).

Physiological Assessment of ADHD and ADD

Neurophysiological studies to differentiate the two groups have had relatively small samples and subjects have been predominantly male; mean IQ scores were similar for both groups; 60% of the studies yielded significant differences between ADHD and ADD; subjects were distinguished by auditory evoked potential studies. Compared to controls, children with ADD had smaller than normal P3 components in both auditory and visual modalities, and longer P3 latencies to both target and novel stimuli. P3 is thought to be closely related to attention, especially to the "relevance" of the eliciting stimulus. Amplitude and latency abnormalities were identified, suggesting deficient preferential processing of attended stimuli. In response to the challenge dose of l-fenfluramine and compared in plasma catecholamine metabolites and platelet 5-HT, the more aggressive ADHD boys had a significantly greater prolactin response, indicating clear differences of central 5-HT functioning implicating decreased serotonin levels (Halperin et al., 1994). An evoked potential study conducted by Robaey et al. (1992) of controlled and automatic processes in boys diagnosed with ADHD yielded evidence that automatic processes are enhanced when higher-order controlled processes are inadequate.

ADD children were slower in responding to tasks requiring them to name similar alternating stimuli as fast as possible. This has been interpreted as related to the deficits in automaticity consistent with learning disabilities. ADD demonstrated sensory-localization deficits associated with parietal lobe dysfunctioning. ADHD children were consistently more impulsive on motor response as opposed to ADD, who were initially impulsive and later able to inhibit their responses. This pattern of performance was consistent with the idea that ADD represents a sustained-attention disorder and ADHD represents a selective-attention disorder characteristic of deficits of frontal processes. The ADD group required more retrieval cues to achieve a performance similar to the ADHD group. The right hemisphere is seen as contributing to the ability to anticipate targets, while the left hemisphere has the primary mediating role in search necessary for selective attention. ADD revealed an inconsistent pattern in the development of reading skills with word-attack skills exceeding word-identification skills. ADD were slower than controls in the search stage of information processing. Overall, a sluggish cognitive tempo was observed with ADD (Holcomb et al., 1985, 1986; Sergeant and Scholten, 1985; Trommer et al., 1988; Hynd et al., 1989, 1991; Goodyear, 1991; Lorys et al., 1990; Schaughency et al., 1990; Satterfield, Schell, and Nicholas, 1994; Prather et al., 1996; Prather, Brownell, and Alexander, 1996). Findings of Shibagaki, Yamanaka, and Furuya (1993) used the method of skin-conductance response to confirm the hypothesis of ADHD and found a lower level of arousal and short attention span. Abnormal plasma catecholamines were significantly identified in children diagnosed with ADHD, supporting the possibility that increased circulatory levels of dopamine and/or epinephrine may be a marker to identify ADHD.

It is proposed that behaviors associated with ADD seem to be more reflective of posterior, possibly right-hemisphere dysfunction. Children with ADHD have deficits in attention and motor regulation similar to frontal lobe-lesioned patients. ADHD is linked to dysfunction in the diencephalic-forebrain inhibitory system (Zametkin and Rapoport, 1987). Heilman, Voeller, and Nadeau (1991) propose that ADHD children have dysfunction in a right-sided, frontal striatal system, which explains symptoms of defective attention, response inhibition, and motor restlessness. Further, inattention, defective response inhibition, and impersistence are more commonly seen in adults with right- as opposed to left-hemisphere dysfunction; children with ADHD not only appear to demonstrate these symptoms, but also neglect the left side and have decreased activation of their right neostriatum.

Clinically, we have observed a clear spatial problem, inattention that is more commonly seen in ADD, and symptoms of ADD would meet the above-mentioned criteria. It appears that ADD has been commonly misdiagnosed as ADHD, and it would seem that those studied by Heilman and associates may meet the criteria of ADD, which would explain the classic inattention and neglect symptoms we have so commonly observed as a repetitive pattern.

Sandler (1995) found one of the key learning disorders of older adolescents diagnosed as ADHD to be a phonological processing disorder, characterized by symptoms that highly resemble the "neglect" seen in ADD, noting the struggle to decode words and strategized means of compensation as the whole-word approach. Spelling was problematic with frequent errors in the inability to sound out a word, utilizing mnemonic means to circumvent these difficulties. Reading, however, remains tiring and requiring such effort that this can eventually lead to a total lack of reading. Sandler, in describing language problems, found constant difficulties with word timing, oral and written expression, and poor passage comprehension, although word knowledge was adequate. Relationships between words was difficult; words with ambiguous meaning, metaphors, and figurative language were seen as partly understood. Again, although diagnosed as ADHD, these patterns related to reading and language are highly descriptive of ADD and demonstrate the inattention to the whole (neglect of space), an inability to see and process the parts, pronounce the whole word (here the need to use memorization and the whole word), difficulty relating parts to a whole concept for abstract-figured meaning, and generally missing the whole picture of things. This can be applied to thinking about a problem, anticipating consequences of one's actions, using numbers and completing mathematical problems, and so on. The more that is demanded, the greater the use of the limited capacity of the

ADD brain, the more apparent the hemineglect becomes. McCarthy, Kirk, and Goff (1996) identified visuospatial abilities as playing a considerable role in early arithmetic performance. ADHD may truly be a disorder of inattention (the "when" construct), whereas ADD may be a disorder of attention (the "where" construct of parietal systems).

Mann (1991) investigated topographic brain mapping as a diagnostic for ADHD and found increased theta and decreased beta when compared with control on EEG measures. Differences were greater when subjects were engaged in reading and drawing tasks than resting states. Decreased theta activity was more prominent for the frontal regions, while beta was significantly decreased for the temporal regions.

The question of developmental anomalies in ADHD impacting the left caudate and right prefrontal, frontal, and/or posterior parietal hemispheric regions has been continuously assessed by MRI morphometry. These areas of brain functioning are targeted as the attentional network, the result being their relationship to frontalstriatal and posterior parietal function and subsequent areas of responsive to stimulant medication.

Filipek et al. (1997) found the volumes of the anterior superior (frontal) and bilateral anterior-inferior (peribasal ganglia) hemispheric regions to be significantly smaller in ADHD, while the total cortical volume remained intact. This confirmed a neurodevelopmental process altering neural system configuration (particularly in the right hemisphere) as opposed to degeneration or processes involving cell death. Smaller white matter volumes of the bilateral retrocallosal (posterior parietal-occipital) and right and left caudate (head) volumes created a symmetry (as opposed to the *left-larger-than-right* asymmetry present in controls) in ADHD being localized to the left and unchanged by treatment with medical management. The ADHD population was then separated by their response to stimulant medication. White matter was measured to be the smallest in medication nonresponders (most prevalent in the genu and splenium of the corpus callosum). Stimulant responders had the smallest and most symmetrical caudate volume and left anterior superior cortex volume as opposed to the nonresponders, who in addition to diminished anterior superior volumes, had reversed normal caudate asymmetry and the smallest posterior (rostrocallosal, parietal-occipital) white matter volumes.

Regional cerebral blood flow computed tomography studies support the conceptualization of the caudate-striatal region as hypoactive in ADHD children as compared to controls. MRI findings reveal that frontal lobes are symmetrical as opposed to the normal pattern of right greater than left for

ADHD children. Further, research has suggested that the genu and splenium of the corpus callosum may be smaller in ADHD when compared to matched controls (Hynd et al., 1991).

Giedd et al. (1994), using quantitative neuroanatomic imaging, found structural brain abnormalities pinpointing the frontal lobe circuitry in children diagnosed with ADHD. Two anterior regions of the corpus callosum, the rostrum, and the rostral body were found to have significantly smaller areas in the ADHD group. The severity of the differences of these areas correlated with parent and teacher self-report findings of hyperactivity and impulsivity dimensions. Authors concluded abnormal frontal-lobe development and function as being present in diagnosed ADHD. They hypothesized that it is unlikely that a single lesion would account for this finding and findings instead pointed to the hypothesis that the disorder more than likely involves a complex interplay between the various neuroanatomical and neurochemical systems in addition to psychosocial and genetic factors.

Castellanos et al. (1994) examined the caudate nucleus and total brain volumes in boys diagnosed with ADHD to investigate the hypotheses that this structure would be implicated in the disorder as it receives inputs from the cortical regions implicated in executive functioning and attentional tasks. The brains of ADHD and controls were examined using MRI and volumetric measures of the head and body of the caudate nucleus were obtained. Findings indicated that mean right caudate volume was slightly, but not significantly smaller in the ADHD patients when compared with the controls and there was no significant difference of the left caudate volume, substantiating the lack of asymmetry usually found in normals. Together these findings accounted for the highly significant lack of normal asymmetry found in the caudate volume in ADHD; the total brain volume was 5% smaller in the ADHD boys, while ruling out the impact of age, height, weight, or IQ. Smaller brain volume, however, did not account for the caudate volume or symmetry differences and, for the normal boys, the caudate volume decreased substantially (13%) and significantly with age, while in the ADHD group, there were no age-related changes. Authors conclude that the results support the developmental abnormalities found for the frontal-striatal circuits in ADHD diagnosis and related to the lack of asymmetry found in dyslexics in such regions as the planum temporale. Significant differences have also been cited in the left perisylvian gyral region for diagnosed dyslexics and ADHD, citing new directions for research, contrary to prior findings of smaller volume of genu and splenium of the corpus callosum. Significantly larger areas were evidenced in comparing ADHD to a normal population. The speculation is presented that larger measurements in these regions represent excessive interhemispheric transmission and the result of overactivity (Hynd et al., 1996; Hall et al., 1996).

This neurodevelopmental process that apparently alters neural connections, and appears to occur specifically with greater impact to the right hemisphere in ADHD correlated with spatial findings and an inattention to the whole (related to right hemisphere dominance for spatial functioning) which is commonly noted in the ADD population. Findings and directions of future research may begin to provide more concrete documentation of the widespread and common existence of ADD without hyperactivity, often misdiagnosed as ADHD due to the overwhelming anxiety that is present on a continual basis. Authors of this study view results as providing confirmation of the right frontostriatal circuits. There was, however, surprise with regard to the impact to parietal areas and clinical deficits of the posterior attentional system. The authors recognize the need for further research to explore the impact of the posterior attentional system. It is proposed that inattentive symptoms of a more focused attention may arise from bilateral posterior parietal cortices. There is additional involvement of the frontal-left striatal dysfunction which is exacerbated by diminished anterior and posterior ipsilateral and contralateral hemispheric interconnections (Filipek et al., 1997).

Whyte (1994) in reviewing the research on attentional processes and dyslexia concludes that reading disabled or dyslexic individuals had problems with specific applications of attention, while the ADHD individuals seemed to have a more-centralized deficit. ADHD vs. ADHD with dyslexia performed significantly worse than controls on measures of sequential memory and attentional tasks involving impulse control and planning and organization, and ADHD individuals specifically tended to have lower scores on measures requiring organized deliberate rehearsal strategies, unsustained strategic effort, and use of self-regulatory or executive processes for consideration of response alternatives. ADHD with reading disability performed worse on measures involving a verbal or linguistic component. Subjects with both ADHD and LD had more pervasive attention problems and more visual/motor problems than ADHD or LD alone (Korkman and Pesonen, 1994).

Other studies with findings that are quite different from the above maybe more indicative of co-morbid disorders underlying the attentional disorder. The anatomic definitions may differ from study to study, and as noted above, there may be a posterior attentional system associated with the inattentive type of ADHD with the hyperactive subtype responding more positively to medication. This becomes rather confounding, however, given that responses to stimulant medication that are considered as nonresponsive could be subject to the effect of undiagnosed underlying disorders quite possibly that of anxiety. The consequence of the stimulant may become overly difficult to maintain at the necessary dosage level that is substantial enough to actually observe results. As noted by many researchers including Heilman (1991), deficits observed in the ADHD population may be related to the disinhibition of the right hemisphere via abnormal development of frontostriatal dopamine connections. Subtypes of this disorder may in fact be differentiated by hyperactivity/impulsivity vs. inattentive symptomotology, anterior and posterior attentional systems, and right frontal bilateral striatal dopamine dysfunction and retrocallosal (posterior parietal-occipital) regions.

Millichap (1997) reported three cases of identical locations of arachnoid cysts in the left middle crania fossa, involving medial aspects of the temporal lobe, with comorbid findings of ADHD, proposing that there is a causal association between the attentional disorder, learning and language disabilities. The children had presented symptoms of partial seizure disorder with complaints of headaches, episodes occurring suggestive of seizure activation, language delay, syncope, tremors, and abnormal neurological signs with findings of slow wave abnormalities in the left temporal region. Cysts appeared as the result of a structural congenital developmental anomaly was correlated to ADHD via cortical-striatal circuit damage, related to temporal lobe and sylvian region pathology, providing evidence of the heterogeneity of this disorder.

In our clinical practice, it is not uncommon for 1 of 10 children seen, to present with symptoms characteristic of seizure activity thus denoting pathology beyond that of the attentional disorder. A child was evaluated recently with this same pathology, symptomotology, and etiology of the tempora fossa subarachnoid cyst. This child was recently evaluated with a full neuropsychological examination at the age of 10 years, which provided evidence of impact to brain functioning significant of seizure disorder (impact to the language and memory systems) and impact to an already weakened area of brain functioning, the parietal area. This demonstrated substantial spatial distortions and neglect phenomenon, characteristic of stroke (sensory evaluation revealed bilateral severe impairment). Motor skills were also diminished for the right hand due to a stroke occurring *in utero*. The site of the cyst was left temporal which had been removed during infancy at the age of 7 months. The child demonstrated the type of emotional lability consistent with seizure disorder and the development of a personality commensurate with this type of continuous impact to brain function. Intellectual levels were highly diminished due to substantial language delay (achievement evaluation indicated math, reading, and spelling within well-below-average limits) and memory deficits revealed delayed retrieval problems significant of his inability to learn due to lack of retention of learned material. It was his emotionality and reactivity that made an earlier evaluation unsuccessful.

This child had been previously evaluated at the age of approximately 5 years. The evaluation at that time, however, was unsuccessful due to unmanaged emotional outbursts, lack of any motoric control as well as absence of any language capacity. In the original assessment, this child was diagnosed with ADHD. This recent evaluation, however, revealed well-developed skills of logical reasoning (within the superior range) and a profile more consistent with the clinical picture of ADD without hyperactivity, confirmed by the substantial weakening of the parietal area. Learning, language, and math delay was the consequence of impairment in areas that would normally have provided compensatory means of coping with reading and math difficulties associated with an attentional disorder, specifically that of memory and the substantial spatial deficits. This further exacerbated the situation.

Neuropsychological Studies

Problems overall with the research to date primarily are the confounding and confusing diagnosis and conceptualizations of the two subtypes of ADD. Neuropsychological measures require a qualitative approach as opposed to a quantitative method, and consequently, results are confusing, not in the expected direction as prior research would predict, and researchers find themselves having to explain their surprising results in a number of ways, ranging from the type of popularized to motivational and psychological factors. One such example that clearly elucidates this problem was the research conducted by Holdnack et al. (1995), with well-educated, highly successful residual adult ADD population. Findings reported extensive verbal learning problems, slow psychomotor speed and integration, slow reaction time, more developed verbal IQ over performance IQ (verbal skills vs. nonverbal skills), and uneven cognitive development in the face of a lack of impairment in executive functioning (that was hypothesized to be problematic). These findings are highly similar to patterning observed in the ADD population. The second issue is that in using neuropsychological measures (unless specifically using means and standard deviations as comparisons), average is seen as adequate, which may not be the case for individuals of higher intellectual potential.

Barkley, Grodzinsky, and DuPaul (1992) review neuropsychological studies of frontal-lobe functions in children with ADD and ADHD. They found that tests of response inhibition more reliably distinguished the two groups. Further, ADD was found to have an additional problem with perceptual motor speed and cognitive processing. ADHD children may have more problems with sustained effort or "resource allocation", especially with tedious and boring tasks, while ADD revealed a more "sluggish" cognitive tempo and impairment in focused attention.

Boucugoani and Jones (1989) found significant differences for ADHD when compared to normal controls for frontal lobe trait deficits of perseveration, self-directed attention, and inhibitory capacity. Tannock, Purvis, and Schachar (1993), using a story retelling task to assess narrative abilities in boys diagnosed with ADHD, found that overall they provided less information and their stories were more poorly organized, less accurate, and less cohesive when compared with controls. Consequently, stories were confusing and difficult to follow and authors attributed this problem to that of poor organization and monitoring of information, functions of executive control. Authors concluded that the deficits observed were reflective of the underlying deficits in executive or frontal processes. Despite the appearance of memory difficulties, memory processes are intact (Cahn and Marcotte, 1996).

The ADHD population has typically been viewed as being highly correlated to learning disability. However, studies do not tend to agree as to the impact and degree of disability when using neuropsychological assessment. Often it does not find tremendous differences between the LD and ADHD groups. Studies generally conclude that ADHD symptoms are the result of the impact upon frontal processes. ADHD is viewed as more of a behavioral disorder, involving the dopaminergic system. Research references ADD as more of an attentional disorder, as difficulties with focused and sustained attentional processes, and with specific targeting of the norepinephrine system. LD and ADHD, however, may be highly related due to the more extensive impact to brain processes rather than merely the attentional aspects. Shapiro et al. (1993) evaluated the social impairment with the ADHD population and concluded that deficits of complex auditory processing and working memory were additional variables in the problematic processing of emotional cues. The ADHD population has been found to be specifically vulnerable to speech and language disorders, in addition to behavioral and psychiatric comorbid diagnoses, constituting an at-risk group (Javorsky, 1993). The ADHD group was found to demonstrate a lower Performance IQ on intellectual assessment, measuring effects of an executive dysfunction present in this population, and neurological soft signs were significantly correlated in a negative direction with Full Scale IQ in 7 to 9 year old children. Neuropsychological evaluation revealed poorer performance on measures of distractibility, verbal fluency, a measure of whole brain functioning, and novel learning task. The ADHD group evidenced visuomotor difficulties as well as problems with sequences and it was hypothesized that this disorder is related to visuomotor, sequential and temporal symptoms of an executive dysfunction disorder (Pineda et al., 1997). Similar findings were obtained with children ages 10 to 12 years, whereby neurological soft signs continued to predict a variable FSIQ, the PIQ was lower as well as scholastic achievement (whether a cause of effect of the executive dysfunction). Although all measures for this older population revealed lower scores, only the WCST perseverative errors and responses provided significant discrimination from the ADHD population and matched controls (Pineda et al., 1997). Presence of neurological soft signs were related to sensory integrative difficulties and a sensory defensiveness (Foodman, 1996). Diagnosed ADHD boys (ages 6 to 17 years old) rated as socially disabled, were more impaired on measures of social functioning and at risk for psychiatric comorbidity (Greene et al., 1996). The types of tasks that Pineda denotes as symptoms of an executive dysfunction, however can be attributed to spatial dysfunctioning (inability to view the whole) and typically children in our research with this type of deficit demonstrate poor performance on the above tasks for this reason. Smoking was investigated as a risk factor for ADHD and 22% of the ADHD child population studied were positive for a maternal history of smoking during pregnancy, significant differences were obtained in IQ values pointed to the negative impact of smoking (Milberger et al., 1996).

Girls diagnosed with ADHD were demonstrated as impaired performance on some measures of attention and achievement (math and reading); however, they scored significantly less impaired on neuropsychological measures of executive function when compared with boys diagnosed with the same disorder (Seidman et al., 1997).

Hoza et al. (1993) reported that ADHD children reported a positive self-image despite clear-cut academic failures and social rejection. Authors question whether this is a defensive maneuver to avoid feelings of failure or may reflect the distorted thinking patterns that are so characteristic of ADHD. Frontal processes dysfunctioning would clearly produce this type of bias and as a result these children do not experience a depression due to failures occurring in their life.

Studies are methodologically sound; however, they often fail to include control groups in their design when comparing the ADD with and without hyperactivity groups. Measures that are supposed to successfully differentiate the ADD group from the control group and its subtypes include behavior-rating scales, sociometric ratings, self-report measures, math ability and achievement measures, long-term memory measures, and measures of acquired automatic processing. There is considerable overlap between the two subtypes of ADD (with and without hyperactivity) and current measurements tend to be misleading and confounding, yielding mixed findings and contributing to considerable confusion in diagnosis.

An example is research conducted by Hooks, Milich, and Couch (1994), which indicates a sustained attention deficit in ADHD boys utilizing a computerized measure designed to assess attentional processes (The Continuous Performance Test). There was no evidence of a selective attentional deficit, hypothesized to be characteristic of ADHD. Performance of the ADHD group that declined over time was explained as a model of energy resources (either not available or not being optimally utilized). Demands on the encoding and/ or arousal stages of information processing were such that these children could not compensate, resulting in sustained attention deficits and omission errors on the tasks utilized for measurement. ADHD boys were also slower on the speeded classification task, seen by authors as a problem of inefficiency or "diffuse" attentional problems. Amin et al. (1993) also report underutilization of resources, resulting in described overall self-regulatory defects and a three-year maturational lag. However, this phenomenon could easily be the consequence of slow cognitive speed, information-processing deficits, a capacity problem, and inability to sustain attention and focus to task, highly characteristic of ADD. This would also result in inefficiency and failure to utilize energy resources noted by authors.

The clinical profiles of the two subtypes of ADD are very different. ADD classifies along the internalizing dimensions as opposed to the externalizing dimension of behavior of the ADHD group. ADD is seen as a more attentional/ cognitive/anxiety type of disorder in contrast to attentional/behavior/impulsive aspects of ADHD (Berry et al., 1985; Lahey et al., 1988; Hynd et al., 1991; Barkley, 1990; Shaywitz et al., 1986). Both groups have been described as underachieving, having impaired learning, and problems of incomplete work. Poor school performance among ADHD children has been linked to attentional/

behavioral problems, while poor school performance among ADD children is linked to more attentional/cognitive disabilities. Barkley (1995) maintains that ADHD includes the disturbance of executive functions that permit such processes as forethought, planning, goal-directed actions, self-discipline, willpower, and persistence. Disruption of the ability to prolong events; work with a sense of time; internalize language for self-governed behavior; possess regulation of affect, motivation, and drive states; utilize problem-solving creativity; and motor-control fluency to accomplish more complex goal-directed behavior.

ADHD is proposed as a multidirectional, evolving concept, providing a diagnostic category for children exhibiting signs of impulsivity, inattention, and motor hyperactivity. Creative children are seen as having similar characteristics, according to Cramond (1994), resulting in a high probability of misdiagnosis and considerable overlap between the two groups.

Seidman et al. (1997) examined individuals 9 to 22 years on several neuropsychological measures to determine the enduring quality of ADHD. The ADHD group was found to be significantly more impaired on measures of attention and executive function, impairment was significant across the age span (in comparing the younger, less than 15 years, to the older population) and impairment was evident regardless of other psychiatric and cognitive comorbid disorders. This study supports findings of underlying neuropsychological issues associated with the attentional disorders, and although authors implicate the frontal attention network, measures may have been subject to the impact of the posterior attentional network.

Jenkins et al. (1996) identified attentional problems and learning inefficiency in diagnosed childhood ADHD for adults. Given that the adults presented themselves to an adult ADD clinic, it is highly suspected that prediagnosed childhood ADHD was due to the anxiety exhibited, appearing behaviorally as overactive. This is a rather common phenomenon that also occurs in our adult outpatient ADD clinic, and we have documented rather extensively the misdiagnosis of ADD as ADHD. Finally, when considering the level of severity and rather poor outcome statistics for the ADHD population, it would inherently confirm the increased presence of the less severe, more anxious and compulsive subtype likely to read up on the topic of ADD and seek help.

Differentiation Using Self-Report Measures

Parents and teachers agreed on self-report measures that ADHD children are viewed as hyperactive, distractible, impulsive, short attention span and an inability to stay on task (Poillion, 1991). This may reflect the identification of five core behaviors with which to define ADHD. The groups failed to identify 11 of the 14 characteristics listed in the DSM-III-R criteria for ADHD. It appears that the defining variables between ADHD and ADD should be behavioral correlates and inattention.

Fischer et al. (1993) reported significant longitudinal continuity of both internalizing and externalizing behavioral pathology for ADHD children over an 8-year period into adolescence. Stanford and Hynd (1994) found that parents and teachers using self-report measures viewed children diagnosed with ADHD as more disruptive than children diagnosed with ADD or children diagnosed with LD. ADD and LD children were described as more underactive and shy and daydreaming more so than children diagnosed with ADHD. Finally, girls with problems of ADHD tend to go unrecognized because they do not present management problems evidencing lower levels of externalizing behavior and hyperactivity, greater intellectual impairment, and less aggression that would result in a lack of any outward problems to warrant an evaluation for ADHD. We have found that girls tend to be seen as not very bright. They themselves see the same picture in their own evaluation and lapse into a thought pattern of simply not being good enough, resulting in gross underdevelopment and, at times, low self-esteem and victimization, actual problems to warrant an evaluation for ADHD (McGee and Feehan, 1991; Gaub and Carlson, 1996). Sherman, McGue, and Iacono (1997) evaluated male twins aged 11 to 12 years, using self-report measures and structured interviews to identify the importance of genetic factors. They found ADHD more prevalent in monozygotic than dizygotic twins. The question of relying upon self-report measures and the necessity of using both parental and teacher information due to the bias present within each reporting source is addressed. Teachers more frequently endorsed ADHD items as well as a variety of other behavioral problems; mothers appeared to under-report the information. Johnston and Freeman (1997) noted that parents of children diagnosed with ADHD tended to view the behavior of the child as stemming from a physical disorder beyond their control, viewing inattentiveness, overactivity, and oppositional-defiant behavior as natural consequences of an internally driven, neurobiological system. Similarly, these parents also viewed prosocial behavior with the etiology as being more internalized, less subject to external control of the child and as a result, less stable over time. Generally, in comparison to parents of children without behavioral disorders, these parents saw themselves as having less responsibility and control over the positive or negative behavior of their child. McDermott, Spencer, and Wilens (1995) cite the necessity of recognizing the adult diagnosed with ADHD based on history and self-report symptoms. Authors point to the confusion and misconception regarding adult ADD and the toll this takes on the individual. In agreement, we strongly advise accurate and specific assessment of adult ADD to differentiate the two subtypes and specifically pinpoint problematic symptoms in a logical, clear-cut manner. The use of our battery, composed of very simple neuropsychological measures, carefully explained to the ADD adult and their family, finally clarifies this rather confusing, vague, elusive disorder.

Clinical Observations

Clinically observed and with the use of self-report measures, we have found certain characteristics that frequently differentiate one disorder from the other. ADHD individuals tend to be more out of control, participating in true impulsivity and low frustration tolerance, i.e., when they quit, they are done and cannot be "talked into" returning. These individuals tend to be extreme in nature, lack internal drive and motivation, and are difficult to reach emotionally due to the lack of connectiveness. ADHD adolescents and adults tend to become those true addicted individuals participating in alcohol or substance abuse, workaholism, alcoholism, overeating, gambling, sexual addiction, and so on. Substance abuse of the ADHD individual tends to be that of cocaine as they are looking for the stimulation. The prognosis is poor, due to the severity and pervasiveness of the disorder in addition to the predominant problem of connection and lack of both internal and external motivation.

ADD individuals are highly different beings. They tend to be highly anxious, there is a clear history of anxiety and anxiety-related disorders in the family, and they want to please. The anxiety creates the hyperactive behavior and the misdiagnosis of ADHD. However, these individuals are very sensitive and may be overly dramatic as opposed to the "not caring" of the ADHD. Instead of being out of control, ADD individuals tend to be overcontrolled and perfectionistic. These individuals may procrastinate, avoid, and manipulate; however, they can be reached, and practice these behaviors not due to inherent tendencies, but rather out of fear of reprisal and a desire to please. They tend to become involved in alcohol use to allow themselves to participate in the social arena more so as a form of self-medication. The substance abuse tends to be that of marijuana, which calms them down and it appears to target the sensory system, thus allowing them to cognitively function better; adults and adolescents will report "clearer" thinking when smoking marijuana. According to Michael and Hall (1994), marijuana is now more potent than ever and people are smoking what are called "blunts". The effect of smoking blunts may exceed marijuana intoxication and there is a more stimulant-like reaction reported. However, we have found that marijuana use results in a pervasive lack of motivation, rendering adolescents and the adult population listless and uncaring about anything and everything.

The picture becomes clearer in understanding the differentiation between the two subtypes, identifying ADHD as related to a left-hemisphere disorder characterized by learning disabilities and emotional, behavioral, and cognitive consequences of the disinhibition and inactivity of the frontal processes and the subcortical loops. ADD is more characterized by inactive right-hemisphere functions, extensive spatial issues (explaining reading and language problems), and deficits related more to deficient parietal information-processing problems with emotional, cognitive, and behavioral consequences that are highly distinct. Based on these clear anatomical differences, comorbid disorders are seen more with one subtype than the other.

CHAPTER 11

Comorbid Disorders and Disorders Associated with ADD

This chapter focuses upon the types of disorders that are comorbid and associated with the attentional disorders. The goal is to also address the occurrence of misdiagnosis of an attentional disorder, due to the overlap of symptomatology between an attentional disorder and other disorders that may produce the same set of symptoms, but the etiology is not that of an attentional disorder.

Allergies and Asthma

It was originally thought that the cure for ADHD was a type of diet that prevented use of any food additives, refined sugar, and so on. The diet was in fact helpful to ADHD children, however, not for relief of the symptoms related to an attentional disorder, but to relief from food allergies. Allergies appear to be quite common for the attentional disorders and may simply reflect a more vulnerable biological system overall as related to the disordered biochemical system. ADHD can often be misdiagnosed for symptoms of hyperthyroidism and ADD for symptoms of hypothyroidism.

McGee, Stanton, and Sears (1993) completed a study with ADHD children and found that both ADHD and allergic disorders do not have the common biological background previously assumed. Utilizing a large sample from the general population, there was no association found between parent, teacher, and self-report measures of hyperactive attention disorder behaviors and a history of allergic disorders (such as asthma, eczema, rhinitis, and urticaria) at the age of 9 or 13 years. Thus, although overlap of symptoms is often observed in the attentional disorder population, the overlaps are not causally related to one another. Biederman et al. (1994) confirmed asthma as a comorbid condition existing independently, but overlapping ADHD in its transmission genetically. Periodically in assessing for ADD, this author finds the comorbid diagnosis of multiple system allergies whereby the individual suffers from extensive allergic reactions to all types of stimuli. When this occurs evaluation indicates heightened distractibility. These individuals, are, however, more susceptible to memory disturbance and seizure activation.

Hypothalamic Pituitary Adrenal Axis

Kaneko et al. (1993) examined the hypothalamic pituitary adrenal axis (HPA) function in children diagnosed ADHD by measuring the diurnal variation and response to the dexamethasone suppression test (DST) of saliva cortisol. Abnormalities were found in HPA function in approximately one half of the children examined. Normal diurnal saliva cortisol rhythm was found in only 43.3% of ADHD children and DST results evidenced suppression in 46.7% of ADHD children. It was concluded that an abnormal diurnal rhythm and non-suppression to the DST test was more frequent for the severely hyper-active as opposed to the mildly hyperactive group of children diagnosed with ADHD. Authors suggest that hyperactivity (particularly in the severe state) may be associated with dysfunction of the HPA and/or that disturbances with the HPA are secondary to the physiological factors in ADHD children (such as disorganized sleep patterns and other habitual patterns) and these factors may result in changing the diurnal cortisol rhythm. Finally, it was proposed that the dysfunction of the HPA may be due to a disorder in regulation by the serotonin mechanism that has been proposed as playing a role in the pathophysiology of ADHD, especially in the area of impulsivity.

Sleep Disorders

Sleep disorders are commonly found in the attention-disordered population and can be observed during infancy. These children are described as the babies who would not go to sleep, would wake up often during their sleep cycle and/or sleep for unusually short periods of time. Clinically, we have observed a subtype of ADD, characterized as being overfocused, who have pervasive sleep problems that persist throughout their childhood and into adulthood. These sleep problems may evidence as either early or late insomnia, problems getting to sleep, all of which result in a degree of sleep deprivation that only further impacts symptomatology in addition to emotional symptoms of being highly irritable and overreactive to their environmental stimuli.

Sleeping can involve passing through two very different states, REM (rapid eye movement) and non-REM (slow wave) sleep. In non-REM sleep, we go through four stages, numbered successively by increasing depth with Stage II characterized with nearly 50% of sleeping time, and the deepest sleep whereby there is little or no conscious experience. Four or five times per night the individual can emerge into a REM state and REM episodes become longer as the night goes on to eventually occupy 20% of the sleeping time, mainly occurring in the early morning hours. Almost all dreaming tends to occur in REM sleep. REM sleep has been found to be an especially constant and inflexible need and, when individuals are deprived of REM sleep, they can become irritable, disoriented, uncoordinated, experiencing difficulty with attention and concentration, and may even develop hallucinations and delusions. The most common type of sleep disorders, with seriously disastrous consequences is an imbalance in the cycle of sleep and waking with an inability to sleep as well as an inability to stay awake (Harvard Mental Health Letter, 1994; Potolicchio, 1994).

Sleep apnea can be a cause of daytime drowsiness. In sleep apnea, the inflow of air is blocked in the pharynx (the passage that connects the nose and mouth with the trachea or windpipe) due to sagging muscles and sometimes excess tissue; the individual stops breathing and awakens with a gasp every few minutes throughout the night. The majority of individuals with this disorder fall asleep again immediately each time and do not even remember the apneic episodes the next day. Often, the problem is initially noted by someone else who hears the loud, irregular snoring that occurs when the pharynx is partially blocked, just prior to the breathing actually stopping. The daytime symptoms are easily mistaken for depression and similar disorders. The individual suffering from apnea awakes unrefreshed, always feeling tired as a result, concentration and memory is poor, and they tend to fall asleep at inconvenient and inappropriate times during the day. Blood pressure and heart rate tend to rise during apneic episodes and, consequently, these individuals may have morning headaches and cardiac arrhythmias, and the continual nightly oxygen deprivation increases the risk for strokes and heart failure as well as brain impairment over a period of time (Harvard Mental Health Letter, 1994; Sher, 1994).

Problems with snoring or sleep apnea often have cardiovascular risk factors such as obesity, hypertension, smoking and/or alcohol abuse. Sleep apnea can be present in as many as 35% to 50% of patients presenting with some form of heart disease (congestive heart failure, myocardial infarction, and coronary heart disease). There appears to be a high correlation between mortality factors related to heart disease and sleep apnea. Similarly, treatment of sleep apnea has been found to improve cardiac function of blood pressure control thus reducing cardiovascular mortality and morbidity factors. Sleep apnea was additionally found to have a high frequency of occurrence in patients in the acute phase of the TIA and stroke process. Sleep apnea was found to be more likely to occur in patients with sleep disturbance, habitual snoring and severe stroke (Bassetti, Aldrich, Chervin and Quint, 1996). In our evaluations I have found a high correlation between individuals diagnosed with ADD at the age of 40 to 50 years, also presenting with symptoms of sleep apnea. The presence of this disorder was reflected in an increased severity in their performance beyond what would be expected of a premorbid attentional disorder.

Another syndrome with similar effects on sleeping and daily functioning is that of restless legs, defined as uncomfortable crawling, tingling, and itching sensations that cause an irresistible urge to move the legs at the onset of sleep or upon awakening in the middle of the night. These movements can be slow rather than sudden. Walters et al. (1996) identified genetic etiology: diabetic peripheral neuropathy and lumbrosacral radiculopathy. The use of Gabapentin provided positive results with almost complete remediation of symptoms for up to 6 months in treatment of Restless Legs Syndrome (Adler, 1997). The positive effect of anticonvulsant medication, e.g., Gabapentin, for treatment of Restless Legs Syndrome may provide evidence of seizure activity occurring during sleep as an underlying etiology in the sensory and motor symptoms of this disorder. Often it is observed that both children and adults suffering from this type of activity at night have substantial impact to spatial areas of functioning and, in some cases, memory impairment is documented, suggesting that seizure activation not observed outwardly is correlated with this type of phenomenon and with deteriorating brain functioning. When this symptom is observed in the newly diagnosed ADD individual, further neurological evaluation is indicated, especially if any signs of tremor are noted. Narcolepsy is another causal factor for sleeping problems and daytime drowsiness, although less common than sleep apnea and its characteristic symptom, is that of sudden, periodic daytime attacks of REM sleep. Narcolepsy can be observed genetically in familial distribution. Narcolepsy can often be confused with symptoms of psychosis and responds well to stimulants (Jackson and Bachman, 1996). We have found comorbid disorders of narcolepsy and ADD resulting in increased severity of ADD symptoms and to progressive impact to brain functioning. Symptoms of daytime sleepiness in combination with a greater severity than would be expected for ADD or cognitive measures is sufficient to warrant referral for sleep evaluation.

Finally, sleepwalking and sleep terror are two forms of parasomnia that tend to occur in the latter stages of the sleep cycle, mostly in childhood. There is a genetic component (the problem is observed more often for boys than for girls), and in adults it can be associated with anxiety, depression, alcoholism, or brain injury. The degree to which sleepwalking is genetic in origin is illustrated by a study conducted by Hublin et al. (1977) who found that 66% men and 57% women of the population engaged in sleepwalking as children. Of this population adult sleepwalkers occurred in 80% of the men and 36% of the women. As this disorder becomes more common, there is a question regarding the impact of environmental issues.

The frightening dreams that follow a traumatic experience are different from ordinary nightmares and may be accompanied by body movements, shouting, sleepwalking, and night terrors, occurring in either non-REM or REM sleep. It is hypothesized that this indicates a malfunction of the biological rhythms that govern sleeping patterns and represent mismatched activation patterns in those relevant areas of the brain. In addition, when people talk in their sleep, fight imaginary foes, jerk their limbs, grind their teeth, wet the bed, and suddenly wake up from a deep sleep in terror, it is obvious this would impact their functioning ability during daytime hours, particularly attention and concentration to task at hand (Harvard Mental Health Letter, 1994).

Thyroid Disorders

Recent research findings indicate a relationship between thyroid status and cerebral activity. A relationship was found whereby peripheral TSH (a marker of thyroid status) was inversely related to global and regional CBF (cerebral blood flow) and cerebral glucose metabolism. Authors are examining the relationship between thyroid activity and its contribution to primary and secondary mood disorders. They are currently replicating their research to continue to study the relationship of brain activity to thyroid indexes (Marangell et al., 1997).

Much has been written relating ADHD to thyroid disorders and it has been hypothesized that evidence of a thyroid disorder may be a predictor for the presence of ADHD. This predictive hypothesis has not been supported by the majority of research studies that generally conclude there is simply a preponderance of thyroid dysfunctioning to be present in the attention-disordered population, more so than that indicated in the normal population. Hauser et al. (1993) examined the relationship of ADHD with generalized resistance to thyroid hormone (a disease caused by mutations in the thyroid receptor gene and characterized by reduced responsiveness of peripheral and pituitary tissues to the actions of the thyroid hormone). Authors systematically evaluated the presence and severity of ADHD in families with a history of generalized resistance to thyroid hormone. Findings indicated that the odds of having ADHD were 3.2 times greater for male subjects with generalized resistance to thyroid hormone, and 2.7 times greater for males than for females not having a history of generalized resistance. Finally, the presence of ADHD was 2.5 times greater in those identified with a generalized resistance to thyroid hormone than those without. It was concluded that ADHD is strongly associated with generalized resistance to thyroid hormone, but not causally related. Subjects diagnosed with hyperthyroidism, prior to treatment, reported significantly worse memory, attention, planning, and productivity, in addition to mood swings, sudden droops in academic performance, and difficulty concentrating, while hyperthyroid (Stern et al., 1996; Eberle, 1995).

Studies comparing thyroid dysfunctioning to ADD have not been prevalent. It has been observed clinically that those diagnosed with ADD have a greater preponderance to hypoglycemia (a low blood-sugar condition) and hyperthyroid disease. The disorder of subclinical hypothyroidism (Kabadi, 1993) is identified as a state of thyroid function characterized by normal serum thyroxin and triiodothyronine concentrations with a slightly elevated thyrotropin concentration and an exaggerated thyrotropin response to intravenous administration of protirelin. It is believed to be a forerunner of primary hypothyroidism and this seems to be the phenomenon most often observed in the ADD population. Symptoms can be easily confused with an attentional disorder of this type evidenced by consistent lethargy, sluggishness, foggy appearance and impact upon general state of arousal and alertness.

Primary Nocturnal Enuresis

Primary nocturnal enuresis (PNE) is a frequent problem associated with both subtypes of ADD that can persist through adolescence and even (in some cases) through adulthood. Current statistics indicate that those suffering from PNE are dry at night by 5 years (81%), by 7 years (90%), by 10 years (95%), and these approximate statistics show a decrease of PNE by 1% for each additional year, leaving 1% persisting into adulthood. PNE is defined as primary urinary leakage at night (the child has never been dry and is past the age for nocturnal control). Secondary nocturnal enuresis (nighttime bedwetting in children dry for over a 6-month period) accounts for 20 to 25% of diagnosed cases. Present theories to account for this occurrence are that of sudden arousal from the non-REM stage of sleep, bladder instability (limited functional bladder capacity), and antidiuretic hormone (ADH deficiency). Delayed central nervous system maturation (affecting urinary control), genetic predisposition (75% have family history of enuresis), as well as social and psychological factors are additional causal variables. An underlying organic cause has been found to occur in only 1 to 3% of diagnosed cases. DDAVP (desmopressin acetate), in oral and nosespray form, based on the theory of abnormal nocturnal ADH secretion, has been found highly effective in the treatment of enuresis due to its antidiuretic effect. The gains made in achieving "dryness" far outweighed the side effects (Milk, Goldberg, and Atkins, 1989; Phône-Poulenc Rorer Pharmaceuticals, 1995; Shortliffe, 1993; Nergäärd and Djurhuus, 1993; Stenberg and Lackgren, 1993).

Developmental Disability (Mental Retardation)

Down's syndrome is the most common, single, biological causal factor of mental retardation with statistics of 1 in 1000 births. Abnormalities on chromosome 21 are generally associated with cognitive impairment. Down's syndrome is associated with selective impairment of phonological processes and inferior short-term verbal memory. Cognitive deficits are diffuse with specific difficulties in language development, memory skills, and the phonological loop (Jarrold and Baddeley, 1997). Down's syndrome has an abnormal aging process that through time develops the same neuropathology as that of Alzheimer's disease. After age 40 the symptoms of the two disorders become indistinguishable. Primarily parietal and temporal cortical areas are impacted in both Down's and Alzheimer's disease (Pietrini et al., 1997).

It becomes important to separate out symptoms due to a lowered level of intellectual capacity and an attentional disorder. Clearly, an individual's intelligence will determine the degree of attentional capacity and produce limits on attentional abilities. Pulsifer (1996), in reviewing mental retardation (MR) from a neuropsychological perspective, found common cognitive deficits (for idiopathic MR, and MR due to genetic or prenatal factors) of inattention; short-term memory; and sequential information-processing, language, and visuospatial abilities or disabilities were more variable and dependent on the type of MR. Fee et al. (1993) addressed the issue of hyperactivity, attention deficits, and conduct problems among the mentally retarded population using self-report measures. They concluded that conduct problems were less strongly associated with hyperactivity and attention deficits among the mentally retarded population as compared to children of normal intelligence. The idea was introduced that attention and conduct problems may be associated with mental retardation in general and not necessarily with ADHD. Authors questioned the validity of self-report measures used to diagnose ADHD in the mentally retarded population and the validity of a diagnosis that is not based on one's functional ability and capacity. Fee, Matson, and Benavidez (1994) confirmed the validity of ADHD in the mentally retarded population, and when diagnosed with comorbid ADHD, had more factors related to anxiety than the higher IQ controls. This may implicate overdiagnosis of ADHD and relate more to ADD (which is highly characterized by anxiety) instead. The mentally retarded population as a whole (with or without the comorbid diagnosis of ADHD) was seen with less social behavioral disturbances. This would appear to confirm the idea of overdiagnosis of ADHD and provide reason for confounding research results regarding the attentional disorders.

Merrill and O'Dekirk (1994) in their research found that subjects who were mentally retarded performed significantly worse than non-retarded subjects on measures of attention. In addition, findings revealed no difference in attentional processing between individuals whose mental retardation was the result of different etiologies. Authors concluded that those diagnosed as mentally retarded exhibit a global attentional processing deficit relative to individuals who are not mentally retarded. Severe anoxia produced variable levels of impairment on brain functioning, particularly cognitive and memory symptoms, while attentional functioning remained perserved (Hopkins et al., 1996). This would confirm our findings of the impact of MR on comorbid attentional symptoms as increased severity on those measures related more to whole brain functioning or association cortex areas.

Learning Disability, Dyslexia, Dyscalculia, Dysgraphia, and Spelling Apraxia

Attention can be oriented to not only the events occurring in one's external environment, but also to internal representations, such as words, images, or memories. Skilled reading would require mastery or ability to manipulate the processed material and then to accommodate the situational demands and constraints inherent in the task, and in this manner would reflect both automatic and control functions. Automaticity would be manifested by the fact that reading itself draws nothing or very small amounts from limited mental resources, while control may be manifested by the ability to ignore a word or inhibit its processing as the prevailing conditions require. The automatic processing of words is what skilled readers indicate makes reading so effortless for them, and here, automaticity is an important aspect of superior performance. Skill, however, needs to be evidenced not only in the unintended reading of the irrelevant word, but also in the ability to inhibit processing when necessary for the task at hand, and the ability to control reading would result in decreased interference. Further, the ability to suppress word-reading processes that are usually automatic is dependent on the degree of language competence, and thus becomes an important aspect of skilled reading performance (Rafal and Henik, 1994). Resta and Eliot (1994) found significant problems with writing, copying, and composition for both subtypes of ADHD and ADD.

Reading problems are highly evidenced in the attention-disordered population. ADHD seems to be more correlated to learning disabilities and a "true" dyslexia, while the language problems of the ADD population seem to be more related to a spatial inattention and/or problems with information processing. A central processing disorder has been found associated with reading problems and ADHD (Riccio et al., 1994; Schuerholz et al., 1995; Moss and Shelffele, 1994; Duncan et al., 1994).

Linguistic processing deficits described as inherent in poor readers parallel symptoms associated with information-processing problems and spatial inattention deficits leading to descriptive markers of problematic phonetic segmentation, rapid naming, and overall deficient phonetic awareness. Phonological processing underlying language production takes place simultaneously in an overlapping and distributed manner, probably characteristic of information-processing circuitry (S.E. Nadeau, 1995). August and Garfinkel (1990) found two functionally different deficits in ADHD and comorbid reading problem: effortful processing and deficits in rapid automatized naming, that result in a complicated cyclical interaction likely to increase problems.

Heilman (1993, 1994) refers to the neglect syndrome as the tendency to neglect or not attend to one part of space. Willinck (1996) identified neglect dyslexia as reading deficits due to symptoms of neglect and evidenced by word-level errors (letter substitutions, additions, and omissions and/or text-level errors). Phonological processing problems were related to decreased activation of central parietal and frontal area in diagnosed dyslexics (Ackerman et al., 1994). The neglect is seen as a consequence of deficits in attentional factors and scanning factors or internal representation deficits. Writing deficits are perceived similarly, characterized by visuospatial deficits observed in margin displacement, superimposed and undulating lines in addition to factors of omission and/or duplication and sentence/paragraph level errors. Paulesu et al. (1996) propose that the defective use of the phonological system is the consequence of a lack of connectivity between the anterior and posterior language areas. Although viewing the reading problem as primarily an issue of disconnection, authors did note a lack of activation specific to those diagnosed with dyslexia for the right hemisphere; however, authors did not attribute this as a causal factor for developmental dyslexia.

Phonological dyslexia is seen as a developmental disorder resulting from a general impairment in phonological representation (Farah, Stowe and Levinson, 1996; Howard and Best, 1996). It is defined as the ability to read at a normal rate; however, substitutions are made. These substitutions increased in diagnosed dyslexic children when they read faster and when they tended to sound out words to a lesser degree. When attention is diffused and distributed over the entire word, it is recognized more quickly (Hendriks and Kolk, 1997). Characteristic symptoms of difficulties with word decoding, particularly nonwords (inability to string letters in a meaningless manner), reflect phonological difficulties. In evaluating children with dyslexia, abnormalities emerged in urine samples and serum analyses which may be related to underlying peptidase deficiencies for the proteins gluten and casein, similar to abnormalities related to syndromes such as Tourette's, Autism, ADD, Schizophrenia and Depression (Knivsberg, 1997). Non-word reading and impairment was identified as related to sight phonological errors. Children with reading difficulties were subjected to phonological processing deficits, demonstrating the strong relationship between reading and spelling problems and phonological skills. Preschool phonological skills have been seen as a predictor of the later development of reading and spelling ability (Snowling and Hume, 1996).

Neglect dyslexia is seen as a reading disorder resulting from visuospatial neglect and is associated with right hemisphere dysfunctioning. Dyslexic error can be seen as a result of neglect in reading text, single words or individual letters. Larger words were more prone to neglect errors (Worthington, 1996). The impact of spatial issues commensurate with a condition of hemineglect is what we have seen as being the single unitary component of ADD symptoms to slowly and totally obliterate language skills in a subtle, but highly deteriorating manner for those diagnosed with ADD. This problem becomes the silent killer, moving softly, but swiftly to destroy reading abilities, unless combated by a driven compulsivity to use mnemonic abilities on a continual basis.

Clinically observed, there is the inability (to a greater or lesser degree) to exercise control over the interference of irrelevant words, to focus on the relevant and process the information (signaling the impact of distractibility). In addition, a spatial inattention or inattention to the whole similar to a hemineglect results in the inability to read down a page without getting lost, find sentences in a page, and visually scan from right to left in a cohesive manner necessary for adequate performance of reading. Further, there is a noted problem in establishing a more comprehensive sight vocabulary, due to the inability to utilize phonetics, and the need to view the word as a cohesive whole and to relate the recognition of the word with its comprehensive meaning using mnemonic strategies. Thus, unless memorized, it has been found that individuals who know the meaning of words cannot spell them correctly in a sentence nor recognize or pronounce them. If the individual hears the word pronounced by someone else, he/she can memorize the sound of that word, but cannot read the word correctly him/herself until using visual memory processes. Finally, spelling is highly problematic unless compensated for by mnemonic devices, and writing skills are poor as well, resulting in sentences running off the page, words running together, some letters smaller and some larger for no significant reason (other than this hypothesized spatial problem, which appears as dysgraphia). Mathematical abilities are also problematic when mathematical calculations demand some type of spatial cohesiveness, either calculations that require some sort of visual entity (seeing the problem in one's head, such as story problems) or complex tasks necessitating compilation in a more spatial format. An example of this is that the ADD individual would have an easier time with algebraic equations rather than the geometric designs and calculations of geometry, which become more spatial in nature. A last final note is that this appears to correlate specifically with ADD being more related to parietal functioning, and thus correlated with the more posterior dysfunctioning of the attentional system.

Kosslyn et al. (1994) found hemispheric bias due to attentional effect, whereby the left hemisphere monitors outputs comprising the more-difficult aspects of the encoding process for high resolution output, while the right hemisphere complements the left monitoring low-resolution outputs. Thus, reading difficulties associated with learning disability are associated with left hemispheric dysfunctioning, whereby the individual is clearly unable to read (to varying degrees) and the impact is greater due to the greater impact of left hemisphere dysfunctioning. The impact is less severe when the involvement is either spatial in nature, right hemisphere-oriented (such as spatial inattention problems as characterized with ADD), thus confirming poor reading skills as opposed to dyslexia and an inability to read.

Asymmetry of the cortical areas has been associated with changes in the volume of architectonic areas, size differences in overall numbers and densities of some neurons, and variation in the patterns of callosal connections. Indirect evidence suggests that asymmetry is determined early during early brain formation (corticogenesis, probably during the time when the neuroblast pools are being established on the two sides of the midline of the neural tube) and the idea that there are not only storage factors differentiating the two hemispheres, but also factors of network size and detailed connectivity (Galaburda, 1994). This finding serves to explain what is now well documented, the asymmetry of the planum temporale associated with left-handedness, developmental disorders, autoimmune disturbances, learning disabilities, and language dysfunctioning (Leonard, 1995).

The planum temporale is located on the superior surface of the temporal lobe and typical architecture indicates the left planum is larger than the right for the human species. It has been known as an auditory association cortex area involved in word generation and language functions (Shenton, McCarley, and Tamminga, 1995). However, Galaburda (1996) maintains that the asymmetry of the planum temporale results from a normal reduction in cortical neurons. Further research needs to be done. Kulynych et al. (1994) address the issue of gender differences, finding a significant difference for males versus females, with males having significantly greater asymmetry than females. Differences have been cited of the perisylvian gyral region and, contrary to smaller volumes of neuronal activity, larger volumes are currently cited as distinguishing ADHD and dyslexia (Hynd et al., 1996; Hall et al., 1996).

The controversy continues. Javorsky (1996), found that 70% of subjects diagnosed with ADHD qualified for a diagnosis of learning disabled. Subjects identified as ADHD performed significantly poorer on measures of language abilities. In studying the speech patterns of learning disabled children, Berk and Landau (1993) found that learning disabled children used more task-relevant private speech than controls, and this phenomenon became more pronounced for the learning disabled group that had a dual diagnosis of ADHD. Only the less-symptomatic ADHD children were able to utilize private speech as a self-regulatory mediation strategy to ameliorate behavioral and attentional difficulties. Private speech was defined as an externalized thought that serves as a self-guiding function, and increases under conditions of difficult and demanding tasks. This would explain why ADD children and adults are more adept at problem-solving and using cognitive processes to cope with symptoms of the disorder than ADHD children and adults. Further, this helps to clarify why ADHD is clinically known as the more-severe disorder in that this type of cognitive coping skill is not available for those diagnosed with this disorder.

Feldman et al. (1993) investigated the developmental, demographic, educational, and psychosocial outcome of adults with third-generation familial dyslexia. Compared with controls, those with familial dyslexia had higher incidences of perinatal complications, left-handedness, right–left confusion, reading and spelling problems, and were more likely to report depression/anxiety symptoms, and to be diagnosed ADHD. Stanford and Hynd (1994) clarified differences between the two subtypes of ADD as it relates to diagnosed learning disability. They found that the identified ADHD group had more behavioral symptoms of impulsivity, while the ADD subtype was more prone to daydreaming, being underactive and shy.

Symptoms related to neurological disorders can easily be mistaken for an attention deficit disorder and further symptoms of ADD need to be separated from symptoms relating to subsequent injury to the brain.

Social Emotional Processing Disorder

Extensive deficits presenting enhanced symptoms of ADD, seizure-like activation, spatial deficits, and emotional symptoms of the overfocused subtype meet the criteria for developmental social emotional processing disorder (SEPD).

This disorder is specifically associated with right-hemisphere abnormalities and early brain injury impacting this area of functioning. The right hemisphere is affected to the degree that it fails to support the adequate development of cognitive, affective, and behavioral functions. The identification of SEPD, characterized by symptoms of poor social skills, attentional deficits, paucity of interpersonal relationships, deficiencies in non-verbal areas (particularly spatial) resulting in poor language development and communication skills offers a clear explanation for consistent findings to explain severity of symptoms beyond that of an attentional disorder without the presence of clear etiology of brain dysfunctioning. There is overlapping symptomatology: schizoid personality, social phobia, and Asperger's syndrome, undiagnosed seizure activity causing sudden bursts of emotion (unprecipitated crying, sadness, or confusion) (Manoach, Sandson, and Weintraub, 1995). DeLuca et al. (1997) documented a right hemisphere learning disability on neuropsychological evaluation, presenting evidence of symptoms of poor arithmetic skills, visual spatial difficulties, diminished deductive reasoning skills and intact reading, spelling, and rote verbal skills. PET scan results revealed a hypometabolism in the right parietal and bilateral superior temporal areas.

Neurofibromatosis

Neurofibromatosis (NF) Type 1 is a common autosomal dominant genetic disorder resulting in approximately 40% being diagnosed with comorbid ADHD and/or learning disability. Research indicates impact to brain functioning occurs due to the presence of tumors and white-matter hypertensities.

Charcot-Marie-Tooth Disease

Charcot-Marie-Tooth disease (CMT) represents a group of genetic disorders that are heterogeneous in nature and affect the peripheral nervous system producing neuropathies. CMT is characterized by a progressive weakness and atrophy of distal muscles of the upper and lower extremities, ranging in severity from severe foot drop to high arched feet (Timmerman et al., 1996).*

---

*To illustrate the genetic role, Haneman et al. (1996) documented a disease stage dependent altered Schwann cell phenotype hypothesized as a direct consequence of the PmP22 overexposed on Schwann cell growth behavior which early in the course of the disease directly or secondarily alters Schwann cell phenotype.

A symptom of the disease can be a delay in walking. The first signs occur around the age of 5 years with early deformities to the feet and spine (Kessali et al., 1977). We have found comorbid ADD with remission of symptoms, with the advent of stimulant treatment and coping mechanisms thus decreasing stress-related symptoms.

Epilepsy

Convulsive status epilepticus may occur in an individual diagnosed with epilepsy, as well as a non-epileptic. Seizure activity can be due to a variety of causal factors, such as head injury, cocaine overdose, and metabolic derangements (high fever, hypoglycemia, CNS infection, tumor, anoxia, alcohol intoxication or withdrawal, and so on). Most epileptic seizures end within 30 to 90 seconds. In clinical practice, treatment is recommended when a seizure lasts 5 to 10 minutes (Dodson, Leppik, and Slovis, 1992; Deonna, 1993; Walsh, 1994). Seizures can be triggered by psychological factors and/ or stress situations. Benign partial epilepsy of childhood with rolandic spikes (BPERS) is a frequent childhood epileptic syndrome and accounts for approximately 20% of the epilepsies occurring during school age (Deonna, 1993). BECT refers to Benign Epilepsy of Childhood with centrotemporal spikes, which has an excellent prognosis with most children having only a few seizures and in remission by the age of 12 to 13 years. Poorer predictions are evidenced with adolescence or adult-age onset whereby there is a more abnormal interictal pattern and etiology is remote and less clear-cut. BECT is characterized by brief, simple, partial hemifacial motor seizures, associated somatosensory symptoms related to sleep, an onset between 3 to 13 years, and spontaneous remission. There are no demonstrable lesions accompanying this disorder, there is a family history of BECT and male predominance (Bouma et al., 1997).

Epilepsia partialis continua (EPC) has been defined as continuous focal jerking of a body part (usually that of a distal limb) which can last for hours, days, or years, as a consequence of impact to the cerebral cortex (Cockerell et al., 1996). Juvenile myoclonic epilepsy (JME) is defined as a hereditary syndrome with symptoms of myoclonic jerks, awakening generalized clonic-tonic-clonic seizures and absence seizures. This disorder comprises approximately 5 to 11% of the epileptic population and appears to impact frontal processes, thus creating emotional instability, inadequate adjustment and the tendency to jump from one place of action to another. Neuroimaging-studies evidence suggests that JME results in abnormal patterns of cortical activation creating subtle cognitive dysfunctioning as a consequence of the disorganization of verbal circuitry, affecting the epileptogenic potential and creating a hypofrontality state (Swartz et al., 1996).

Childhood absence epilepsy (CAE) is found occurring in school age children with prior normal development. Peak onset occurs at 6 to 7 years of age. Numerous absence seizures can occur daily and EEG findings depict bilateral synchronous, symmetric 3-Hz spike and wave discharges with normal background rhythm. A proportion of the population of children diagnosed with CAE (approximately one-half to one-third) develop generalized seizure activity during adolescence. Absence seizures can also occur in 10 to 34% of those children diagnosed with JME and 43% of those children who did not have remission developed JME. (Wirrell et al., 1996). When tonic-clonic seizures present years after the onset of absence epilepsy, the prognosis becomes worse than if absence seizures remain the only type of seizure activity evidenced (Bouma et al., 1996; Wirrell et al., 1997).

Febrile seizures occur in approximately 2 to 4% of the child population and 2 to 10% diagnosed with this type of seizure activity, develop subsequent unprovoked seizures. Factors predictive of development of seizure activity is a familial history of epilepsy, presence of complex and/or recurrent febrile seizures, and neurodevelopmental abnormalities. Febrile seizures typically do not result in unprovoked seizures or present as a causal factor for impact to brain functioning (Berg and Shinnar, 1996.) Febrile seizures occurred generally in the first year of life usually ceasing by approximately 11 years. A generalized epilepsy syndrome with a genetic etiology was hypothesized as responsible for this type of seizure activation. It was proposed that a single genetic syndrome, entitled *generalized epilepsy with febrile seizures plus (GEFs+)* was responsible for the emergence of a whole spectrum of types of epilepsy including febrile seizures (Scheffer and Berkovic, 1997). The occurrence of seizures during a critical period of neural maturation (onset before age 5 years and seizing occurring regularly before age 5 years) poses the greatest risk to normal cognitive development, more so than such factors as the total duration of seizures, history of severe convulsive episodes, and/or the occurrence of another neurological issue, which were not seen as contributing significantly to impaired cognitive development in the temporal lobe epileptic population (Glosser et al., 1997).

Those who continue to evidence seizures on an indefinite or continuous basis manifest the "running down phenomenon" significant of temporal-lobe epilepsy. A history of head trauma, encephalitis, post temporal localization and bi-temporal spiking, had worse outcomes than those with a history of febrile seizures. The area of epileptogenesis can lead to secondary epileptogenic areas in the same hemisphere by recruiting adjacent cortex via hypoexcitability and hypometabolism leading to a pathological hyper-synchronization facilitating a kindling process and interictal spiking (Merlet et al., 1996; Salonova et al., 1995). Schlaug et al. (1997) identified possible epileptogenic zones and a pattern of distinctly abnormal metabolic brain regions. Patients diagnosed with temporal lobe epilepsy and a unilateral interictal spike location were more likely to have consistent ictal onset patterns than patients with bilateral interictal spike location. Interictal spike location significantly influenced the reliability of the seizure activity and unilateral interictal determined more consistently localized temporal lobe seizures, thus providing confirmation that bilateral provided a sign of independent bitemporal excitability (Sirven et al., 1997). Acharya et al. (1997) identified seizure symptomatology and correlated symptoms with the location of the epileptogenic zone. Seizures evidencing a decrease in motor activity with minimal or no automatisms and indeterminate level of consciousness were found to arise from temporal, temporoparietal, or parieto-occipital areas as opposed to those seizures with localized or bilateral clonic, tonic, or atonic accompanying motor phenomena arising generally from the frontal, frontocentral, central, or frontoparietal areas.

van Domburg and associates (1996) present evidence of a progressive neurological disorder that ends in early death. With the initial stage being a severe sensory neuropathy, with its onset in adolescence, and later stages evidencing a myoclonic epilepsy with the etiology being that of multisystemic involvement of the nervous system. Rasmussen's Syndrome is a rate, progressive neurologic disorder with intractable, focally originating seizures and the presence of chronic encephalitis. Etiology may relate to persistent herpes virus in the CNS (McLachlan et al., 1996). Right temporal epilepsy can result in the impact to spatial and figural aspects of nonverbal memory. Symptoms of depression and psychosocial difficulties are a consequence of complex partial seizures. Alterations of a sense of reality, recurrent thought patterns, mystical religious experiences, alterations in the sense of time, and distortions of body image are also factors contributing to symptoms of depression evidenced in this population (Breier et al., 1996; Mendez et al., 1996). Mendez et al. (1997) identified characteristics to define a *cognitive aura* with distinguishing features of being stereotypical, out of context, occurring for only a brief duration of time and observed in the context of other seizure symptomology. Symptoms describe the disordered thinking that occurs subsequent to seizure activation, specifically that of intrusive thoughts or forced thinking, derealization, depersonalization, dreamy state, compulsive urges, and an altered time sense.

Seizure activity varies in the traumatic brain injury (TBI) population. There are worse outcomes for post traumatic seizure activity that occurs within the first year, subsequent to the injury. The presence of seizure activity is seen as reflective of the severity of impact to brain function. Seizure activity can result in the presence of olfactory and gustatory hallucinations, visual distortions and misperceptions, depersonalization, derealization, and sudden and unexplainable fears. Post ictal phases may present symptoms of decreased alertness, confusion, lethargy, and fatigue, similar to symptoms of an attentional disorder. Children and adolescents diagnosed with a range of mild to severe TBI were found to respond to anticonvulsant medication which decreased symptoms of staring spells, memory gaps, and temper outbursts. Episodic symptoms can persist 2 to 3 years post injury and provides explanation for the chronic disruptive behaviors, social inappropriateness, and mental inertia observed as common sequelae to TBI. Such symptoms easily parallel an attentional disorder and it becomes difficult to differentiate. Staring spells, characteristic of seizure activity need to be discriminated from symptoms of an attentional disorder, such as distractibility (Haltino et al., 1996; Hernandez and Naritoku, 1997; Roberts et al., 1996; and Hines, 1996).

Clinically, seizure activity is often seen with the attention-disordered population, particularly those with a familial history of other disorders involving altered brain functioning and more-severe psychopathology. The QEEG or quantitative analysis techniques utilize a method of mathematical processing of EEG to provide a *finer* measure of the data obtained, often revealing abnormalities not seen otherwise. QEEG analysis has been the subject of considerable review and debate (Nuwer, 1997). In our clinical practice, we find that this method is quite helpful and adept in correlating with neuropsychological test findings to isolate seizure activation not seen otherwise. Research conducted with QEEGs have found particular brain-wave patterns that responded to antiseizure medications and other combinations of antidepressants and antiseizure medications. This research will be the forerunner of more-specific research examining the attention-disordered population for a vulnerability to seizure activation that appears to be a mild, absent-mal type. We have observed a particular combination pattern of seizure activity with some regularity with the overfocused subtype of the ADD population, with concomitant features of early irritability in infancy, clear sleep problems, a general intolerance for change, and a tendency toward overdramatization, thus denoting a more fragile individual. These individuals also tend to exhibit tic-like symptoms that are characteristic of Tourette's Syndrome. Often inappropriate behavior is observed in the classroom setting — swearing, name calling, hitting, oppositional behavior, and an inability to remain seated.

Brief partial seizures characteristic of mesial temporal-lobe epilepsy were found to mimic symptoms of panic disorder, which can be accompanied by concomitant symptoms of anxiety, phobia, and true panic attacks, making it difficult to differentiate from true psychiatric symptoms. Differentiation would depend on the brevity of symptoms (with seizure episodes of anxiety lasting only a few seconds) sporadic seizure activity, presence and rapid shift of ictal symptoms (Young et al., 1995; Herbert and Devinsky, 1995).

Tremors are produced by oscillation of either central neuronal networks or sensory motor loops with the origin and underlying pathology being both complex and diverse. Tremor is distinguished from other movement disorders as a periodic movement about an axis. Tremors are defined by behavioral classification (rest, action, postural, kinetic, isometric) etiology (physiological and essential) (Parkinson's, dystoric, cerebellar, midbrain, neuropathic, drug induced, and trauma) (Deuschl, Krack, Lauk, and Timmer, 1996; Findley, 1996). We have found a correlation between evidence of observed hand tremor and seizure-like activation, hypoglycemia, and/or motor neuron disorder commonly observed in the adult ADD population.

A final note is that in normal EEG findings, generally there is a 15% detection rate for simple, partial seizures without motor activity as well as other neurological measures, do not necessarily mean that there is an absence of seizure activity. The use of quantification and the QEEG, specifically, is not impervious to this phenomenon as well. Epileptic discharges are variable pathophysiological events, subject to all kinds of internal and external influences, and thus are not constant in time. An example is that of deeply situated epileptic foci, such as limbic foci, which would not always show up on a surface EEG. Thus, in order to properly document and determine seizure activity, several strategies must be employed, such as videotaping, 24-hour EEG, neuropsychological evaluation, response to antiseizure medication, observation of behavior in school and at play, and questionnaires to parents and teachers (Sisodiya et al., 1995; Deonna, 1993). Additional techniques utilized to measure seizure activation, e.g., MRI, MRS, SPECT, and FDG-PET, allow for further understanding of this elusive phenomenon. The MRI is utilized in defining structural abnormalities while the functional MRI can identify the functional brain areas responsible for specific cognitive traits.

The MRS (magnetic resonance spectroscopy) investigates cerebral metabolites and some neurotransmitters, while SPECT (single photon emission computed tomography) identifies regional cerebral blood flow (Duncan, 1997). FDG-PET (providing evidence on regional cerebral blood flow and the binding of specific ligands to receptors) is thought by some researchers to be a very useful method, delineating a 60 to 90% incidence of hypometabolism in the temporal area occurring interictally in both children and adults with the diagnosis of TLE. This remains in debate and Duncan (1997) advocates the use of this technique, indicating that the FDG-PET tends to provide evidence of the major cerebral metabolic associations and consequences of epilepsy. However, it does remain nonspecific with respect to etiology. Investigations with specific ligands provide identification of the neurochemical abnormalities associated with epilepsy. SPECT studies can provide information occurring at the time of seizure activation.

Powell et al. (1997) identified lateral and bilateral orbitofrontal hypoperfusion utilizing the Brain 99mTc-HPAO SPECT, that specifically targets nonconclusive epilepsy, in a father and son who outwardly displayed considerable symptoms of ADHD (inattentiveness, impulsivity, poor concentration, and motor restlessness). This also presented symptoms of seizure disorder (nonresponsive staring, complex automatic behavior, amnesic periods and specifically in the son, atonic drop-attacks) responding quite well to antiseizure medication.

The disorder of autosomal dominant nocturnal frontal lobe epilepsy can begin in childhood, persist into adulthood, and, due to considerable variation of symptoms, be misdiagnosed as benign nocturnal parasomnias, psychiatric and medical disorders (Scheffer et al., 1995). Seizure activity can account for symptoms related to both the overfocused subtype of ADD, as well as the "out of control" emotional dysregulation of ADHD (characteristic of lack of inhibition of frontal processes). Symptoms of ADD and continuous seizure activity can appear in an interchangeable manner and lead to misdiagnosis.

Parkinson's Disease

Another example of disordered attentional processes due to brain dysfunctioning is that of Parkinson's disease (PD). Parkinson's disease is classically based on a motor symptom triad of tremor, bradykinesia, and rigidity, and originally there were no indications of intellectual impairment. Research has clearly indicated intellectual impairments, particularly that of the attentional processes, inability to maintain internally directed control, sustain attention to task, self-directed planning, and compromised supervisory attentional system (SAS). Stam et al. (1993) identified a deficiency in the SAS with PD implicating a disturbance of the frontal regulation of attentional processes and degeneration of the dopaminergic mesocortical enervation of the frontal cortex. Research points to the disturbance of the regulation of attentional processes under novel, non-routine conditions and further indicates the complexity of this neurodegenerative disorder. Parkinson's patients clearly show an abnormally rapid disengagement of attention, which resulted in numerous perceptual errors made in attempting to target specific stimuli. These findings suggest a deficiency in maintaining covert attention, which may underlie the visuoperceptual impairment symptomatic of the disorder (Filoteo et al., 1994). Bennett et al. (1995) did not find a problem of the covert orienting of attention in examining Parkinson's patients, finding instead the intact ability to orient attention toward the expected source of stimulation and the problem was more that of allocation of resources and managing more than one attentional task. These deficits were observed in the relationship between task-related distribution of attentional resources and time efficiency of processing, pointing to the impact on the basal ganglia system as a modulating influence. Attention and sentence processing deficits observed in Parkinson's suggest a defect in anterior cingulate cortex, which was confirmed using PET scan studies (Grossman et al., 1992). The use of attentional strategies and visual cues was helpful to elicit a normal stride length in Parksonian patients, implicating the effects of attention as a means of overcoming a habitual pattern based upon dysfunctioning and disregulation of the basal ganglia system (Morris et al., 1996). Gait difficulties were exhibited due to the impaired postural shifts that mediate changes from one posture to another. The greatest difficulty noted with Parksonian patients was when they start to walk. This was due to timing, sitting, and rising from a chair. Error deviations in their postural shift of gait initiation was responsible for steps being aborted prior to the first step (Elble et al., 1996). This phenomenon, similar to that observed in the Parksonian patients is seen with ADD children. Specifically in the ADD without-hyperactivity population, we have found the greatest disturbance in this area. The gait of these children tends to be disturbed to one side or the other. There can be an imbalance created from the inability to maintain the body physically in space. This phenomenon tends to occur when the spatial functioning is more impaired than what would normally be observed in the ADD population. Often, this relates to specific impairment to that area of brain functioning subsequent to seizure activation (on a continuum from tics to absence seizures) resulting in a general weakening. Bondi et al. (1993) demonstrated frontal lobe deficits in non-demented Parkinson's patients confirming the striatofrontal outflow model of neuropsychological impairment (a complex loop whereby it emanates from widespread projections of cortical association areas, funnels into and through the caudate nucleus, and relays back to the prefrontal cortex via thalamocortical projections). Due to the issue of Parkinson's disease causing changes in the nigrostriatal system, authors suspect that the dopamine deficiency in the caudate nucleus would have implications for behaviors dependent on this loop and thus impact frontal functioning. Thus, the idea that the combination of disturbed caudate outflow and reduced availability of dopamine places at even greater risk those functions that depend on the prefrontal region, as proven by the tests administered.

Ebersbach et al. (1996) suggest a model of attentional neglect, the disease process impacting the anterior and posterior attention system, producing deficits of hemineglect leading to cognitive and visuospatial abnormalities characteristic of ADD, which explains the responsivity to the dopamine agonists.

Alzheimer's Disease

Researchers have consistently reported significant reductions of brain volume and biochemical changes (revealing neuronal losses) in the temporal and parietal areas. Significant reduction of regional cerebral glucose metabolism was found in Alzheimer's patients in the posterior temporal, parietal, and frontal lobes when compared to same-age counterparts. Sensory impairment affected the ability to read or hear in these patients. Apathy and loss of insight was found related to right hemisphere dysfunctioning. Deficits presenting with a more progressive mental impairment may be associated with Lewy body disease. Prominent deficits overall for this population presents early evidence of attentional difficulties, diminished problem-solving skills and notable visuospatial abilities that impact reading with the neglect type of inattention. Memory tasks, tasks of verbal and nonverbal recall, disorientation, constructional ability, and executive decision-making skills are all compromised. Distinctive for the Alzheimer's versus frontal types of dementia is the clear deficits of impaired memory and language functioning as well as visuoconstructional issues. Whereas with the frontal types of dementia, impairment occurs more with behavioral-emotional disturbances and dysfunctioning of the executive system, producing abnormalities in planning, set shifting, sequencing, and judgement, and displaying more intact language, memory, and visuoconstructive abilities (Aglioti et al., 1996; Bowen et al., 1996; Hooten and Lyketsos, 1966; Meltzer et al., 1996; Mendez et al., 1996; Ott, Noto, and Fogel, 1996; Pachara et al., 1996; Saffron and Coslett, 1996; Tedeschi et al., 1996). Similar to that evidenced in the ADD-without-hyperactivity population and characterized by distortions significant of impact to brain processes, this population displays a type of hemispatial neglect that predominately impacts the left hemispace and is consistent with right hemisphere impact to parietal functioning (although a subgroup of this population evidenced difficulty attending to the right hemispace as well). Hemispatial neglect is viewed as an attentional problem and may relate to difficulty in disengaging attention or in visual exploration which can significantly impact such routine tasks as driving, as well as contribute to wandering, disorientation, and the tendency to become easily lost in formerly familiar surroundings. These characteristics are symptomatic of the disease process (Mendez, Cherrier, and Cymerman, 1977).

Multiple Sclerosis and Huntington's Disease

Recent research suggests the role of autoimmunity to glutamate receptors as involved in the pathophysiology of many neurodegenerative diseases such as epilepsy, stroke, Huntington's disease (HD), amyotrophic lateral sclerosis, and progressive olivopontocerebellar atrophy (OPCA). Glutamate dysregulation is viewed as a primary participant in the disease process. It operates as an important excitotoxicity neurotransmitter and is believed to produce excitotoxic neuronal death. The question remains if autoantibodies initiate or are a consequence of the disease process (Gahring, Rogers, and Twyman, 1977). Infectious agents may play an additional role in triggering the autoimmune process in the susceptible individual, and although the agents that initiate multiple sclerosis (MS) may be heterogeneous in nature, the final pathway leading to the microglial activation and demyelination process is actually more specific and common. Issues contributing to the pathogenesis of MS reside within the CNS, that of microglia activation, the target is the oligodendrocyte myelin unit. The oxidative free radicals and excitatory amino acids may exacerbate toxic factors (Sriram and Rodriguez, 1977).

Widespread slowing of information processing was found to be associated with the cognitive deterioration of MS, which may be the consequence of diffuse demyelination changes (Kujala, Portin, Revonsuo, and Ruutiainen, 1994). Understanding that in the early stages this slowly evolving disorder is difficult to diagnose, symptoms can easily appear as an attentional disorder. MS patients exhibited substantial deficits under more demanding dual task conditions and dual task performance indicated impairment in the speed of information processing. This reflects cerebral inefficiency and the inability to allocate sufficient attentional resources (D'Esposito et al., 1996). During relapse, verbal skills and overall left-hemisphere functioning improved as opposed to the stability of right hemisphere functions (Rozewicz et al., 1996). The degree of cognitive impairment correlated with the degree of the impact of the MS. On a task of logical skills (switching a set and main-taining a set), cognitive improvement was noted with the use of interferon; attentional measures, however, remained relatively stable (Pliskin et al., 1996). Problem-solving deficits were found to parallel that of dysfunction with executive processes (Beatty and Monson, 1996). This is subject to question, due to the type of measurement utilized and measures thought to identify frontal-lobe dysfunction are subject to the complexity of the area of functioning and are thus not readily explained by singular issues. Individuals presenting symptoms of MS may also have comorbid ADHD or both MS and ADHD (Penn and Salloway, 1995). Attentional deficits present early in the disease process, specifically the vulnerability to being distracted. MRI findings correlated with neuropsychological test data and present evidence of varying degrees of diffuse deficits. These findings provide evidence of the widespread impact of the disease process affecting general functioning subsequent to the disconnection between prefrontal, limbic, and association cortices (Foong et al., 1997). This disease is highly variable. Intact cognitive functioning may remain quite stable and/or cognitive decline may be widespread and highly progressive which can be predictive of further deterioration (Kujala, Portin, and Ruutiainen, 1977).

Huntington's Chorea

A number of higher-level cognitive deficits relating to attentional factors is also a consequence of disturbances neurologically due to HD. The self-generated maintenance of attention, divided attention abilities, simultaneous monitoring of the various sensory input channels and operating in an integrative manner is disturbed as a consequence of the impact of this disease on the limbic system and its connections affecting both the posterior and anterior attentional systems (Sprengel et al., 1995). Executive and problem-solving disturbances characteristic of schizophrenia distinguished HD from PD (Hanes, Andrews, and Pantelis, 1995). Symptoms can easily mimic both subtypes of ADD as a result. Neeper et al. (1995) presented a case study of a 13-year-old male presenting symptoms of HD with a familial history of HD; however, throughout childhood he had been diagnosed ADD. Prior to the onset of major motor symptoms of HD, symptoms presented and treated were characteristic of Tourette's syndrome and obsessive-compulsive disorder.

Toxicity

Research is beginning to address the impact of toxic substances and attentional deficits (due to the high vulnerability of the cortical and subcortical systems that subserve attentional processes) that are quite commonly indicated. Morrow, Kamis, and Hodgson (1993) found that subjects exposed to mixtures of organic solvents exhibited symptoms of depression, anxiety, fatigue, confusion, and somatic concerns. Cognitive changes and emotional liability were seen as central components of solvent encephalopathy (Morrow, Steinhauer, and Condray, 1996). Morrow and associates (1997) noted that chronicity and acuteness were critical determinants of the impact of solvent exposure upon learning and memory abilities when evaluating chronically exposed journeymen painters on a variety of neuropsychological measures. Morrow (1994) assessed attentional processes in individuals with mild solvent neurotoxicity and found reaction times significantly slower, implying a disruption in the early stages of orienting attention and the alert operation, as well as an impairment in the disengage operation. Toxicity due to chronic elemental mercury poisoning impacted intellectual functioning, non-verbal short-term memory, visuospatial perception, used judgment of angles and directions visually sustained, and selective attention, manual dexterity, information processing, and psychomotor speed. Often there are personality changes and motoric signs of seizure activation (Hua, Huang, and Yang, 1995). Personality changes included depression, anxiety, the desire to be alone, lack of interest and sensitivity to physical problems. Follow-up 1 to 5 years later indicated recovery of cognitive and personality factors indicting transience of the above symptoms.

Exposure to cocaine (*in utero*) was found to impact the dopamine system, selectively impacting attention and language processes typically mediated by the left hemisphere. Cocaine-exposed fetuses (ages 8 to 40 months) were found to exhibit a slower orientation to stimuli in their right visual field despite repeated trials (especially after attention was initially cued to the left visual field) and were less likely to orient to the right when given the choice, implicating impact to the left hemivisual attentional system (Heffelfinger, Craft, and Shyken, 1997). The toxic effects of alcohol and its metabolites have been well demonstrated, resulting in impairment to brain functioning (memory, visuospatial, motoric speed) via cellular changes, nutritional deficits and impact of liver disease (Koob and Nestler, 1977; Rothstein, 1996; Sher et al., 1997).

The presence of meningitis in children results in an increased vulnerability of the immature CNS to generalized neurological insult. By the time this disorder is evidenced clinically for diagnosis, the inflammation of the cerebral blood vessels has already occurred and neurological complications of vascular occlusions, cerebral edema, hydrocephalus, and subdural effusions have become possible. Children whom experience this illness were divided into two groups before and after 12 months of age. Overall findings on evaluation (intelligence, language function, memory, learning, and reading ability) indicated that although the children were within average ranges on measures of intelligence, linguistic ability, and learning scores, their performance was consistently below that of the controls. The children who had onset prior to 12 months of age evidenced greater deficits. On measures of reading rate, accuracy, and comprehension, children that were post meningitis performed worse on a consistent basis. These children were four times more likely than controls to be unable to read at all and were more likely to evidence reading 2 years or more behind age peers. Language skills, comprehension of instructions, and verbal fluency were reduced as well as difficulty retaining complex material 6 years post illness (Anderson et al., 1997).

When presenting for evaluation for ADD, survivors of meningitis present a more severe picture and are often subject to seizure activation and impact to brain functioning. They present a severity beyond that usually evidenced with an attentional disorder.

There is a question of diagnosed ADD, individuals being at greater risk for the development of a cutaneous marker for predisposition to melanoma and/or a genetic influence or response to environmental toxins resulting in the onset of cancer.

Closed Head Injury

Closed head injury can easily present symptoms commonly seen in an attentional disorder and it becomes quite critical to differentiate (as much as possible) the effects of ADD and subsequent impact of injury to the brain. Clinically, it becomes less difficult to differentiate the two as time goes on, and in the adult population it is easier, using historical data, to hypothesize what symptoms are due to the presence of an attentional disorder and what symptoms are the result of insult to the brain. In children, this becomes a very difficult task, due to the difficulty differentiating specific symptomatology with the developing brain, much less attempting to determine the impact of variables of ADD. Further, children are different from adults in that injury to the brain disrupts normal development. The most common changes observed with moderate to severe closed head injury is that of sustained attention, attentional deficits during dual task demands, impulsivity, inability to regulate responses, memory, effortful or controlled cognitive processing, and processing speed, learning ability, and overall neural efficiency. Often, the presence of injury will serve to exacerbate the deficits of ADD, resulting in a more profound and severe picture of attentional deficits. Characteristic of ADHD and closed head injury are the personality traits and changes with the onset of injury to the brain involving depression, increased psychopathology, disinhibition, apathy and irritability (Arcia and Gualtier, 1994; Burns et al., 1994; Cicerone, 1996; Donders, 1993; Geffen et al., 1994; Speech et al., 1993).

MRI findings suggested a concentration of frontal lobe involvement in addition to scattered, diffuse deficits. Significant symptoms of Obsessive Compulsive Disorder were reported in a pediatric head-injured population. Children with severe injury and a familial history of psychiatric disorders were at greater risk to develop psychiatric symptoms 3 to 6 months post injury. Attentional deficits and impulsivity were seen as persistent sequelae of head injury with the lower ages of injury presenting the greatest risk (Brady and Gerring, 1997; Grados et al., 1997; Gerring et al., 1997; Max et al., 1997). Those suffering from head injury were found to be significantly slower in their response time which reflects the diminished ability to allocate resources, operate efficiently, and sustain attention. The presence of TBI can result in decreased signal processing efficiency, decreased attentional capacity, and increased latency and variability of motoric response. The variability and inconsistency in TBI is a primary issue and is related to the allocation and control of attentional factors (Segalowitz, Dywan, and Unsal, 1997).

Garth, Anderson, and Wrennall (1997) noted changes in children suffering from moderate to severe head injury, differentiating a younger and older age group (before or after the age of 6 years). Overall findings indicate that frontal lobe injury disrupts the development of executive skills. While the earlier age of injury did not impact the child's overall ability to carry out executive tasks, there was a significant impact upon the rate of performance on abstract reasoning and problem solving tasks, which confirmed that this type of injury at younger ages does not imply a more positive recovery. Injury at earlier ages primarily impacted the efficiency as opposed to skill acquisition (Garth, Anderson, and Wrennall, 1997). Younger children with severe injuries evidenced slower growth as measured on visuospatial and motor tasks when compared to older children with similar severity of injury or same-aged children with less severe injuries, all of which points to the vulnerability of rapidly emerging skills in children due to insult to the brain (Thompson et al., 1994). Children severely injured at preschool age often evidenced greater learning difficulties. Cognitive deficits were found to occur with restricted educational capacity, and the biological deficits were due to the intracellular changes which occur with TBI providing confirmation of the limitation of the young brain to ever fully recover. Presence of pre-morbid ADD clearly complicates this process and would exacerbate the situation.

As a result, TBI occurring at earlier ages has a more severe effect upon future social and vocational outcome, and thereby, negates the earlier theory of the plasticity and recovery of function (which has been suggestive of the greater possibility of rehabilitation with early TBI) (Asikainen, Kaste, and Sharna, 1996). Typically with the theory of plasticity, it was maintained that the earlier the injury the less the impact on brain functioning as the brain has a greater ability to recover. However, that does not appear to be what is actually occurring. The problem becomes a loss of skills, specifically if the injury occurs during elementary school years — "building block" years. It is during these years that the learning of skills specific to academic abilities of reading, writing, math, and spelling occurs. The child who is recovering from brain injury and working on reacquiring lost skills will be unable to attain new skills at the same time. Thus, what is missed is the ability to acquire age appropriate new-skill learning and the child remains continually behind age peers as a result. When there is pre-morbid ADD and the individual suffers from head injury the combination is particularly devastating. Typically head injury, impacting memory and logical-reasoning processes, results in a diminishing of the two compensatory mechanisms that the ADD (specifically ADD without hyperactivity) individual utilizes to compensate for deficits as a result of the pre-morbid attentional disorder.

Generally, mild TBI can result in abnormal cerebral metabolism (predominantly midtemporal, anterior cingulate, precuneus, anterior temporal, frontal, and corpus callosum areas) as confirmed by PET data findings and pointing to the impact of those brain areas responsible for the integration and registration of new information, correlation of that information with prior learned material, and the planning and motoric execution of that response. Anterior and posterior brain regions were seen as functionally organized neuronal networks, subserving attentional processing with the anterior cingulate and temporal areas serving as links connecting these two attentional systems. A process of excitotoxicity resulting in excess glutamate is seen as a major etiological factor in setting off the cascade of events involving both biochemical and intracellular components resulting in neuronal degeneration (Gross et al., 1966; Rothstein, 1996). Review of the research suggests that mild trauma can trigger the release of cytokines and excitatory amino acids and points to the hippocampal region as being more vulnerable to such changes. Subsequently, the impact is to the cholinergic function of this region, providing evidence of the consistent short-term memory deficits following TBI (Silver and McAllister, 1997). As a result of the common presence of posttraumatic seizure activity, TBI becomes a risk factor for the development of psychiatric disorders, primarily that of depression as well as bipolar disorder, generalized anxiety, borderline, and avoidant personality disorders (Van Reekum et al., 1996).

TBI subjects demonstrated impaired visuospatial attentional abilities and a lack of efficiency in the allocation of attentional resources. Geldmacher and Hills (1996) identified decreased speed or efficiency in the ability to redirect one's attention in space, and impaired processing of information, which would contribute to the distractibility and spatial attentional deficits noted in this population. In our evaluative process, a common observation is the severe impact upon parietal processes when ADD without hyperactivity is a premorbid diagnosis, confirming the idea that this area, already weakened due to the presence of the premorbid attentional disorder, becomes a target for the intracellular cascade of events leading to neuronal degeneration. Attentional deficits typical of TBI were not found to be associated with hyperactivity. The TBI population was found to be inattentive when involved in self-directed tasks (Whyte et al., 1996). The loss of pragmatic communication skills negatively affected the ability to negotiate, hint, or describe a simple procedure and to use sarcasm (Turkstra, McDonald, and Kaufman, 1995).

In studying a group of young adults with TBI for conversational assessment, Snow, Douglas, and Ponsford (1997) found that all subjects had some type of discourse error (more commonly that of nonspecific vocabulary, linguistic nonfluency and revision behavior) associated with information transfer. TBI subjects made errors in parameters not evidenced in the normal population: insufficient information was provided; information was redundant; information was not appropriate to the situation; messages were inaccurate; and structure to the discourse was lacking. Those who were more severe in their injury, evidenced errors associated with the more fundamental rules of conversational interaction. Tendencies of excessive talkativeness, circular and tangential thinking, fixation on specific topics, diminished turn taking skills, difficulty contributing to and sustaining conversation, as well as the reduced ability to present their ideas in a logical manner, were common problems evidenced in the TBI population. Competent communication requires the use of language in an everyday capacity to allow the individual to address the variety of possible interactions in their environment, ranging from the more superficial and social in nature to the more complex and educational in academic and work settings. Conversation impacts an individual's daily life and the head-injured population (from children to aged) was unable to express themselves, to address their needs verbally, and to simply exchange feelings and/or information in a competent manner, on a daily basis.

Children diagnosed with TBI were found to generate fewer positive, assertive responses and more indirect responses to peer group entry situations when compared to controls. Social information processing deficits were identified in these children. TBI children generated fewer total solutions to entry situational problems. Provocation situations elicited more negative assertive, help-seeking and non-confrontative reactions and overall they experienced greater difficulty than their peers (Warschausky, Cohen, Parker, Levendosky, and Okun, 1997). In investigating TBI adults Lubinski, Moscato, and Willer (1997) found significant speech and language pathology that created chronic communication difficulties and limited the individual's ability to work and to create new opportunities for themselves, thereby, it impacted their interpersonal relationships. Language areas, specifically verbal fluency and lexical difficulty were clearly negatively affected by dysfunctioning in the attentional areas, impacting the processing of information and abstract thinking (Jordan et al., 1996). Cognitive skills are thought to have a critical impact upon the development of language competency which becomes severely impacted by injury to the brain. Key issues will be to ascertain the affect of the impact to brain functioning vs. any premorbid language skill deficits.

Minor head injury, which can typically result in the presence of post concussive symptoms (PCS), occurs in 50% of this population. The presence of PCS tends to correlate with the presence of seizure activity. Those who have suffered a head injury are often subject to outbursts of anger and rage significant to seizure activation. Symptoms range over both degree and presence and include the following; constant headache, dizziness, fatigue, irritability, reduced concentration, insomnia, sleep disturbance, double vision, alcohol intolerance, short-term memory problems, emotional liability, anxiety, depression and sensitivity to heat, noise, temperature, and light. Psychiatric syndromes lying dormant can be activated and re-activated. PCS was found to be an internally consistent syndrome. Despite the variance of complaints (71%) they are related to a common etiological factor. Depression was not found to influence PCS as a premorbid variable. Anxiety was found to increase the subjective response of children, who reported more symptoms, despite the degree of neurological insult. Irregardless of the fact that these symptoms are related to the head injury, parents report symptoms as attention deficits, hyperactivity and/or conduct disorder, rather than PCS. There is an overlap of PTSD and PCS and, therefore, it is necessary to separate out the symptoms (Cicerone and Kalmar, 1997; McGrath, 1997; Mittenberg, Wittner, and Miller, 1997; Mooney and Speed, 1997). PTSD was found to occur in some cases after minor or severe TBI with attentional complaints similar to that of PCS, other symptoms of excitability, emotional problems, and sleeping difficulties are nonspecific and can be found in other conditions as well (McMillan, 1996).

It is the symptoms of PCS that results in the mild head-injured population frequently being dismissed as not having a significant head injury and/or resolution of issues previously observed. In my practice, it is rare that symptoms observed post injury actually abate and unfortunately because the individual outwardly appears intact, they are often dismissed as cured and it is only that individual and their significant family members that are aware that the problems actually continue to exist and interfere with daily functioning. If a child or adolescent is bright they will perform within average ranges in the academic setting and it is mistakenly believed that this means they are intact and no longer suffer from the sequelae of head injury. It is the PCS symptoms that eventually, over a period of time, produce a personality that has formed around the continual (often undiagnosed) seizure activation with the result of extensive emotional issues that often remain undiagnosed as well. To truly understand the impact of head injury, the individual's premorbid functioning needs to be comparatively analyzed with their post-morbid skills. Many evaluators are utilizing norms that are either not appropriate and/or with such a wide range (from one to two standard deviations either side of the mean) that comparisons are no longer appropriate nor relevant.

The difficulty of assessing the mild TBI population, whereby brain imaging does not support evidence of injury, does not necessarily mean that there is an absence of injury. Often survivors report persistent sequelae 6 to 12 months (or longer) of post injury symptoms characteristic of PCS (e.g., sleep disturbance, headache, decreased energy, dizziness, somatic complaints, and sensitivity to noise and light). Professionals, trained to examine for evidence of head injury may report no findings or significant findings depending which side of the litigation they are. The trained evaluator needs to address issues of malingering, pre-morbid status, environment, motivation, physical and emotional health, impact of medications, errors in scoring and misinterpretation (Silver and MacAllister, 1997). Leathem and Body (1997) report a low level of agreement between peers, teachers, and parents concerning behavioral and cognitive difficulties that TBI students were experiencing. They were generally not identified as having problems, in a review of 25 years (1970–1995) on mild head injury involving children and adolescents, Satz, Zaucha, and associates (1997) noted that 98% of this population revealed mild effects that were transitory with the academic measures indicating no immediate or long-term effects. Variability of findings increased with the severity of the injury. Outcomes of individuals 5 years posttrauma indicate that the most frequent area of residual impairment was that of headaches. Balance difficulties and fatigue or weakness were observed secondary to that of headaches as common complaints (Hillier, Sharpe, and Metzer, 1997).

TBI and PCS clearly result from different factors and present a different etiologic pathway. PCS can occur in the absence of head injury or years subsequent to the head injury. PCS tends to occur subsequent to the changes occurring within the brain subsequent to the head injury and can be significant to the presence of seizure activity. The presence of PCS can be used as an indicator to determine the individual's ability to cope with stress factors following the injury. Pre-injury factors (i.e., age, education, occupation, personality, emotional adjustment) and post-injury factors (i.e., pain, family support, compensation, stress, expectancy) interact with cognitive factors and directly impact PCS (Kirby and Long, 1997). PTSD is actually an uncommon phenomenon in TBI patients and does not provide adequate explanation for amnesia for the events of the injury. Failure to recall events prior to or subsequent to injury are primarily due to neurological factors. Of the proportion of their subjects meeting some qualifications of PTSD, Warden et al. (1997) found the majority suffering from genetic mood disorder and/ or anxiety and the posttraumatic amnesia was their method of protecting themselves again disturbing memories.

SPECT spans are emerging as the most sensitive measure, especially with persistent PCS. They have demonstrated abnormal findings in 53% of a TBI population as opposed to abnormal findings on an MRI (9% of the population) and abnormal findings on a CT scan (4.6% of the population) (Kant, Smith-Seemiller, Issac, and Duffy, 1997).

In examining individuals with mild TBI only and mild TBI with repeated incidents of sexual abuse, the latter group revealed the most significant deficits in working memory and executive function and exhibited poorer performance on tasks of learning and memory. Those diagnosed with mild TBI demonstrated the most deficits with working memory (as well as deficits in executive function) while those who had been sexually abused had deficits with executive function when compared to controls, although not when compared to the TBI groups (Raskin, 1997).

Sports-related injuries of the mild-concussive type demonstrate deficits (despite resolution of outward neurological symptoms) that appear more related to speed as opposed to processing deficits, which may provide an index of severity of the trauma (Maddocks and Saling, 1996).

Tourette's Syndrome

Tourette's syndrome (TS) is a chronic familial disorder that is characterized by motor and phonic tics that wax and wane in severity, accompanied by an array of behavioral and emotional problems. Once thought to be a rare condition, it is now estimated to be one case per thousand boys and one case per 10,000 girls. Age of onset is approximately 7 years, although there are children who may exhibit these symptoms as young as 2 and as old as 20 years. The syndrome tends to have a gradual onset with one or more transient episodes, followed by more persistent motor and phonic tics toward becoming severe enough to diagnose the clinical syndrome. Compulsive behaviors appear first and, initially, it is difficult to discern the rituals of OCD (obsessive-compulsive disorder) from TS. Neuropathological, neuroanatomic, and neuroradiologic data have consistently implicated the basal ganglia along with related thalamic and cortical structures. The mesencephalic monoaminergic (dopamine, norepinephrine, and serotonin) projections that modulate these circuits are repeatedly implicated for both OCD and TS. OCD patients were found to evidence problems of delayed recall of nonverbal information, in the face of normal recognition. Results were interpreted by Savage and associates (1996) as providing initial evidence of a nonverbal memory retrieval deficit consistent with theoretical cortiostriatal system dysfunction seen in this disorder. OCD, whether acquired or idiopathic, was found to have similar neuropsychological deficits, impacting functions of attention, memory, word retrieval, motor and executive abilities, and affecting global intellectual assessment. Both groups were shown to have a common etiological pathway, that of the frontal limbic subcortical circuits, whether due to structural damage or dysfunction related to neurobiological issues (Berthier et al., 1996). An overall review of investigations of the orbital frontal cortex (OFC) related to specific psychopathological features of OCD noted the following relationship between brain functioning of this area and behavior. OCD symptoms involving the aversive valuation of specific stimuli would be due to the OFC's close anatomical and functional link with paralimbic regions and the amygdala that allows for the processing and coding of the behavioral significance of stimuli, specifically the aversive attributes that trigger OCD symptoms. This heightened sense of awareness faciliates the process of fear conditioning and specific awareness of the adversity of stimuli. OFC's involvement in this aspect of processing related to anxiety and the experience of negative emotions which results in increased vulnerability to experience anticipatory anxiety or distress, and is more specifically implicated in the role of internally generated thoughts, images, and expectations observed in OCD symptomology. The OFC is involved in mnemonic characteristics and the repeated performing of behaviors aimed at reducing anxiety associated with the internally maintained representation that continues to be maintained thus necessitating repeated behaviors. The presence of error detection abilities of the OFC provides the physiological basis for the OCD perception that things were not performed adequately and need to be perfect or repeated. The OFC involvement in neural circuits mediating reinforcement and regard suggests the basis for craving and initial behavior displayed in the OCD individual. Finally, the excessive concern for how actions will affect significant others as well as consistent feelings of guilt, shame, anxiety, and concern for social norms suggest the OFC impact upon social affiliative behavior (Zald and Kim, 1996). OCD patients who demonstrated frontal-lobe deficits were found to have greater serotonin dysfunction. Hollander and Wong (1996) indicated the relationship between abnormalities of the serotonin system and executive function impairment, suggesting this system as highly implicated in the pathology of OCD.

Clinical assessment tends to point to attentional and activity problems characteristic of ADHD. Often the ADHD symptomatology presents greater problems than the tics, particularly in the area of social functioning (Sherman, Janzen, and Joschico, 1996). It has been proposed that many children have these difficulties before the onset of their tics, and it is suggested that ADHD-like problems are prodromal or the earliest manifestation of the biological vulnerability to the eventual tic disorder.

Yeates and Bornstein (1994) found distinct patterns of neuropsychological dysfunctioning and ADD children displaying more-severe complex tics and obsessive-compulsive symptoms, as well as significant deficits in areas of attention (more specifically that of encoding, sustaining, focusing, and executing) and academic achievement. Executive function or dysfunction seen as the link of ADHD and learning disability was found more often for ADHD alone, and ADHD and TS, than TS alone. The finding is of poor timed performance, slowing of mental search, and linguistic productivity and efficiency suggestive of impact to left frontostriatal pathway (Denckla, 1995; Harris et al., 1995; Schuerholz et al., 1996).

Reading disabilities were not found to be intrinsically related to TS while arithmetic disabilities were, indicating that math functions may be more closely linked to the underlying nature of TS. Generally, however Yeates and Bornstein (1996) found that the presence of LD in the TS population is more idiosyncratic and that the specific learning problems in neuropsychiatric disorders may be more related to the specific underlying pathology of each disorder and therefore not providing a global correlation with LD. Further indicated was the difficulty with the liberal criteria utilized for the classification of LD. LD was not found to be present in a TS-only population. This group, however, had a significantly poorer performance on a measure of letter word fluency. Other research pointed to the finding of specifically poorer performance in timed linguistic efficiency tasks for the TS population as opposed to LD. Findings were related to the pathophysiology of a left frontostriatal pathway as a factor involved in the slowing of mental search and linguistic productivity, linked to linguistically based executive dysfunction. Findings also lent support to the impact of abnormalities of the basal ganglia and its interconnecting pathways which would also support the relationship between TS and ADHD as associated with striatal thalamocortical dysfunction. Given the idea of cognitive slowing as a function of TS, the issue of medication may need this problem and not further complicate things with side effects creating further suppression (Schuerholz et al., 1996). The morphology of the corpus callosum in both TS and ADHD was investigated with the finding of no interaction between TS and ADHD factors and indication that the total area of the corpus callosum was larger in children with TS. The hypothesis was supported that both ADHD and TS have similar neurobiologic mechanisms involving the frontal subcortical circuits. Basal ganglia abnormalities were reported in both TS and ADHD with a significant loss of the normal globas pallidus asymmetry (Baumgardner et al., 1996). Other research indicated that the presence of TS did not differentiate the ADHD group which evidenced a loss of asymmetry substantiating the similarity, but not the predictability of the two disorders (Castellanos et al., 1996).

Moriarty et al. (1997) measured the cross-sectional area of the corpus callosum using volumetric MRI techniques and noted an increase in this area distinct from intervening variables of age, handedness, comorbid ADHD and the intracranial area. The consequence of the increase of this area is a loss of the normal asymmetry of the caudate nucleus. Eidelberg et al. (1997) used a quantitative FDG/PET (a marker to characterize abnormal metabolic topographies associated with neurodegenerative processes) to calculate global, regional, and normalized rates of glucose metabolism in an effort to identify specific patterns of metabolic use with TS. Instead they found overall global and regional metabolic rates to be commensurate with the normal population. However, further analysis identified two TS related brain networks, one involving a nonspecific pattern of increased motor activity and the other involving the decrease in activity of the limbic system basal ganglia thalamocortical projection system. Shucard et al. (1997) demonstrated attentional deficits in boys diagnosed with Tourette's Syndrome, who evidenced a significantly slower reaction time (when compared to their normal counterparts) although their ability to discriminate targets from nontargets on the Continuous Performance Test (i.e., measurement of sustained attention requiring the subject to press a response key when the target stimulus is presented) was within normal limits. The severity of tics was predictive of more impaired reaction time which confirmed the impact to brain functioning as a consequence of this disorder. Abnormal motor activity in the absence of problematic overall thresholds provided evidence that the tic symptomology observed in TS is the result of a subcortical disorder that impacted the motor cortex and/or an impaired inhibition that resulted in disinhibited afferent signals and rendered this disorder as separate and distinct from dopaminergic disorders of the classical motor loop of the basal ganglia (Ziemann, Paulus, and Rothenberger, 1997). Initial research identified monoclonal antibody D8/17 as a marker signaling the susceptibility to the development of childhood onset OCD, TS, Rheumatic fever, and Sydenahm's chorea, and further that the emerging presence of OCD and TS in childhood may represent an interplay between environmental, genetic, and developmental factors (Murphy et al., 1997). TS is seen as related to OCD, ADHD, and disorders of affect and social conduct but not to schizophrenia or types of thought disorders (Lichter, Diegelman, and Jackson, 1997).

Adults diagnosed with ADHD were compared with adults diagnosed with TS or attentional measures. The ADHD population performed significantly worse than normal counterparts on tests of mental flexibility and psychomotor speed. Among the TS population, those with comorbid ADHD, performed worse, similar to that of ADHD and had increased OCD symptoms. The presence of this resulted in increased variability in attentional functioning. Results point to the need to identify the impact of tics, comorbid ADHD, and OCD on the functioning of the TS patient (Silverstein et al., 1995). Cognitive deficits found in both TS and Huntington's disease were found to stem from abnormalities of the major pathways interconnecting the basal ganglia and frontal lobes, creating primarily difficulties in attentional shifting (Georgiuos et al., 1995).

Research is inconclusive with some studies supporting and some not supporting the comorbidity of ADHD, and TS with ADHD occurring no more often than that of chance. It was concluded that more precise diagnostic methods were required to further differentiate the presence of ADHD. Aspects of the syndrome may simply reflect a "spontaneous discharge" of microcircuits or breakdowns in the holistic regulation of the functioning of one or more circuits. Symptoms such as the sudden thought, the intrusive gesture, the throat-clearing sound or loud whopping noise may reflect seizure-like activation of a small, tightly organized cluster of cells that are liberated from the normal functional organization and operation of the brain (Cohen and Leckman, 1994). This seizure-like activation may also apply to the clinical symptoms evidenced for the attention-disordered population, in particular the overfocused subtype of ADD. Leckman et al. (1994) addressed the "just right" perception associated with the compulsive behavior evidenced in TS. His team concluded that the presence of these perceptions is common for TS and reflects a similar neuropathological origin for both OCD and TS. When addressing the syndrome of TS, the symptoms characteristic of OCD need to be considered. Spencer et al. (1995) view tics and TS as part of the same continuum representing different forms of severity. Similar to other findings, TS was significantly associated with OCD, ADD, and phobia. TS has been observed in a clinic in both diagnosed ADHD and ADD.

The most interesting research to emerge recently is the idea that TS is not always represented in the form of the tic behavior we so commonly associate with it. The idea was introduced of nonobscene, complex socially inappropriate behaviors as symptoms manifested in TS. Behaviors of insulting others, usually directed at a familiar family member or person in a familial setting or in the home, and resulting in overall social difficulty. TS is seen as representing poor impulse control, the urge to carry out behaviors normally suppressed, and being seen more often in younger males in an adolescent to adult population. Less common was the behavior being directed at a stranger or taking place in a public setting. Nearly one third of those individuals reporting socially inappropriate behavior resulted in social difficulties involving verbal arguments, fist fights, school or job problems, removal from a public place, and legal difficulties or arrest (Kurlan et al., 1996).

Adolescents diagnosed with both OCD and TS were found to be more violent and aggressive with OCD symptoms and were richer in violent impulses and sexual images/obsessions than with OCD alone. Males were predominant at a ratio of 14 to 1 for presenting with OCD and TS. This study included both subclinical forms of OCD and individuals with at least one motor or vocal tic that were defined as TS. This provides a more applicable example of what would be evidenced in the typical clinical treatment setting as opposed to continued measuring of the more severe forms of both disorders (Zohar et al., 1997). A patient with severe TS developed self-injurious behavior, including self-attempted strangulation, eye injuries, and the attempt to pull out their tongue in response to watching similar violent scenes on television, suggesting a stress-induced echopraxia. It was suggested that such stereotyped echopraxia was designed to neutralize the anxiety experienced over the unpleasant experience. Findings supported the limbic regions (anterior cingulate gyrus) and interconnected subcortical motor centers (caudate nucleus) as responsible for self-injurious behavior (Berthier, Comps, and Kuliseusky, 1996).

Autism

Autism is seen as having a characteristic course, defined by social deficits, communication abnormalities, and sterotyped or repetitive behavior. The etiology is mainly genetic, with a rate of occurrence of 6 to 8% in families and up to 200 times the risk in the general population. There is a high rate of social and communication deficits noted in the families of autistic children with multiple-incidence autism (families with a minimum of two autistic children). In these families, there were autistic characteristics noted in the parents and extended family members with 20% of the mothers having a communication deficit. Genetic lability is evidenced in the symptomotology of the nonautistic relatives who reveal characteristics that are present quantitatively but in a more mild and qualitatively different form (Piven et al., 1997).

Autism is characterized by movement and gait abnormalities, and symptoms are attributed mainly to faulty modulation of sensory input and motor output that is thought to arise from disturbed processing in lower levels that then impacts higher-level functioning (Kalivas and Barnes, 1993). Smith and Bryson (1994) propose the idea that symptoms of autism, particularly the imitative deficit, is the consequence of basic information-processing problems rather than a social dysfunction.

Current behavioral and neurophysiological evidence suggests that the neural systems mediating the modulation of arousal and attention are inherent in the development of autism. It is further suggested that the symptoms of autism, the abnormalities of movement and action, are diagnostic of attentional and perceptual processes and, further, that social deficits stem from problems within the complex information-processing requirements of social stimulation. Autism has typically been viewed as a consequence of abnormalities attributed to a dysfunctional parietal system which presents spatial deficits in attention. It has been suggested to be a spatial neglect syndrome. Townsend, Harris, and Courchesne (1996) confirmed the presence of a neglect type of inattention as being present only when there are parietal abnormalities. In studying autistic adults with no parietal abnormalities, evidence of cerebellar damage was found to account for another type of attentional problem, that of being slow to shift attention and within modalities. Siegel et al. (1993) found a variable pattern of abnormal activity consistent with difficulty with the striatum and cinguate cortex, and on an attentional measure, autistic subjects did not perform as well as controls.

MRI and PET scan studies noted that the right anterior cingulate area was significantly reduced in relative volume and was less active in autistic adults. Increased cell density rather than cell loss was provided as explanation for the decreased volume and accounted for reduced dendritic fields associated with a smaller total structure as well as lower metabolism. Anterior cingulate regions, heavily involved in serotonin receptor density may suggest medical management possibilities (Haznedar et al., 1997). MRI and PET scan data additionally yielded a significantly smaller size of the body and posterior subregions of the corpus callosum which is consistent with volume abnormalities of the posterior (temporal/parietal/occipital) rather than anterior, frontal involvement in autism. The corpus callosum (identified as the largest and most prominent axonal pathway) is heavily involved in the interhemispheric transfer of information and cortical connectivity in the brain. Local, ipisilateral cortical connections triumphing over more distant connections from the contralateral hemisphere, resulted in the selective elimination of callosal projections and the decreased callosal size. Abnormal cortical connectivity was suggested as the underlying pathophysiology observed in autism. Findings provide confirmation of this in addition to increased brain volume that is unrelated to the size of the corpus callosum (which may reflect increased volume of nonneural cortical tissue or cortical neurons that do not project axons to the callosum). Authors suggest interpreting findings with caution given overall prior research of mixed findings and a question of directionality of the size differences that would normally be hypothesized for the corpus callosum area (Piven et al., 1997). Research also points to enlarged total cerebellar volume as related to autism and generally the underlying pathology of autism involves the abnormal development of several regions of the brain that are part of a distributed neural network (Piven et al., 1997).

Finally, Asperger's syndrome has been referred to as a high-functioning autism, whereby the clinical presentation is that of social isolation in combination with odd and eccentric behavior. Social impairments are characteristic of the disorder and tend to pervade all aspects of the individual's functioning to reveal a pervasive lack of responsiveness with clear deficits in communication and socialization and a persistent inability to decode non-verbal social information, as well as an inability to use vocal intonation to communicate effectively. Symptoms are similar to that of pervasive developmental disorder (PDD). Evaluation indicated neuropsychological functioning characteristic of non-verbal learning disability, emphasizing impaired right-hemisphere deficits of weak visuospatial abilities and poor visual tracking (Huntzinger, 1995; Szatmari, Bremner, and Nagy, 1989). Asperger's syndrome, similar to that of autism, is highly genetic. Parents of children diagnosed with Asperger's syndrome evidenced cognitive symptoms of the disorder and deficits in social cognition (specifically that of mind reading and the ability to make sense of and/or to predict social behavior) in a milder form (Baron-Cohen and Hammer, 1997). Clinically, Asperger's syndrome has been observed with ADD, and it is difficult to differentiate between the social isolation and difficulty with communication characteristic of the attention-disordered individual from the diagnosis of Asperger's syndrome.

Addictions

Symptoms demonstrating an addiction fall into three classes: patterns of use (taking more and for longer than intended), impairment caused by the habit (continuing to use the drug despite ill effects), and tolerance (needing more for the same effect) (Harvard Mental Health Letter, 1992). Recent developments in genetic research have identified increased risk for alcoholism in the offspring of alcoholics with the dopamine receptor gene identified, and the dopaminergic neurotransmission may represent a common pathway for both serotonergic and opioidergic effects of alcohol consumption. Early onset alcoholism has been linked with serotonergic transmission. There is growing evidence for a dichotomous typology of alcoholism whereby one subtype is characterized by greater depression, binge drinking and antisocial behavior. Antisocial personality is emerging as the only distinct predictor of an individual's risk for alcoholism.

Specific drugs act on specific neurotransmitters and their receptors (e.g., dopamine, opioid peptides, serotonin, GABA, and glutamate). The reinforcing effects may result from the multiple neurotransmitter interactions producing subtle changes in neurochemical function and signal transduction thereby altering the neurobiological substrates of reinforcement. The mesolimbic dopamine system and its connections provide a focal area for activation by nicotine, opiates, cocaine, amphetamine, and ethanol. A subsystem of the basal forebrain (the extended amygdala) appears to play a specific role in the motivational aspects of drug reinforcement (Koob and Nestler, 1977). Schlaepfer et al. (1977) researched the effects of cocaine with human using positron emission tomography, and provided evidence of an impact to the dopamine system and higher concentrations of dopamine competing at the receptor site. Cocaine vasoconstriction is associated with cardiovascular problems and stroke.

Biederman et al. (1995) examined the relationship between ADHD and substance abuse in adults, finding a pattern whereby the ADHD population had higher rates of substance abuse (drug use alone, and drug and alcohol abuse). The diagnosis of ADHD alone increased the risk for substance abuse. The diagnosis of antisocial disorder increased the risk for substance abuse (separate and distinct from ADHD), and the presence of mood and anxiety disorders increased the risk for substance abuse in both the ADHD group and the control group. Interestingly, the authors noted the more common use of marijuana (67% for the ADHD population and 72% for the controls) to a considerably greater degree than that of the stimulants or cocaine and suggested that the research provided support for the idea of self-medicating symptoms of the attentional disorder with substance abuse. A drawback to this study was the determination of diagnosis based on self-reported symptoms and in all probability due to confounding differentiation of ADHD and ADD without hyperactivity. The picture, however, is a complex one and it is suggested that alcoholism be thought of not as a single disease entity, but as a group of illnesses in which the influences of genes and environmental variables interact with one another over the course of one's lifetime (Devor, 1994; Kranzler and Anton, 1994; Schukit et al., 1994). de Wit (1996) isolated a "priming" effect to explain why even a small amount of a previously abused drug would trigger a relapse.

Schuckit et al. (1994) found that with the exception of antisocial personality, it is difficult to identify a reliable personality profile with which to predict alcoholism. This supports the clinical finding in the attention-disordered population, whereby with ADHD it appears to be highly linked to that subtype of alcoholism that is more extreme in nature with a true loss of control of one's behavior, as opposed to the ADD individual who seems to turn to alcohol use to self-medicate primarily symptoms of anxiety.

Data could well support the clinically observed tendency of ADD: self-medicating usage of alcohol (for anxiety symptoms) and marijuana (for anxiety symptoms and enhancement of sensory areas of the brain), providing (via self-report) temporary amelioration of ADD symptoms. There are residual cognitive effects of heavy marijuana use implicating the attentional executive functions. Memory processes appeared intact and isolated attentional problems, namely that of the inability to shift sets and sustained attention, were noted in researching the effect of usage with college students (Pope and Yurgein-Todd, 1996). The measure used in this study may reflect problems related more to sustained attention, distractibility, and information-processing deficits experienced by the ADD with Hyperactivity population. We have not found that marijuana exacerbates symptoms of the attention disorder (similar to that of alcohol abuse), but rather creates a pervasive amotivational syndrome, resulting in a total lack of caring about anything and lack of follow-through.

High-sensation seekers were more likely to report both a lifetime history of antisocial personality, attention deficit disorder, and conduct disorder (Ball, Carroll, and Rounsaville, 1994). Wexler and McClelland (1996) indicate a lifetime interplay of cyclical factors of ADHD, conduct disorders, juvenile delinquency, depression, antisocial personality, alcoholism, substance abuse, early aggressive behavior, and eventually criminal behavior. Volkow et al. (1994) reported significant increases in brain metabolism during initial alcohol withdrawal and documented persistently low levels in the subcortical (basal ganglia) structures of detoxified alcoholics, suggesting differences in recovery rate, depending on the amount of time abusing the substance. It is suggested that the pathophysiology underlying the basal ganglia dysfunction could involve the disruption of the dopaminergic neurotransmission as a result of chronic alcohol use. What this means is that the ADHD individual abusing alcohol would only succeed in creating increased symptomatology of the attentional disorder, thus creating a cyclic need to continue abusing drugs due to inability to function, low self-esteem, and need for escape.

There is an association between alcoholism and the advent of seizure disorder. Alcohol has been found to be a risk factor for seizures and seizures are more frequent in the alcoholic population than in the general population. Findings are similar for both sex and race, for ages fifteen years and upwards. A trend is evidenced whereby the risk is decreased when exposure to alcohol is removed. The idea is that there is a toxic affect and/or common genetic predisposition of alcohol on seizure generating structures (Leone et al., 1977). Alcohol is believed to act on GABA and glutamate receptors which is highly related to an excitotoxicity process documented in the head-injury research to result in seizure activation (Koob and Nestler, 1977; Rothstein, 1996). Documented neuropsychological findings reveal the impact of alcohol abuse, specifically in the areas of visuospatial and motor speed with increased impairment for those abusers who were more dependent upon alcohol use, thus demonstrating the direct toxic effects upon brain tissue (Sher et al., 1997). Ethanol and pentobarbital (barbiturate hypnotic) were compared for behavioral and subjective effects, evidencing comparable results on neuropsychological evaluation of impaired short- and long-term memory and psychomotor performance and similar subjective reactions (although at the highest dose, pentobarbital was experienced as more sedating). Evidence suggests that ethanol elicits a more barbiturate-like effect than a benzodiazepine-like effect similar to that of alcohol (Mintzer et al., 1997). Fillmore and Vogel-Sprott (1997) documented in their research that the impairing effects of alcohol can be resisted (on a task involving information processing) provided that subjects are given an immediate, informative monetary reward conveying information regarding performance adequacy. Subjects were adult male social drinkers which may have impacted findings in that their resistance occurred subsequent to the absence of any type of toxicity and/or genetic liability.

In our research over the past 10 years we have isolated an undiagnosed attentional disorder. It is subsequent to chronic substance abuse and has become a situation that has exacerbated beyond control due to the addition of undiagnosed seizure activity. Presence of the seizure activity in this population does not necessarily target the spatial area, rather the temporal functioning is impacted and both short- and long-term memory processes become impaired. Often, the alcoholic becomes subject to rages and temper outbursts that are rather disconcerting for family members and which are directly related to seizure activation. Seizure activity impacts learning by negating a primary compensatory mechanism used by the ADD population — memorization — and with impaired memory functioning, any type of learning decreases automatically. For those individuals who begin drinking heavily in the latter portion of elementary years, by high school they will have already significantly hindered any learning ability. Intense alcohol use is not always a comorbid factor for ADHD, rather the anxiety, frustration, overfocused thinking, and intense derogatory thought patterns of ADD without hyperactivity, overfocused subtype, will create the need for escape in early years that cannot be denied due to the enormous discomfort created by these thinking patterns. The only relief becomes the use of alcohol, often accompanied by daily usage of marijuana. This combination becomes the necessary *cocktail* to get through the day. Addictive factors result from the intensity of the thinking, the overwhelming fear and anxiety, and the hopelessness and futility, without belief in a future. This is created by years of previous failure subsequent to the impact of the undiagnosed ADD symptoms upon academic functioning.

Fetal Alcohol Syndrome

Nanson and Hiscock (1990), in comparing children diagnosed with fetal alcohol syndrome (FAS) with ADD children and controls on reaction time and vigilance tasks, found that the attentional deficits were similar for both FAS and ADD. It was proposed that the central nervous system insult caused by prenatal alcohol exposure and the postnatal environment disruption resulting from the alcoholic lifestyle appears to interact to produce the problems with hyperactivity and attention. FAS typically occurs with other risk factors for developmental delays, such as low socio-economic status, poor maternal nutrition, prenatal care, maternal substance abuse (cocaine), and cigarette smoking. Individuals with FAS are at risk for congenital heart disease; cleft lip and palate; limited joint movements; seizures; auditory and visual deficits; delayed motor and language development (receptive and expressive deficits); impaired abstract thinking, problem-solving abilities, motoric skills, attention, and short-term memory. Difficulties with abstraction and problem-solving lead to social interactions that are often inappropriate. Authors proposed that treatment to facilitate learning in children with ADHD may also benefit FAS children. There is the need for extensive assessment in this population to rule out other factors related to biological risks and neuropsychological development (Pulsifer, 1996; Klove, 1995; Troland, Sommerfelt, and Ellersten, 1995).

Lupus/Antiphospholipid Antibody Syndrome

Antiphospholipid Antibody Syndrome (APS) is defined by the presence of lupus anticoagulant or anticardiolipin antibodies and recurrent fetal losses as well as vascular changes. Deficits include decreased cognitive efficiency, impaired attention, impaired semantic fluency, problematic memory and visuospatial functions, and cognitive deterioration, which suggests subcortical-frontal system involvement (Aharon et al., 1996; Beers et al., 1996). We have found that the diagnosis and subsequent treatment of comorbid ADD results in positive relief of symptoms, slowing down the progressive process, and providing remission of symptoms in some cases.

HIV/AIDS

Stern et al. (1996) followed a group of intravenous drug users for 3.5 years, measuring changes occurring with respect to their neuropsychological status related to HIV status and disease severity. Findings reflected that the disease process of HIV affects cognition early, even when the patient is not showing outward signs. Difficulties increase with an increase in the disease process affecting memory, executive functioning, language, attention, and motor speed. Attentional difficulties were confirmed in HIV positive intravenous drug users (Hestad et al., 1996).

Chronic Fatigue Syndrome

Significant differences were found only for one attentional measure and a measure of incidental memory when patients suffering from chronic fatigue were compared to normal counterparts. The failure to demonstrate appreciable deficits other than the above measures despite reports of altered cognition, suggests that many complaints may be related to the high expectations these patients have of themselves (Kane, Gantz, and DiPino, 1996).

Plioplys (1997) acknowledges the variability of studies, presenting no evidence to confirm the ongoing theory of circulating autoimmune antibodies and reactivity to CNS antigens. CFS is defined as a physical and mental fatigue that may be causally related to immunologic abnormalities (although this also remains variable).

Related Comorbid Disorders

Kusche, Cook, and Greenberg (1993) compared neuropsychological and cognitive functioning of children diagnosed with anxiety, conduct disorder (CD), attention problems, and learning disability (LD) and anxiety, comorbid psychopathology. Findings indicated that regardless of type, children with psychopathology were found to have significantly lower IQs as compared to non-pathological controls. These differences were also observed in measures of executive functioning. More specifically, children diagnosed as anxious with somatic symptoms demonstrated problems in the temporal and parietal areas. Conduct disorder-diagnosed children had more problems with right-hemisphere than left-hemisphere processing. The combination group of comorbid pathology demonstrated dysfunction that was severe and global. This study could become confusing in that CD (determined via externalizing behaviors) was linked with attentional problems not defined as either ADHD or ADD. Thus, anxiety could be correlated with attentional problems as well as learning disability in a respective fashion, whereas linking anxiety and CD can be confounding and certainly not consistent with research on CD.

McConaughy and Skiba (1993), in investigating the impact of comorbidity in children, identified the following:

1. Depressed children with comorbid CD had worse short-term outcomes and were at higher risk for adult criminality than depressed children without CD.
2. Children with ADD and comorbid CD/ODD (Oppositional-Defiant disorder) had worse outcomes than children with ADD alone.
3. Children with comorbid LD and anxiety had fewer social problems than children with LD alone.

Cohen et al. (1993), in examining the developmental aspects of psychiatric disorders, found age-specific prevalence patterns:

1. Overanxious disordered rates were comparable for both boys and girls. By late childhood, there was a strong linear decline for boys 10 to 20 years of age.
2. Separation anxiety rates were comparable for both boys and girls and there was a 23% decline in prevalence for each year after the age of 10.
3. For the diagnosis of major depressive disorder, prevalence patterns differed for both boys and girls. Rates were low and comparable between the sexes until adolescence, whereupon girls indicated a very sharp increase.
4. Prevalence rates for ADHD was nearly twice as high for boys as girls up to the age of 17 years, at which age prevalence declined nearly 20% per year on the average for boys. (It is important to take into account that statistics are probably based on clinical evaluation that is more heavily based on self-report measures and observed symptomatology that can be highly confusing and subject to misdiagnosis).
5. For the diagnosis of CD, the prevalence rate was twice as high in boys as in girls and rates were more prevalent at younger ages, declining from 10 to 20 years of age. For girls, there was an increase in prevalence, peaking at the age of 16 years, followed by a sharp decline.
6. The same prevalence pattern was indicated for ODD for both boys and girls with low levels among the 10- and 11-year-olds, rising to high levels from 13 to 16, followed by a sharp decline.
7. Alcohol abuse increased over the age span and was especially high in post-high school years. In the 17- to 20-year-old group, the prevalence rate for boys at about 20% was twice as high as that of girls.
8. Marijuana abuse increased with age as well, and rates for girls were not as high as that for boys.

A follow-up study by Cohen, Cohen, and Brook (1993) indicated that for almost all combinations of diagnosis and severity levels, one third or more of the cases diagnosed at ages 9 to 18 years were still at an equivalent diagnostic level 2-1/2 years later (Cohen et al., 1993). The genetic familial transmission of ADHD, major depression, and generalized anxiety was seen as distinct, although overlapping disorders that are not causally related to one another. These distinct disorders are separate entities with symptomatology that persists through the developmental life cycle (Milberger et al., 1995).

Anxiety and Depression

There tends to be a high comorbidity between anxiety and depression for both children and adolescents. Research findings suggest that there is a general negative tendency that is common to both disorders, whether it be in the form of low self-esteem and negative feelings toward the self or negative feelings in the prediction and anticipation of the future. Beidel, Christ, and Long (1991) found that the concurrently depressed and anxious population tended to be older and more symptomatic. The presence of panic disorder with major depressive disorder was identified by them as a more-severe illness. In the particular group that they studied, the anxiety symptoms tended to predate the depressive symptoms. Grunhaus et al. (1994), in their research, found that those individuals diagnosed with major depressive disorder and panic disorder were significantly different from individuals diagnosed with major depressive disorder. The concurrent population, diagnosed with both disorders, reported symptoms occurring earlier in life, sought treatment at younger ages, and required hospitalization earlier and more frequently. The severity of each illness episode was greater with more "core" symptoms of depression (such as insomnia, guilt, suicidality, retardation, and lack of reactivity in mood) and greater feelings of inadequacy, somatic anxiety, and development of phobias.

Commonly found in clinical experience, is that the depression lies underneath the rather apparent anxiety, and it is the anxiety that serves to blanket the unresolved and inconsolable depression. Anxious children were found to experience a broad range of somatic complaints, more so than normals with a more-pervasive symptom pattern. When feeling nervous, anxious children endorsed significantly more experiences of choking, flushes and chills, palpitations, fainting, shakiness, headaches, and feelings of dying. Whereas normal children had an average of 3.5 somatic symptoms, anxious children had an average of 5.8 to 6.9 symptoms under identifiable conditions.

Surprisingly, ADHD children were found to have a greater incidence of depression and anxiety. Children diagnosed as ADD/anxiety/depression had higher levels of co-existing stress and parental symptoms than those who had the single diagnosis of ADD. Again, these results may be due to a problem of diagnosis, as clinically ADD tends to correlate rather highly and consistently with anxiety and depression. It is the presence of generalized anxiety (usually a familial disorder) that produces the constant state of movement that appears as "overactivity", when, in fact, it is truly anxiety, and results in the misdiagnosis of ADHD for ADD. It stands to reason, from a logical perspective, if we are talking about ADHD and the true loss of control as well as motivation, these individuals would not hypothetically care enough to be either anxious or depressed (Beidel, Christ, and Long, 1991; Brady and Kendall, 1992; Grunhaus et al., 1994; Katon, Sheehan, and Uhde, 1992; Lonigan, Carey, and Finch, 1994; Jenson et al., 1993).

Lonigan, Carey, and Finch (1994) investigated symptoms of depression and anxiety in children and adolescents and found that depressed children related more problems to having a loss of interest in activities and low motivation, in general, and they were found to have a more-negative view of themselves and their capabilities. Anxious children, on the other hand, reported to be more worried about their future, well-being, and the reactions of others toward them. Authors purport the difference between these two disorders that so frequently overlap is that of positive affectivity. If applied to the attention-disordered population, findings would confirm the clinical findings that attention-disordered individuals without hyperactivity (characterized by a high degree of anxiety that typically can be evidenced in the familial history), though anxious in childhood, do not evidence symptoms of depression until adolescence or adulthood, whereby hopelessness and repeated failures have contributed to a more-negative outlook and attributes characteristic of depression. The depression evidenced clinically in this population appears to be secondary rather than primary, and both subsequent to and a consequence of the attentional disorder. Frequently, this population is diagnosed with primary depression due to the underlying attentional disorder and its ramifications not being considered.

There is considerable controversy as to the inheritability of depression and the impact of the environment. Functional and quantitative measurement of the G protein in the mononuclear leukocytes is currently being researched as a biochemical marker for the diagnosis of depression. Abnormal levels of the G protein is seen as playing a central role in the etiology of bipolar disorder as well (Avissar et al., 1997; Mitchell et al., 1997). Kendler et al. (1994) found the estimated heritability of depressive symptoms to be between 30 and 37%; genetic factors were found to account for only half of the stable variance in depressive symptoms; and there was no evidence that the liability for depressive symptoms was environmentally transmitted from parents to offspring. Nigg and Goldsmith (1994) found mixed support for the genetic influence of depression, obsessive-compulsive and borderline personality disorders. Early expressions of girls (as young as toddlerhood) indicate that they are more prone to be overcontrolled, to inhibit their emotional and behavioral problems, and to channel problems into more internalized forms often resulting in anxiety-based disorders. Girls, as opposed to boys, are encouraged to develop adaptive skills in prosocial behavior (Keenan and Shaw, 1997). Anderson and Hammen (1993) found that children of women with unipolar depression displayed significant deficits in psychosocial functioning when compared with children of either bipolar diagnosis, medical illness, or defined psychiatrically "normal" women. Children of depressed mothers were rated as being less socially active and displaying less competency, in addition to school behavior problems and poor academic performance. Authors speculated that the psychosocial problems experienced by these children were chronic in nature and continued to be in evidence over the 2-year follow-up, due to the stressful environment created by the depressed mother and the child's own deficits, which interfered with future development of competency. Thus, these children remained perpetually behind their peers in social skills. Taking into consideration the difficulty of learning social skills and developing the ability to fit in with one's peers as a particular problem for the attention-disordered population, the additional factor of maternal depression would create a comorbid factor that would serve to exacerbate these problems. Patients diagnosed with psychotic depression evidenced deficits on neuropsychological tests of attention, learning, memory (retention), psychomotor speed, and motor skills similar to that of schizophrenia (Jeste et al., 1996).

There was a high rate of comorbidity found in children and adolescents with major depressive disorders or diagnosis of dysthymia. Comorbidity with conduct disorder and oppositional-defiant disorder ranged from 21 to 83%, comorbidity with anxiety disorder as a diagnosis ranged from 30 to 75%, and comorbidity with attention deficit disorder ranged from 0 to 57.1% (Angold and Costello, 1993). Jensen et al. (1993), in examining the validity of ADHD, found that children who had the diagnosis of ADHD were similar to those children being seen in a psychiatric clinic in reporting significantly more depression and anxiety than normal cohorts. In fact, those diagnosed with ADHD had more externalizing symptoms than the psychiatric population. Children diagnosed with ADHD as well as symptoms of anxiety and depression had higher levels of co-existing life stresses and similar symptoms present within their parents. Findings coincide with the idea of ADD, comorbid anxiety, and familial history of anxiety, and lend credence to the overdiagnosis of ADHD, as well as the impact of comorbid disorders.

Nolen-Hoeksema, Girgus, and Seligman (1992) found that the best predictor of childhood depression is that of depression experienced in the past. Children with higher levels of identified depressive symptoms had more pessimistic explanatory styles, and this rather stable pessimistic attributional style tended to place children who had a bout or bouts of severe depression in the past at risk for future depressive episodes. Remission of depressive symptoms diminished in adulthood when the individual employed an explanatory style that was more optimistic.

It is likely to assume that failures of the attention-disordered individual occurring as a consequence of the presence of the disorder would prevent the development of a more-optimistic explanatory style. This would explain why those individuals with comorbid depression are unable to utilize cognitive strategies to move symptoms into remission and develop alternative thinking.

Bipolar Disorder

Bipolar disorder is characterized by manic-like and hypomanic-like symptoms intermixed with episodes of depression for rapid cycling of a minimum of four episodes within a 12-month period. Bipolar I is distinguished from Bipolar II by severity and recurrence rate.

Young et al. (1994) found evidence for abnormalities in G-protein levels and function in the pathophysiology of bipolar disorder, but not for major depressive disorder. Recent research is now implicating the G protein as a biochemical marker for both unipolar and bipolar depression (Avissar et al., 1997; Mitchell et al., 1997). Bipolar disorder is frequently misdiagnosed for ADHD when the individual is in the manic phase, and clinically the presence of bipolar depression and ADHD occur more frequently as opposed to the less-severe disorder of ADD that is more often seen with unipolar depression. Winokur et al. (1993) found that bipolar patients had traits of hyperactivity as children. The disorder had an earlier onset, more acute with more episodes, was most likely to occur in males, and alcoholism and mania were frequently found in the familial history. Adolescents diagnosed with both mania and ADHD were found to exhibit more severe symptoms of mania, and common to the bipolar group were diagnoses of conduct disorder, substance abuse, ADHD, and psychosis. Genetically, there is evidence to support ADHD and bipolar disorder as a diagnostic entity. Finally, the unipolar group was found to exhibit increased levels of anxiety prior to diagnosing mania, as the two often overlap in their symptomatology (Borchardt and Bernstein, 1995; West et al., 1995; Wozniak et al., 1995).

The language performance of diagnosed bipolar disorder and schizophrenic subjects were evaluated for language skills. The manic population was found to display a higher lack of overall connectiveness in their speech. They introduced multiple topics in a continual elevated frequency with poor connections between the ideas presented. The schizophrenic population was found to produce less information, although they had equal levels of disconnection during episodes of clinically impaired speech; yet due to the paucity of information presented, their speech appears more vague and with less substance (McPherson and Harvey, 1996).

Social Phobia

Social phobia goes beyond shyness to present a fear so intense and pervasive that it limits the individual's life in general, prevents taking opportunities, results in considerable constriction and overall loneliness. Any situation that may result in the individual being judged or criticized evokes crippling anxiety. These individuals are constantly aware of being scrutinized and constantly worried about being made to look foolish for the simplest activities. The anxiety of social phobia can be so intense that it provokes blushing, stammering, sweating, stomach upset, a racing heart, trembling limbs, and at times a full-scale panic attack. In its most-severe form, generalized social phobia, there may be a total absence of social activities or involvement with others. A more-limited form is that of discrete social phobia or performance anxiety that would permit a more or less normal social life, but would subtly impair the quality of one's life. Social phobia is one of the more common psychiatric disorders and community surveys have found rates ranging from 1 to 13%, depending on the definition. Social phobia is usually associated with other psychiatric disorders: 59% of individuals with social phobia had simple phobias, 49% had panic disorders with agoraphobia, 19% were alcohol abusers, and 17% suffered from major depression. People with social phobia often use alcohol as self-medication, and it was found that 15% of socially phobic individuals had an alcohol problem at one time or another. If they have used alcohol for a long period of time, the original symptoms of social phobia will be obscured and it will re-appear when the drinking or drug use has abated (Harvard Mental Health Letter, 1994). Stuttering is often a sign of the social anxiety significant of social phobia (Stein, Baird, and Walker, 1996).

Attention-disordered individuals are known to have a misrepresentation of appropriate social skills and often they are unaware of the overlearned social rules nor how to apply them in the generalized setting. Due to the problems of anticipating social consequences and being unable to "think on one's feet", this characteristically anxious population, particularly that of attention disorder without hyperactivity, finds it easier to retreat and withdraw from social activities. It is quite common to find that these naturally shy, anxious, ADD, individuals self-medicate with either alcohol or marijuana use on reaching adolescence and such use continues to increase during these precarious social years. The social phobia connected with ADD often goes unnoticed. In addition, ADHD individuals may also be shy, sensitive, and socially phobic, who, rather than retreating will be aggressive as if to offset their tendency to withdraw. ADHD individuals tend to be more rejected by their peers, while ADD are isolated, neglected, and withdrawn.

Post-Traumatic Stress Disorder

Warshaw et al. (1993) studied the effects of the quality of life associated with post-traumatic stress disorder and found that those individuals diagnosed with PTSD had the worst functioning when compared to those without trauma or trauma without symptoms of the disorder. It was concluded that PTSD has a profound and severe impact on the quality of life in virtually all areas, and further, that this disorder was associated with such symptoms as high levels of depression, suicide attempts or gestures, and alcohol abuse. The research confirmed the long-lasting effects of this disorder. Neurological soft signs were found using neuropsychological evaluation of individuals diagnosed with PTSD, as well as problems of attention and memory, implicating the role of hyperarousal and dysfunction of the frontal-subcortical systems. Bremner et al. (1995) identified a smaller right-hippocampal volume in PTSD associated with severe deficits in memory functioning. The hippocampal area, associated with the function of binding memories for long-term storage, may explain the specific memory deficits related to PTSD and separation of specific memories (Gurvits et al., 1992; Sutker et al., 1994). PTSD was found to be a long-lasting phenomenon in research conducted by Solomon and associates (1994) with POWs and veterans who were still suffering from symptoms of PTSD almost two decades later.

A variety of factors, including the child's individual disaster experience, age, gender, parent's functioning, and general atmosphere in the home, were predictive of PTSD in a community sample of children. The strongest predictor of the number of PTSD symptoms was an irritable family atmosphere, followed by a depressed family atmosphere, and the overall functioning of the parents, particularly that of the mother (Green et al., 1991). Symptoms of PTSD begins soon after exposure, with hyperarousal as the first symptoms to occur, followed by the natural self-medication course of substance abuse (Bremmer et al., 1996). Research provides preliminary support for the existence of a pre-morbid dissociative subtype of PTSD whereby individuals exhibit diminished physiological reactivity and are unable to process traumatic experiences which only serve to exacerbate symptoms of trauma. Such individuals respond with a suppression of their own autonomic responses that is trauma specific and a larger proportion of these individuals (97%) had symptoms of PTSD as well as a discrepancy between self-reported stress and objective physiological indicators of stress (Griffin, Resick, and Mechanic, 1997). Simeon et al. (1997) present evidence of a depersonalization disorder that is a distinct entity with a specific course that is continuous, can be episodic, characterized by severe stress and high levels of interpersonal impairment with common comorbid factors of unipolar depression and anxiety, accompanied by a nonresponsiveness to therapy or medical management. Many individuals were found to suffer from a subsyndromal form of PTSD, appearing less impaired than individuals presenting symptoms of the full syndrome (although still exhibiting clinical levels of functional impairment subsequent to symptoms of PTSD) with the subthreshold form evidencing itself to a greater degree in women. Lifetime exposure to serious traumatic events were noted as 74.2% for women and 81.3% for men with lifetime trauma exposure in the range of 39 to 84% (Stein et al., 1997).

The question of the impact of divorce as trauma to the child resulting in PTSD is continually debated. Barber and Eccles (1992) found studies to be both inconsistent and inconclusive regarding negative outcomes and the impact of divorce on cognitive performance, delinquency, and self-esteem. Some of the negative outcomes were hypothesized by the authors to be due to economic struggle or parental conflict. Divorce and an attentional disorder can become problematic simply due to the extra time and energy required for the attention-disordered child.

PTSD symptoms can be observed in either ADHD or ADD; however, symptoms will more often resemble those of ADD, in that these individuals often appear quite "spacey", withdrawn and "out of it", thus missing information from their environment and responding with a slow cognitive speed. Misdiagnosis can occur in that outwardly they can easily resemble symptomatology of the attention-disordered population.

Dissociative Identity Disorder (Multiple Personality Disorder)

The course of multiple personality disorder (MPD) has been known to be that of a childhood sexual trauma so horrible and repulsive that it has to be split off (dissociated) from the host consciousness and lodged in the alters (McHugh, 1993). MPD is defined as the existence in the person of two or more distinct personalities or personality states. According to Spanos (1994), individuals with MPD behave as if they possess two or more selves, each self having its own characteristic mood, memories, and behavioral repertoire. Under different names, this phenomenon can be observed in different cultures. In examining MPD from a sociological perspective, it was concluded that it is socially constructed, context bound. There is goal-directed social behavior that is geared to the expectations of significant others and characteristics change over time to meet the requirements of the external environment.

MPD does not appear to be more correlated to either ADHD or ADD. MPD can be more prevalent in the ADD population due to the associated trauma, possibility of adoption and its ramifications (the adopted population tends to be associated with a greater number of disorders simply due to the origins of the adoption and/or reasons for the adoption occurring in the first place).

Child Abuse/Adult Children of Alcoholics

Malinosky-Rummell and Hansen (1993) investigated the long-term consequences of childhood physical abuse and reported varied findings ranging from impact on academic performance, vocational problems, substance abuse, and aggressive and violent behavior. Similarly, Kendall-Tackett, Williams, and Finkelhor (1993) found in their research that sexually abused children had a greater incidence of fear, PTSD symptoms, behavior problems, sexualized behaviors, and poor self-esteem.

Adult children of alcoholics (ACOA) are often traumatized and suffer from symptoms of PTSD. They were abused (sexually, physically, emotionally) or neglected as children and their childhood experiences were seen as similar to that of a war-like situation (chaotic and lacking in stability). Children tend to be rather sturdy and can survive most situations, however it is the continual surprise and lack of consistency that they cannot survive. ACOA individuals who emerge from this type of environment find themselves frightened by their emotions and feelings, they have survived their childhood environment by employing the defense mechanism of denial. They have a need to avoid people, avoid situations that may trigger emotion, keep their feelings repressed, and present an outward picture that is quite different from what they might be experiencing internally, often unknown to themselves. These individuals are excellent actors or pretenders, or are just wearing a mask to protect their internal vulnerability. They operate as overachievers and are never satisfied with their performance. They are critical of themselves and of others and project blame and responsibility outward but are easily hurt by criticism and in need of continual acceptance and love as narcissistic supplies. ACOA individuals are distrustful of themselves and others, function as caretakers to ensure love and stability of others, are divorced from their inner emotional life, enjoy and crave, excitement, crises, and problematic situations, and overeat and over-do in an addictive manner.

Domenico and Windle (1993) found that ACOAs reported higher levels of depression and lower levels of self-esteem. They also found that ACOAs felt higher levels of marital conflict and lower levels of perceived social support, family cohesion, and marital satisfaction. A greater degree of parental role distress was indicated as well as the perception of seeing themselves as powerless to control the behavior of their children. ACOAs thus were more likely to drink for coping purposes, although alcohol consumption did not exceed that of controls in the study. Chassin et al. (1993) reported in their research a strong association between parental alcoholism and child substance abuse due to factors of poor parental monitoring practices and a high degree of negative affect.

ACOA can occur with either ADHD or ADD and the additional variable of either emerging from an alcoholic home and/or a home where abuse occurred, exacerbates the communication problem of the attention-disordered individual. Typically, if the comorbid disorder is that of ADHD, the individual will develop full-scale alcoholic traits, including the rigid thinking, perseveration, lack of problem-solving and the out-of-control absence of inhibition characteristic of the dysfunction of the frontal processes. Thus, the symptoms of both the ADHD and the ACOA serve to interact with one another to such an extreme and overlapping degree that it can become difficult to differentiate between them. This contributes to the poor prognosis for treatment as a result of the combination of ACOA and ADHD.

When ADD is the comorbid disorder, the symptoms can resemble that of the alcoholic; however, abusing some type of substance is more related to fears of intimacy and self-medication than anything else. This combination results in clear difficulties in interpersonal relationships, and the tendency to avoid and deny, which only increases the procrastination tendencies already inherent in the attention-disordered population. Symptoms of the attentional disorder prevent positive experiences in terms of mastery and goal attainment, which only confirms the feelings of hopelessness and lack of power one feels emerging from an alcoholic home. It becomes very difficult to remediate symptoms that are so interrelated as the attentional disorders and ACOA. Unfortunately, either the ACOA or the attentional disorder goes undiagnosed due to the extreme nature of both of these disorders.

Obsessive-Compulsive Disorder

Obsessive compulsive disorder (OCD) is an illness that involves endless cycles of repetitive thoughts (obsessions) and feelings of the need to repeat certain actions over and over again (compulsions). Individuals with OCD may have only obsessions or compulsions (about 20%), while most have both obsessions and compulsions (80%). Obsessions may be frightening, disgusting, painful or trivial, and common obsessions include the fear of germs, harming a loved one, or constant doubt about anything and everything in an attempt to predict the future. These individuals tend to be able to explain in great detail the degree of their obsessions; however, they tend not to know the root cause. Typically, the obsessions are constant and, although the individual will call them "annoying", they continue to be well enmeshed in maintaining them. The idea is that if one stops predicting and anticipating gloom and doom, then something terrible will happen and one will not be prepared for it. The element of surprise is more disturbing than the obsessions, and will cause extreme anxiety and feelings of discomfort and dread that build to unbearable levels.

Compulsions operate to provide relief for the tremendous anxiety and build-up of fear occurring within the individual by providing something for them to do. Consequently, rituals are developed, such as handwashing or continual checking and re-checking in a specific sequence of behaviors, and such compulsions serve to stave off the dread of some unpredicted or predicted occurrence happening. Rituals may have rules and be incredibly elaborate or very simple in nature. Typically, they are very time consuming and interfere with the daily routine of life and task performance in particular. Rituals only briefly lessen the anxiety, and they need to be repeated on a continual basis as the only means the individual has of lessening the discomfort. Typical obsessions and compulsions are that of fear of contamination, fear of harming self or others, checking, counting or repeating, collecting or hoarding.

There is believed to be a biological basis for OCD and it is treated with medication. Patients with diagnosed OCD were found to have frontal and prefrontal abnormalities. Harris et al. (1994), using SPECT and MRI studies, confirmed increased frontal function, increased perfusion for the right-middle frontal gyrus area and cerebellum, continuing the theory that the arbitofrontal hypermetabolism localized primarily in the right hemisphere and could be reflective of serotonergic dysfunction. Aronowitz et al. (1994) relates the presence of neurological soft signs to the neurobiological foundation for OCD placing individuals at risk for development of further psychopathology, such as asocial schizophrenia, emotionally unstable character disorder, ADHD, or anxiety disorders. Evaluation of specific neuropsychological measures indicated findings as predicted substantiating what the authors perceived as primarily deficits of frontal-lobe functioning and that of its connectors. Notable were deficits in visuospatial analysis and synthesis, immediate visual recall and visual discrimination implicating more specifically limbic/right hemisphere or temporo-parietal cerebral structures. Performance was compromised by slow cognitive speed hypothesized as a psychological remnant of the disorder. However, findings are quite similar to the clinical picture of ADD, coincide structurally with the definition of this subtype, and together with the link of OCD to anxiety (neurotransmitter system of serotonin) may provide a different neurological viewpoint of OCD.

However, it is important to separate the diagnosis of OCD from the defense mechanism of being obsessive-compulsive, such as obsessive-compulsive personality as opposed to the disorder. There is a very distinct difference; generally extended college-degree programs are primarily composed of obsessive-compulsive personality types. The defense of being obsessive-compulsive tends to be a reaction to anxiety, a generalized anxiety state and/ or a childhood trauma. As a result, the person becomes highly rule-oriented (to provide stability and clear order to one's life, thus warding off the chaos), rigidly adhering to a particular way of doing things "the right way", and determined to be perfect in performance of each and every task.

Individuals with an attention disorder, usually ADD, who are bright are well aware of their deficits. They attempt to compensate for these deficits by performing in a perfect fashion on the tasks they can do well and avoiding and procrastinating the tasks they feel less secure about. By maintaining this system, the individual is able to compensate for the disorder, more or less, or at the very least prevent others from becoming aware of its devastating effects. They utilize rules in a rigid manner to organize their lives, and prevent and or attempt to control the distractibility and tendency to become distractible. Thus, an attention disorder can lead an individual to develop an obsessive-compulsive personality and/or its traits. Secondary gains are that the anxiety is treated with the symptoms of this personality type, i.e., the rigidity, specificity of functioning, and so on.

Aronowitz and associates (1994) identified interesting research in their attempt to determine a neuropsychological impact and/or relationship to OCD. Evaluating OCD patients, they found significantly poorer performance than the controls utilized in the study on visuospatial, visuoperceptual, and visual discrimination tasks in addition to that of set shifting, sequencing, and tracking tasks. However, performance was measured more so on speed than on errors, which would indicate that problematic performance was not due to an inability to complete the task, but rather, slow cognitive speed. Authors hypothesize that this slow speed is due to the traits of the OCD individual: to ensure accurate performance, he/she spends a greater amount of time completing the task at hand. However, it is not unreasonable to also hypothesize that perhaps an attentional disorder could have confounded the results as an unknown variable. The authors conclude that the question remains unanswered and suggest further research.

Schizophrenia

Fronto-striatal dysfunction has typically been implicated in schizophrenia, and generally does not provide any confounding results in the genetic research indicating that it is a genetic disorder of biochemical origin. Left frontal and right parietal regions are also suggested as areas of dysfunction related to schizophrenia using EEG recordings based upon nonlinear dynamics, entitled, dimensional complexity (Hoffman et al., 1996). Recent findings are suggesting abnormalities in the superior temporal region and/or the temporoparietal region as implicated in the symptoms of schizophrenia. Debate continues as to the areas of brain functioning responsible for the symptoms observed in this disorder. Schizophrenia is being seen as a higher-order attentional disorder, stemming from executive frontal systems being dysfunctional. The symptoms of thought disorder and auditory hallucinations are seen as a derivative of dopamine imbalance and a failure to control the executive attentional network, specifically activation of competing or disturbing ideas (DiGirolano and Posner, 1996). Attentional inhibition for spatial information was deficient suggesting the difficulty of focusing upon relevant stimuli while ignoring the irrelevant in diagnosed schizophrenic and schizotypal subjects with a more pronounced effect for women, suggestive of the possible influence of gender (Park et al., 1996). Recurrent episodes of postictal psychosis can eventually develop into chronic psychosis, reflecting progressive cerebral dysfunction as a result of continuous seizure activation (Szabo, Rankman, and Stagno, 1996). Paranoid schizophrenic patients diagnosed with Freguli syndrome (characterized by the delusional belief that a familiar person is able to take on different physical forms and adapt another's appearance) was found to have right hemisphere processing impairments of a more sustained as opposed to a transitory nature. The pathology associated with schizophrenia appears to be more diffused than localized, and suggestive of impact upon posterior attentional systems as well (Edelstyn et al., 1996). Capgras syndrome (the belief that a very significant person has been replaced by an exact double and psychologically altered while retaining their physical identify) was found to be related to more frontal executive deficits than visuospatial or perceptual deficits (O'Connor et al., 1996). Undifferentiated subtype as opposed to that of paranoid schizophrenia produced different results on an attentional measure of the interference and/or vulnerability to distractibility from the environment. Carter, Robertson, and Nordahl (1992) reported that the paranoid subtype of the disorder revealed greater interference and generally that schizophrenia subjects revealed a reduced ability to suppress interference, and thus, a vulnerability to distractibility. Findings of reduced thalamic activity is significant of the filtering deficits of sensory information (Buchsbaum et al., 1996). Impaired sensory gating and increased distractibility are seen as key issues to explain information processing deficits (Karper et al., 1996).*

---

*Distractibility in psychotic patients were hypothesized to represent a failure to filter out irrelevant stimuli and/or an inability to appropriately allocate attentional resources. Karper and associates (1996), using a measure of distractibility and lateralized attention, found gating problems supporting the cortical striatal-pallidal thalamic circuit as dysfunctional and producing the cognitive deficits seen in this disorder. Schizophrenia is viewed as a deficit of right hemisphere mechanisms responsible for sustained attention, suggested by a saccadic latency deficit implicating the left visual field and disturbing the process of detection and recognition, pre-attentive and attentive processes (Evans and Schwartz, 1997). Overall IQ values were found to be a marker for psychiatric morbidity, implicating impact to brain functions as the discriminating factor (Hackerman et al., 1996).

Schizotypal patients display characteristics similar to that of schizophrenia with abnormal attention being one of the more prominent indicators of their biological susceptibility to schizophrenic related disorders (Roitman et al., 1997). In our practice we often see what we characterize as the *fragile* individual, whereby symptoms can be observed as young as two years of age and as old as 80 to 90 years of age. Generally, these individuals tend to have symptoms of the Overfocused subtype of an attentional disorder, and thus are more biologically sensitive (allergies and asthma as well as other anxiety related conditions), emotionally reactive, prone to distractibility, and subject to attentional problems in general. Environment determinants as well as adequacy of coping mechanisms determines their sturdiness and ability to survive. When this type of personality is seen in combination with a premorbid attentional disorder, the combination can become particularly devastating with the result being such an overwhelming degree of stress that the individual becomes hopeless and lapses into their own internal dreamworld, rendering them even more fragile and vulnerable. Research has identified that schizotypal subjects were more distractible and demonstrated a diminished ability to inhibit irrelevant distracting stimuli. Individuals with schizotypal personalities share some of the cognitive difficulties with those who develop psychosis and if schizophrenia does develop and compensatory mechanisms are no longer effective, it is at that point that this difficulty with distractibility becomes apparent (Watson and Tipper, 1997). There is a substantial percentage (7 to 8%) of patients diagnosed with schizophrenia or schizoaffective disorder that have symptoms meeting the criteria of obsessive compulsive disorder (Eisen et al., 1997).

O'Donnell et al. (1996) identifies impaired visuospatial representation and perception. Schizophrenic subjects evidenced slowing and impaired accuracy on measures of visual perception, immediate visual recognition, deficit in accuracy of location and trajectory deficits in the perception or representation of spatial relationships, motion, and orientation, in addition to severe deficits in trajectory processing produces the high degree of sensitivity to transient stimulation luminance contrast and low spatial frequencies. It is not difficult to imagine the consequences of ADD as a comorbid disorder, whereby the spatial deficits would be continually exacerbated by symptoms of schizophrenia in a continual cyclical manner.

The idea of preexisting structural brain deficits prior to the onset of symptoms being manifested supports the theory of disturbed neuronal development. The neurochemical pathology of schizophrenia was found to produce a focal change specifically confined to the hippocampal region and dorsolateral prefrontal cortex. This is consistent with research specifically identifying impact to the prefrontal-temporo limbic neural system. Despite the observed reduction in decreased cortical volume, this is not seen as due to a neurodegenerative process (Bertolino et al., 1996). The question remains if gray-matter depletion seen early in this illness represents an active continuing process or overdevelopment of a more static nature (Lim et al., 1996). A reversed planum temporale asymmetry was found in schizophrenic patients when matched with controls with the right being larger than normal, suggesting reduced grey matter volume (Barta et al., 1997). Prenatal nutritional deficiency was found to be associated with an increased prevalence of risk of the development of schizoid personality disorder in males at the age of 18 years (Huek et al., 1996).

Schizophrenic individuals tend to have sleep-wake disturbances in the form of reductions of stage 3 and 4 slow-wave sleep and reductions in REM latency. There are also identified motor abnormalities and postural aberrations in addition to smooth pursuant eye movement, deficits in sensory gating, and increased blink rate. There is a hypothesis that there is enhanced cholinergic activities (Kalivas and Barnes, 1993). Benes et al. (1992) conducted postmortem investigations of schizophrenics to investigate a defect in associative information processing in the upper layers of limbic cortex. The schizophrenic group evidenced considerably smaller caliber glutamate immunoreactive vertical fibers when compared to controls; authors hypothesized that the fibers showing an increased density in schizophrenics may be glutamatergic afferents, possibly ones that are associative in nature. These data support the hypothesis of alterations of associative information processing in the anterior cingulate cortex as a component of the pathophysiology of schizophrenia. Siegel and associates (1993) found evidence of decreased metabolism in the medial frontal cortex, cingulate gyrus, medial temporal lobe, corpus callosum and ventral caudate and a generally lower or hypofrontality when compared to controls. Hypofrontality was more prominent in the medial than the lateral frontal cortex implicating emotional cognitive distortions and an explanation of the thinking problems so prevalent in this population. Findings also supported a cortical–striatal thalamic pathway as the physiological explanation for schizophrenia. The thalamus has been found to have a central role in cortical–striatal thalamic theories of schizophrenia and there is the emphasizing of this structure in the regulation of cognitive and sensory input into the cortex correlating with findings of abnormalities of sensory gating demonstrated in schizophrenic patients.

Aloia et al. (1996) in measuring the use of semantic space (the ability to spontaneously cluster exemplars from a specific category during a fluency task) found semantic networks to be disorganized in a population of early-onset schizophrenic patients. They suggested the possibility of temporoparietal dysfunction as responsible. Verbal memory has been found to be highly impaired among schizophrenic patients and when compared with normals, schizophrenic patients demonstrated a diminished ability to organize their recall of semantic material according to its semantic category. Results identified anatomical abnormalities underlying these findings as related to prefrontal and temporal-parietal cortical areas, resulting in reduced semantic processing, reduced proactive inhibition, and defective memory processes in this population. Proactive inhibition is defined as a declining ability to recall words and successive similar lists of words being presented (Moberg and Gur, 1996).

Geriatric schizophrenic patients were compared with Alzheimer counterparts on the degree of their cognitive impairment and while both groups evidence deficits, the schizophrenic population performed worse on tests of naming and revealed constructional praxis, revealing less impairment on a test of delayed recall. Findings support the role of the midline circuits (prefrontal cortex, temporal and parietal association areas, pontine reticular activating system) in the etiology of cognitive deficits. Deficits may also be related to a fundamental problem of the basic gaiting mechanism linking these structures together (Davidson et al., 1996). Schizophrenic patients who were ascertained to be a stable condition and maintained in an outpatient treatment setting were evaluated on a number of neuropsychological tests and compared with elderly patients without any known etiological disease. The performance profile of the schizophrenic patients was highly similar to that of the normal aged population excluding measures of motor speed. The pattern of deficits was that of generalized impairment with specific issues of verbal learning and memory. The evaluation did not include specific measures of frontal functioning. Results may also have been related to medication and the disruption of memory by the anticholinergic compounds (Cutler et al., 1996). Levitt and associates (1996) identified an association between poor premorbid adjustment scores and visual memory span, implicating the possibility of premorbid impairment in spatial working memory in schizophrenia. Strong left temporal and central region correlations were noted in relating premorbid adjustment scores with schizophrenic patients. It is suggested that psychobiological abnormalities preceding overt symptoms, and persisting after treatment, would relate to overall attentional problems and the problem of working memory. Evaluation of higher-functioning and more-intact schizophrenic patients yielded findings of severely impaired verbal recall as well as impaired familiar-face naming in comparison to more intact abilities in areas of executive function, visual recall, recognition memory, naming and unfamiliar-face processing. Differences were hypothesized to relate to a Supervisory Attentional System and that this population has a difficult time relating unrelated items to aid in retrieval from memory storage (Laws, McKenna, and McCarthy, 1997).

Researchers have differentiated deficit and nondeficit schizophrenia as a categorical means of determining severity levels of this disorder. Nondeficit patients are viewed as having negative symptoms although such symptoms are secondary to other factors. The deficit syndrome, however, represents the more enduring and chronic disorder whereby negative symptoms are primary and the deficit diagnosis is associated with an overall poorer outcome in areas of pre- and post-morbid social adjustment, presence of social and physical anhedonia, insight abilities, quality of life, substance abuse, social and occupational impairment, neuropsychological impairments, and structural abnormalities. Negative symptoms have been significantly implicated in the cognitive inferiority of schizophrenic patients and those with negative symptoms have been noted to have more impaired performance on selected neuropsychological measures, demonstrating deficits in higher order attentional processing or complex mental control (difficulty with efficiency and the ability to mentally track and coordinate ongoing behavior at a sufficiently rapid pace). Studies point to a different type of pathophysiology characterizing each of these subtypes (Buchanan et al., 1997; Hawkins et al., 1997). Nondeficit schizophrenics were found to respond better and to be more amenable to intensive social skills training, (demonstrating observable learning and acquisition of skills subsequent to training) as opposed to the deficit population who displayed significant difficulties with skill acquisition and ability to learn (Kopelowicz et al., 1997). The diminished ability to experience affect and general indifference towards one's future associated with deficit symptoms, creates a shield protecting these individuals from any type of painful self-awareness that would otherwise prompt thoughts of suicide. Factors associated with nondeficit and paranoid schizophrenia are that of a late onset, preservation of affect, more intact cognitive capacities, and an intermittent course, rendering this population more susceptible to the emergence of a dysphoric or hopeless state (Fenton et al., 1997).

Deficit and nondeficit schizophrenics were comparatively assessed on a measure of covert (shifts of attention in the absence of eye movements) visuospatial attention. The nondeficit group emerged having difficulty processing visual information in the left hemisphere which was substantially slower than that of the right cerebral hemisphere. The idea that although utilizing cues appropriately for orientation in both visual fields, the processing of the information was slower to alert and activate the left hemisphere as opposed to the right hemisphere, similar to that of a right hemispatial arousal neglect. The deficit group revealed no evidence of this type of neglect and findings confirmed the existence of a more global pathology as opposed to left hemisphere dysfunction formerly hypothesized as present with schizophrenia. Findings support a differentiation between deficit and nondeficit types of schizophrenia (Bustillo et al., 1997). It may be that the deficit type of schizophrenia which represents a more severe form of this disorder would be more correlated with the less severe form of ADD — that of ADD without hyperactivity. The finding of a right hemisphere neglect is commensurate with findings of spatial problems and/or an inattention to the whole evidenced in the attention disordered population. Hypothetically, the nondeficit type may be highly represented in the ADD without hyperactivity population and exhibit symptoms of this characteristically weakened spatial area. Given that the right hemisphere subserves both the left and right hemisphere for spatial functions and in this manner is more involved in this function, these findings may also represent the global pathology described in schizophrenia targeting an already weakened area (spatial functioning, parietal area) to result in the failure to activate the left hemisphere in a timely manner and slower visual processing. The nondeficit group is seen as a higher functioning group and in this particular study had a higher socioeconomic status.

Buchanan and associates (1997) using different tasks from the above research to measure attention/information processing impairments in schizophrenia, and also differentiating the two subtypes of deficit versus nondeficit, found very different results. However, this may reflect and confirm the above hypothesis as well as provide some insight as to many of the discrepancies in the research on this population. Utilizing the continuous performance test and a forced choice span of apprehension task, deficit patients were found to have a significantly more impaired performance on the continuous performance test, thought to reflect their inability to activate and to allocate attention or an impairment in their ability to perceptually organize visual information. The poor performance of the deficit population was thought to reflect an impairment in the early stage of visual information processing and it was the span of apprehension task that created increased demands on attentional capacity. The nondeficit group, experienced no difficulty on the continuous performance measure, but did experience difficulty on the span of apprehension task. The authors indicated that this may reflect information overload produced by the use of multiple stimuli and demand of rapid scanning. The continuous performance test via positron emission tomography studies reflects impact specific regions of the prefrontal and superior and inferior parietal cortices and basal ganglia (including the caudate). These areas have also been implicated in the deficit syndrome and therefore share a common anatomical substrate (Buchanan et al., 1997). The deficit syndrome may be represented as a more severe attentional disorder whereby individuals could not utilize logic to compensate and/or may reflect ADHD and an attentional deficit that impacts frontal processes. The nondeficit group, had less severe symptoms and were able to utilize logic processes to compensate on the continuous performance test but not on the more demanding span of attention task, whereby the attentional demands, exceeding their capacity also exceeded use of their compensatory mechanism.

Gold, Goldberg, and Weinberger (1992) used regional cerebral blood-flow studies to demonstrate that schizophrenia patients fail to normally activate prefrontal cortex during performance on the Wisconsin Card Sorting Test, a measure that supposedly utilizes predominantly prefrontal processes. This failure to activate the dorsolateral prefrontal cortex was suggested to relate to ventricular enlargement and dopaminergic hypofunction. Findings correlated with the hypothesized relationship of schizophrenia to the mesocortical dopamine system, and the frontal lobe dysfunction accommodating both the positive and negative symptoms of schizophrenia. However, Axelrod et al. (1994) investigated the Wisconsin Card Sorting Test (WCST) performance with schizophrenics and found that performance was not different from the patient comparison groups and authors conclude that the WCST may have other cognitive processes involved and/or multiple cognitive processing. Palmer et al. (1997) found that 30% of the schizophrenic population did not suffer from any neurological impairment. In fact, they socialized more, were less negative, were not as likely to have a recent psychiatric hospitalization, evidenced less extrapyramidal symptoms, and were taking less anticholinergic medication. Findings identified a different subtype of schizophrenic patients suggesting that the pathophysiology is different for cognitive versus psychiatric symptomotology.

The findings of Axelrod and his associates substantiate our clinical findings that performance on the WCST is due to a variety of factors and an individual may rely on prefrontal processes for performance and/or parietal processes, namely that of information processing, and even more importantly, poor performance on the WCST can be due to the confusion that occurs when the individual has lost focus, experienced a capacity setback (only has so much energy to complete task), got distracted and/or needed to rely on information processed from the external environment and could not do so. Thus, there are a number of variables to explain poor performance on this measure other than prefrontal processes. Finally, this hypothesis accounts for the variability of the diagnosis of the attention-disordered population, particularly in differentiating ADHD from ADD, using this measure and regional blood-flow studies, PET, and SPECT scans.

Erlenmeyer et al. (1993) found individuals at greater risk for the development of schizophrenia if symptoms of attentional dysfunction are present. Anhedonia (an inability to experience pleasure in activities that normally produce it) found in adolescence for individuals at risk for schizophrenia was related to attentional dysfunction in childhood. Thus, childhood attentional dysfunction was found to be linked to poor adjustment in adolescents at risk for schizophrenia. Childhood behavior characterized by withdrawal predicted poorer performance on adult neuropsychological measures. Attention and social problems evidenced in childhood were correlated with poor motor performance in an adult schizophrenic population. In comparison, childhood anxiety and depression predicted better adult neuropsychological performance. Schizophrenic patients evidenced earlier onset of symptoms and premorbid problems were found to result in increased problematic adult neuropsychological functioning. The idea of CNS maturation was proposed to have influence in determining when a particular problem in functioning would appear predictive of schizophrenia. Thought disorder problems therefore was not manifested until higher-order cognitive ability comes into maturation (Neumann et al., 1996). Pine et al. (1993) found atypical neuroleptic-refractory psychotic patients able to respond positively to stimulants implicating the presence of comorbid ADHD and the need to rule out an attentional disorder in cases of what appears as atypical psychosis. Bellak (1994) confirmed the complete interaction of ADD and the schizophrenic syndrome.

Conversely, we have found schizophrenia to be linked generally to ADD and the problems of information processing contribute to the cognitive distortions that make up the thought disorder. Further, other symptoms of an attentional disorder, such as distractibility, result in the tendency to isolate and protect against the oncoming stimulus from the external environment.

Oppositional-Defiant Disorder

Developmental patterns of oppositional-defiant disorder (ODD) typically appear during preschool years. Temper tantrums reach their peak when children are 2 to 3 years of age. During preschool years, negative and oppositional behavior is common, resulting in angry outbursts and ensuing conflicts with parental authority about matters that vary with age from toilet training and hygiene to household chores. Destructiveness, bullying, and fighting decrease after preschool years. Early adolescence is associated with increased rebellious behavior. Teachers indicate that oppositional symptoms of arguing, screaming, disobedience, and defiance peak between the ages of 8 to 11 years and then decline, while parents find screaming and argumentative behavior more prevalent during adolescence (particularly in girls). Symptoms increase in adolescence (and boys take on characteristics of conduct disorder—skipping school, drug and alcohol use, stealing, etc.) and become more aggressive. ODD is differentiated from conduct disorder by the degree of aggressiveness. ODD was diagnosed more often in boys than in girls under the age of 12 years and the diagnosis for girls increased in adolescence (Rey, 1994).

Conduct Disorder

Szatmari, Boyle, and Offord (1993) found that there generally is a familial aggregation of emotional and behavioral problems associated with conduct disorder (CD). ADHD was found to have a considerably lower aggregation than that of CD and emotional problems. This indicates that although familial aggregation of attention deficit disorder does exist within the community, the mechanism may be different from that of emotional or conduct problems. Genetic factors account for a large proportion of the phenotypic variance and it is hypothesized that both the genetic and environmental factors operating in an additive fashion produce aggregation of conduct and emotional problems. McBurnett et al. (1993) examined the association of "frontal lobe" functioning and electrodermal activity (EDA) with symptoms of inattention, overactivity, and aggression-defiance factors. They found no significant interaction of aggression and hyperactivity supporting the additive model of comorbidity (consequence of genetic and environmental factors).

Conduct disorder was examined for subtypes by Shapiro and Hynd (1993), who identified the subtype of UACD, (undersocialized aggressive conduct disorder) associated with such characteristics as serious and persistent physical aggression, deception, violation of property rights and societal norms, disturbed interpersonal relationships, and school adjustment problems. According to their review, CD was found to be cross-generational, with the parents exhibiting antisocial personality, substance abuse, and criminal behavior. Neuroanatomical studies attempting to link the problems of the frontal area of the brain with behavior were found to be inconsistent. Biochemical studies point to norepinephrine and serotonin as implicated in CD most often. Studies reported by the authors suggested a clear relationship between UACD and the decreased level of norepinephrine and no relationship to socialized CD. Neurohormonal research implicated the HPA axis, linking testosterone with physical aggression. It was suggested that cortisol may be a biological indicator of arousal associated with behavioral inhibition and withdrawal in children with CD.

Psychophysiological studies examining the autonomic nervous system functioning found that modulation of biological arousal mechanisms may play a role in the experience of childhood psychopathology. Pharmacological studies point to the question of the efficacy of drug therapy with CD. Lahey et al. (1993) found that despite inconsistencies evidence points to abnormal serotonin activity, several indices of the sympathetic (ANS) system, and neurohormonal activity, as well as some features of event-related electroencephalographic potentials, as indices to isolate abnormally severe and persistent physical aggression. Halperin and associates (1994) found a differentiation between aggressive and non-aggressive children with ADHD with serotonergic functioning, comparing both groups on a prolactin response to a challenge dose of the 5-HT agonist D,L-fenfluramine, plasma catecholamine metabolites and platelet 5-HT.

Raine, Venables, and Williams (1995) identified biological factors that would predispose an individual not to commit criminal activity. They found that high rates of autonomic arousal and orienting were factors discriminating adolescent offenders from developing adult criminal behavior patterns that would suggest either the impact of anxiety as a deterrent to crime and/or more proficient and information-processing abilities to prevent the predictive events leading to criminal activity.

Behavioral research supports a two-factor model of Gray (1987) that antisocial behavior is the product of both excessive reward-seeking behavior and insufficient inhibition. It has been argued that boys diagnosed with undersocialized aggressive CD suffer from a predominance of Gray's reward system (REW) relative to their behavioral inhibition (BIS). However, other researchers counter this proposal with the argument that timing and contextual factors can actually affect one's neurobiology. Findings of a research project designed to test Gray's theory of brain function and hypotheses of the BIS and REW system failed to find empirical support (Daugherty, Quay, and Ramos, 1993).

Theories of attachment and attachment-related processes have been used to explain CD, the idea that the child's internal representation of the attachment figure will promote or foster inappropriate antisocial behavior, whether as a model for such behavior and/or a means to secure a relationship, proximity and closeness by using disruptive behavior for a parent they view as unavailable. The mother's internal representation of the parent-child relationship may also foster CD behavior almost as a self-fulfilling prophesy, confirming her beliefs about the child (Richters, 1994). The impact of the family system on CD was examined by Frick (1993), who, based on the research review, found three specific dimensions most consistently linked to the disorder: parental psychological adjustment, parental marital adjustment, and parental socialization practices. Similarly, Short, and Shapiro (1993) advocate interventions for CD to address such factors as family, school, individual, and peer dimension; and viewing conduct disorder as a class of chronic antisocial and disruptive behaviors that interfere with effective interaction with the environment. Conduct disorder is seen as being more stable over time than other disorders and, in its more serious form, onset begins in early childhood and persists into serious delinquency in adolescence and antisocial personality disorder and criminal behavior in adults. As a result, prognosis for treatment remains guarded.

Haapasalo and Tremblay (1994) found that the developmental pathways of physically aggressive behavior for boys from low socio-economic environments were related to family adversity and poor parenting, and suggested that these factors could be used to predict delinquency. Pettit, Bates, and Dodge (1993) sought to identify aspects of family interaction that would be predictive of children's externalizing problems (significant of conduct disorder) during the kindergarten-to-first-grade transition. They concluded that the strongest relationship was found between negative–coercive family interaction styles and later externalizing problems. In addition, their research found that early positive involvement predicted lower levels of externalizing problems in kindergarten and first grade. These findings are consistent with prior research pointing to the combination of high negative control and low positive involvement that provides a critical socializing context for the development of externalizing problems. Authors suggested that parents need to address not only providing a high degree of control of their child's behavior in addition to acquiring proactive skills to anticipate their children's social needs, understand their frustration, and encourage behavioral change. Negative maternal behavior emerged as a powerful factor in predicting non-compliance across a variety of settings (Anderson, Hinshaw, and Simmel, 1994).

Brook, Whiteman, and Finch (1993) found childhood aggression to be a precursor of adolescent drug use and delinquency. Early adolescent drug use was found to be associated with delinquency as well as later drug use and delinquency. According to Short and Shapiro (1993), characteristics of CD may appear as early as 2 years of age with symptoms such as resistance to discipline beyond what would be developmentally appropriate and irritability in general in response to rules and regulations. They also noted developmental cognitive and language delays and early aggressive behaviors. Also associated, although clearly not as well documented, are related neurological functioning problems, tendency toward sensation-seeking behaviors, problematic social cognitive development, and different temperament. Antisocial children were found to exhibit a cognitive response bias in which they interpreted ambiguous interpersonal stimuli as being hostile. Further, these individuals tend to be different in problem-solving skills, cognitive flexibility, particularly in generating multiple solutions to problems. Thus, these children tend to be limited and inflexible in solution-generation. resulting in a narrow repertoire of behaviors for responding to conflict situations. Authors cautioned that not all children who exhibit these behaviors grow up to become significantly antisocial. However, most adolescents and adults diagnosed with antisocial behavior had exhibited symptomatology in childhood. Earliest onset of these characteristics is typically associated with increased potential for subsequent negative behavior. Finally, these characteristics interact with parent and teacher requests to exacerbate and intensify problem behaviors. Children who exhibit antisocial behaviors tended to be poor readers, did not do well academically, and were frequently rejected by their peers.

When examining the characteristics of CD, it can easily be seen how it would correlate with ADHD, reduced functioning of the frontal processes resulting in perseveration, poor problem-solving ability, lack of control, absence of rule-governed behavior, diminished cognitive flexibility, absence of time sense or temporal issues and sequencing problems. Hindshaw (1992) found that in childhood the strongest correlates of academic problems was that of inattention and hyperactivity as opposed to aggression; however, by adolescence antisocial behavior and delinquency were found to be clearly associated with underachievement.

Fergusson, Horwood, and Lynskey (1993), in addressing the comorbidity of CD and ADHD on school performance, confirm the hypothesis that CD and ADHD are two separate disorders resulting in specific symptoms. Early attention deficit was found to be a predictor of later problematic cognitive development, but not of the offending behaviors characteristic of CD. Early

CD was found to be a specific predictor of problematic behavior, but not of cognitive development problem, and it is only the combination of ADHD and CD that produces the cyclical pattern of school failure and poor cognitive development. ADHD and CD emerge as being highly correlated despite the fact that they are two distinct syndromes following different pathways.

Abikoff and Klein (1992) maintain that ADHD and CD share a common dysfunction that maximizes interpersonal conflict, which in turn facilitates the development of aggressive behavior. Impulsivity was found to be the key to the development of CD in ADHD children. Minor antisocial features in ADHD boys, such as defiance, may signal increased risk for later antisocial behavior (Satterfield et al., 1993). Physical or sexual abuse, familial explosiveness or violence, and familial and maternal depression differentiated ADHD boys with CD from ADHD boys without CD (Levine and Pincus, 1996).

ADHD tends to overlap with other areas of learning problems. By adolescence, delinquency is often clearly associated with school failure. As a result, early intervention is critical to attempt to ward off what appears to be a predetermined negative course. The overlap between externalizing behaviors and underachievement ranges from under 10 to over 50% (Hinshaw, 1992). Hinshaw recommends multimodal treatment programs to address issues and long-term interventions to break the pattern of school failure and externalizing behavior. ADHD was found to be the link between aggressive behavior and underachievement, and intervention was suggested to address the learning problems that begin during preschool years. Inattention and impulse control problems are correlated with readiness difficulties early in development. Externalizing behavior problems and severe learning failure combine to create a rather resistant cyclical pattern. Hinshaw recommends instruction in precise academic skills that are deficient.

Conduct disorder and ADHD are two syndromes that clearly overlap to such an extensive degree that CD as a comorbid syndrome is one of the most detrimental and difficult syndromes to remediate due to its cyclical, consistent, and pervasive interaction with the attentional disorder. As time continues in a developmental progression, the impact of the interaction of both disorders becomes increasingly resistant to change and treatment.

Impulsivity

Serotonin is the neurotransmitter primarily indicated in impulsivity and impulsive aggression (Stein, Hollander, and Liebowitz, 1993).

Clinically, we have found it very important to differentiate from the true impulsivity, implicating the serotonin system, and associated with ADHD from the impulsive behavior evidenced in the ADD population whereby, although they appear impulsive, this behavior occurs only in the face of either repeated failures and/or after considerable effort has been expended and by that point in time the individual is tired and adopts an "I don't care" attitude. After a pattern of repeated failures, attention-disordered individuals may race through projects or assignments simply to get them done and to avoid the shame, embarrassment, and trauma associated with the difficulty in performing the task due to symptoms of the disorder. Frequently, this type of "impulsive" behavior will occur only in the gap or detrimental areas that are symptomatic of deficits related to the attentional disorder.

Borderline Personality

Wender (1995) found that ADHD adults share common attributes with that of the borderline personality (BPD): impulsivity, angry outbursts, affective instability, and feelings of boredom. However, the two disorders are still viewed as distinctly different from one another.

Parents of patients with borderline personality disorder had significantly higher rates of psychopathology, particularly in the areas of depression, substance abuse, and antisocial disorders. Neglect (specifically by both caretakers) is viewed as a highly significant risk factor in addition to the issue of abuse in the etiology this disorder, 60% of those diagnosed with BPD reported childhood sexual abuse, 91% reported some type of childhood neglect, and 75% reported emotional abuse in their background. Factors found as most significant were that of female gender, sexual abuse by a male noncaretaker, emotional denial by the paternal object and inconsistent treatment by the maternal object. Abuse, in combination with the atmosphere of general chaos and neglect, creates the pivotal causal effect for the development of this disorder. Patients significantly reported that their maternal caretakers were more likely to deny their feelings, treat them with inconsistency, place them in the role of parent, (symbiotic relationships) and overall fail to provide them with the necessary protection from abuse (Zanarini et al., 1997). Goldman, D'Angelo, and DeMaso (1993) also concluded that BPD is associated with a history of significant family pathology. Maternal inconsistency in the upbringing of a child predicted a persistence or an emergence of BPD, but not of any other axis II disorder. This effect occurred only in the presence of high maternal overinvolvement (Bezirganian, Cohen, and Brook, 1993). In examining the presence of personality disorders in adolescent inpatients diagnosed with major depression, substance abuse or both, BPD was significant for the dual diagnosis when compared to the single diagnosis of either depression or substance abuse, 86% of dually diagnosed major depression and substance abuse met the criterion for BPD (Grilo et al., 1997). Demonstrating the variability of this disorder, Cornelius and associates (1993) found no clear pharmacological treatment of choice for the therapy of BPD. Indeed, BPD appears to be a watershed diagnosis and symptoms range from neurotic depression, psychosis, intense rage, and aggression based on highly irrational thinking. When combined with an attentional disorder, irrational thinking and misassumptions are only enhanced.

CHAPTER 12

Follow-Up Studies: Development Span of the Disorder

ADHD Children: Follow-Up Studies

McGee et al. (1991) studied hyperactive preschoolers over a 12-year period and found that they continued to evidence poorer cognitive skills, lower levels of reading ability, disruptive and inattentive behaviors at both home and school, and higher rates of the disorder according to the DSM-III in preadolescence and adolescence. By age 15, only one fourth of the original group met any sort of recovery criteria and were regarded as "problem free". The problematic cognitive performance of the hyperactive group in primary school was seen as the result of lower preschool language skills more so than hyperactive behavior. Preschool hyperactivity places the child at general risk for difficulty at adolescence. Thus across a 12-year period, these children continued to show cognitive and language problems, particularly with respect to literacy. This pattern was repeated for identified ADHD children who reported continuing symptoms of ADHD (with no gender differences) and experienced more adverse educational and social outcomes at age 15 and 18 years of age (Schaughency et al., 1994). Those who had a history of behavioral problems were seen as similar to the ADHD group, while those without a history of behavioral problems exhibited more diverse pathology in adolescence not related to behavioral issues revolving around ADD. The presence of deficits in attention, motor control, and perception contributed to poor outcome on follow-up measures 9 years later (Hellgren, Gillberg, and Gillberg, 1994).

Wallander (1988), utilizing a Danish population in an 8-year longitudinal study, found a significant, although weak correlation between other problems in males and their arrest eight years later. She concluded that in the general male population attentional problems in childhood are related to antisocial behavior in adolescence and early adulthood; however, this relationship can be moderated by the individual's intellectual functioning and alcoholic behavior of the father.

In a position paper written by Walid Shekim, M.D., psychiatrist, (1990), UCLA, Neuropsychiatric Institute in Los Angeles, she refers to a small but growing body of evidence that shows that ADHD–residual state occurs in adults and that one third to one half of children with the problem may continue to have symptoms suggestive of the disorder when they reach adulthood.

Weiss and Hechtman and their colleagues (1979, 1986, 1992) investigated long-term outcome and impact of ADD beginning in approximately 1962 with 104 children, ages 6 to 12 years, diagnosed as ADHD. Studies revealed a good degree of similarity in their findings, particularly half or more of the children diagnosed as hyperactive had varying degrees of continuing symptoms of the hyperactive child syndrome in adulthood. At different stages, there were different complaints and symptoms of hyperactivity that predominated. The majority of hyperactive children had some continuing difficulties characteristic of the hyperactive syndrome in adult life, especially impulsivity, restlessness, and poor social skills. The high rate of antisocial behavior seen in groups of hyperactive subjects during adolescence (25 to 50%) diminishes as young adulthood is reached. Finally, long-term stimulant medication does little to improve the outcome of hyperactive childhood. Weiss suggests that other modalities of treatment must be sought if adult outcome is to be affected. Stimulants are effective for symptom suppression, but not of the symptoms of the syndrome.

Weiss et al. (1979) indicated that even though overall family ratings did not predict hyperactive adolescent school success or emotional adjustment, it was important in exerting influence over overt antisocial behavior in adolescents. A good family situation was correlated with good outcome in adolescence as measured by academic achievement, emotional adjustment, and absence of delinquency. Thus, family factors are important in both specific and overall outcome at 13-year follow-up assessment. There were no significant differences in the EEGs of hyperactive as opposed to matched normal controls. This supports the hypothesis that EEGs of hyperactive individuals normalize with age and that the mild diffuse scoring viewed earlier reflects an immature pattern that normalizes with age. This normalization is most significant toward the end of adolescence.

Results of the 1986 Weiss study are summarized below:

1. More than half of the hyperactive adults (66% compared to 7% of normals) still had at least one disabling symptom of the hyperactive child syndrome. Almost half of the hyperactive group (44%) was viewed as restless (fidgeting and changing sitting position frequently), compared to 10% of normals.

2. There is no evidence that adult hyperactives are predisposed to psychosis or alcohol abuse. Antisocial personality disorder was the only diagnosis distinguishing hyperactives from normals and 23% met the criteria for the disorder. Hyperactives had less formal education, scored below normals on a general functioning measure, and had more diagnoses (phobic anxiety, somatization, and sexual problems) than normals. Hyperactive subjects made significantly more suicide attempts than matched controls. Follow-up studies indicated that most of the improvement with ADD or ADHD characteristics occurred between the ages of 13 and 19 years.

3. ADD and ADHD increases with age up to 12 years with the greatest percentage of symptoms occurring between 4 and 12 years of age (Weiss, 1986). Statistically, 50 to 65% of children diagnosed as having ADHD also revealed characteristics of ADHD in adulthood. Further, 44% of those adults were seen as restless, exhibiting fidgeting behavior, with changing and shifting of position being notable, and this appears as the remnant of the motor characteristics of the disorder. Antisocial behavior was seen in 20 to 45%, substance abuse in 12%, and only 11% of those adults in follow-up studies were found to be free of any psychiatric diagnosis and symptoms of the disorder. Complaints of anxiety, sadness, and somatic illness affected 79% of those adults, 75% had interpersonal problems, and 10% had attempted suicide.

4. Accidental injury or suicide affected 5% of the population, 30% had dropped out of high school and only 5% went on to study at the university level, compared to 41% of the controls. Finally, 18% had had contact with the court system, primarily traffic violations, and 20% had participated in acts of physical aggression (Weiss, 1986).

Wender (1995) felt that the Weiss study was indicative of problematic follow-up research in that, by the time of a 10-year follow-up in 1974, Weiss et al. (1979) were only able to interview 75 of the original sample. The study, when completed with a 15-year follow-up, included only 61 subjects. The Mamuzza and Klein study (Mamuzza et al., 1993) began between 1970 and 1975 with 103 Caucasian males, ages 6 to 12 years, diagnosed with ADHD. At adolescent follow-up (average age of 18 years), information was obtained on 98% of the original sample, 40% of subjects were still diagnosed as ADHD. At adult follow-up with 88% of the original sample, an average age of 26 years, one third of the group was diagnosed with an ongoing mental disorder and only 8% with ADHD. Studies with such discrepant results are due to numerous variables and Wender aptly sums up the issue by estimating that approximately one third minimum will show continuing ADHD symptoms at follow-up in adulthood (Wender, 1995). Finally, the prevalence of persisting ADHD in the adult population is roughly estimated at ranges from 2 to 7% of those originally diagnosed in childhood.

Researchers have investigated the hypothesis that adults involved in treatment for alcoholism would reveal an increased comorbidity of ADHD and indeed found that 33% of childhood ADD identified in this population. Wood et al. (1983) noted that for many alcoholics the attentional disorder continued to impact their life via symptoms of hyperactivity and attentional deficits as evidenced by an inability to complete tasks efficiently, affective liability, impulsivity, and abnormally poor or low stress tolerance (Horton et al., 1990). Similar findings to a greater or lesser degree have been found for opiate and drug addicts and a tendency toward association with criminality.

Although ADHD may operate as an exacerbating factor, conduct disorder and presence of conduct problems are the predictors of criminality. More severe substance abuse, earlier onset of cocaine abuse, more frequent and intense cocaine use (intranasal rather than freebase or intravenous use of cocaine), and higher rates of alcoholism were correlated with childhood ADHD, conduct disorder, and antisocial personality disorder. ADHD individuals who have comorbid issues of mental retardation, psychosis, or cerebral dysfunction present an even more problematic prognosis (Carroll and Rounsaville, 1993; Eyre et al., 1982; Klein and Mannuzza, 1991; Lie, 1992; Lilienfeld and Waldman, 1990; Rugle and Melamed, 1993; Vaeth, Horton, and Abadpour, 1992). Pihl and Peterson (1991) explored the connection between ADHD, childhood conduct disorder, and the development later in life of alcoholism and/or substance abuse. The importance of aggression was seen as a critical factor delineating those children with ADHD who are at increased risk to develop alcohol or drug abuse.

Kaplan and Shachter (1991) suggest the presence of undiagnosed learning disabilities in ADHD adults. Denckla (1993) further investigated this question and found that learning disabilities persist into adult life and there are characteristics of linguistic inefficiency, executive dysfunction or spatial disability. Combinations of linguistic or spatial dysfunction with executive dysfunctions were encountered more commonly than pure linguistic or spatial impairments, suggesting that executive function is a key factor in the continued compensation for learning disabilities experienced by adults. By the same token, executive dysfunction was found to underlie learning disability decompensation and thereby represented the phenomenon of underachievement for the learning disabled adult.

In our clinical practice, we have found the same pattern and it has become quite apparent that the language problems involving spared executive function are those related to ADD and due to pure spatial and inattention issues, while the more-severe and problematic learning disability of the ADHD individual is seen less often. Thus, in a clinical practice setting, the professional is more likely to see the less-severe ADD who is able to compensate and maintain employment, as opposed to the more severe ADHD individual. College students diagnosed as ADHD in childhood had higher levels of nonconscious processing and poor inhibitory control (Shaw and Giambra, 1993).

Mannuzza et al. (1988) noted that only 48% of previously diagnosed hyperactives qualified for a non-ADHD diagnosis in adulthood. Also noted was an increased prevalence for substance abuse and psychiatric disorders. Greenfield et al. (1988) found two subgroups of ADHD outcomes characterized by alcohol use, antisocial behavior, and emotional problems, and the presence or absence of these syndromes. Findings suggest that adult symptoms are due, at least in part, to the severity of the original diagnosis and the comorbidity of conduct disorder and oppositional disorder. Adults with more positive outcomes are not symptom-free; they appear instead to have managed their symptoms more efficiently and have not fallen prey to environmental hazards. Denckla (1991) reviews retrospective and longitudinal data that suggest a residual type of attention deficit hyperactivity disorder.

A recent evaluation of the clinical profile of ADHD adults using the DSM-IV criteria yielded considerable misdiagnosis (47% ADHD vs. 53% ADD vs. 51% no ADD at all). Major presenting symptoms were that of decreased attention and concentration, disorganization, distractibility, and forgetfulness. Comorbid diagnoses were more commonly substance abuse

(70% marijuana and alcohol), major depression (44%), neurotic depression (33%), personality disorder (23%), and learning disability (50%). IQ assessment revealed a discrepancy greater than 15 points between verbal and performance in 32% of diagnosed ADD subjects (Chang et al., 1995). This study clearly elucidates the multiplicity of ADD as a syndrome. Its varying symptomatology and impact of individual comorbid diagnoses result in a very complicated picture that needs to be accurately assessed for proper treatment to occur, whether coping mechanisms and/or medical management.

Adult ADD Characteristics

By the time the attention-disordered individual reaches adulthood, life has become a series of crises due to numerous problems: accomplishing things, keeping promises, meeting life's daily demands, or just keeping up with day-to-day organization. As life becomes more complex with the occurrence of job, family, and marriage problems, anger and hostility also build up both within and outside of the family structure from the repeated failures and attempt to cope with life and being ill prepared to do so.

Characteristics observed more often in the adult attention-disordered population are low frustration tolerance; emotional lability; highly sensitized; overall fragility; confusion; problematic task completion; continually being overwhelmed by life; self-medicating substance abuse; and subject to hypertension, immune system disorders, generalized anxiety, panic attacks, depression, thyroid, digestive, and sleep disorders. They are constantly worried, overfocused, and driven to perfectionism. There is a difficulty with new situations or experiences, following directions, follow through, completing longer-term projects and planning, general paperwork and note-taking, and difficulty thinking clearly. The distractibility results in wandering from one unfinished task to another, interrupting others lest one forgets one's thought, and inability to complete thoughts, which can resemble a thought disorder. The low self-esteem and negative view of self promotes the tendency to project blame onto others, a fear of failure, labeling of everything as boring and overall fear of failure, which limits any new learning situation and negates the possibility of a learning curve necessary for new task performance.

These individuals are subject to mental restlessness and an inability to sustain ideas in their mind. Adults tend to be late for appointments, misplace things, have poor listening skills, and a general outward lack of empathy. There can be either a restless life style characterized by frequent job changes or extensive stability without any possibility of changes due to the intense dislike of transition. Sustaining relationships are problematic for this population due to missing information (appearing as poor listening skills), inability to maintain eye contact, and highly problematic social skills. Conversations are concluded prematurely and glazed over due to distractibility, and there is an inability to take another person's perspective, which contributes to the social inadequacies.

Zametkin et al. (1990) investigated whether cerebral glucose metabolism differed between normal adults and adults with histories of hyperactivity in childhood who were found to have continuing symptoms. PET scans measured regional glucose metabolism during attentional task performance and were found to be reduced in those individuals who were diagnosed hyperactive in childhood. This was a breakthrough study that began the research to develop the current biochemical theory of ADD. Unfortunately, there have been problems with the use of PET scans and replicating this study as well as measuring effects of medication. Problems, however, appear to be due to the task itself, with neuropsychological measures the area of the brain that one thinks is being measured is not always what is actually being measured. Lou (1991) suggested that the discrepancies in the SPECT studies with adults vs. children was due to adults being less hyperactive.

Statistics for the adult outcomes of ADHD were reported by Mannuzza et al. (1993). They found that adult ADHD individuals had completed less formal schooling, approximately 25% had never completed high school (as compared to 2% of the control population), 10% were more likely to have antisocial personality disorder in adulthood, significantly higher rate of substance abuse, and lower occupational ranking with the largest discrepancies occurring among the higher ranking positions. There were no differences found as to the rate of employment.

Biederman et al. (1993) interviewed adults who had been diagnosed as ADHD in childhood and findings were then compared with prior referred children with the diagnosis of ADHD, adults with the diagnosis of ADHD who had not been referred for treatment, and adults without the disorder who were relatives of normal children. All groups were evaluated on a comprehensive battery of psychiatric, cognitive and psychosocial assessments. Results indicated that the referred and nonreferred adults with ADHD were similar to one another and significantly more disturbed and impaired than the comparison subjects without the diagnosis of the disorder. The pattern of psychopathology, cognition, and functioning among the adults with ADHD closely approximated the findings for the children also diagnosed as ADHD. Research thus supports the validity of this diagnosis in adulthood. Specifically, a significantly greater percentage of the adults with ADHD were male, divorced or separated, and of a lower socioeconomic status. Adults with ADHD had significantly higher rates of the diagnosis of antisocial personality disorder, conduct disorder, oppositional-defiant disorder, substance abuse, anxiety disorders, enuresis, stuttering, and speech and language disorders. Adults with ADHD were found to have significantly higher rates of repeated grades, tutoring, placement in special classes, and reading disability. Adults with ADHD had significantly lower than estimated full-scale and freedom-from-distractibility IQs with lower vocabulary, arithmetic, and reading scores.

Adams and Curtin (1990) refer to ADD as the inability to marshal one's energy in the face of a difficult task that is the hallmark of an attention deficit. The marshaling of energy may take the form of inhibiting one's impulses, fighting distractions, paying attention, concentrating, and allocating effort to complete tasks, even when the reasons for completing the tasks are not intrinsically motivating or provides a short-term reward. Ratey and Miller (1992) discuss adults with an attention disorder who frequently experience a state of internal disorganization that leads them to crave high stimulus situations. Such situations may carry a high emotional charge or a high intellectual charge, whether it be positive or negative. The exact nature of the stimulus is unimportant when compared to the experience of high intensity. Thus, it is the intensity of the experience that organizes the individual and produces an inner state of calm.

According to Ratey, Hallowell, and Miller (1996), it is the disorganization, emptiness, and boredom due to the lack of directness that follows the resolution of conflict and trauma and leads to the internal state that adults with ADD find intolerable. Consequently, there is a need for new and more compelling conflict and/or repetition of old traumas.

Information taken in from the environment through the limbic system classifies and sorts emotional information and then transfers the data to individual data banks comprised of similar information, thus making it likely that the appropriate emotion stored is chosen based upon its affective quality. It may be that the person with an attentional deficit has only a few large memory areas with which to store that experience. The affective quality that defines those areas are intensity, excitement, and crisis as opposed to the more differentiated categories of love, joy, sadness, remorse, and so on. Whether the lack of highly differentiated cognitive–affective structures is that of the attentional disorder or a cause of it remains the question. What appears to be true is that the need for high stimulation becomes hardwired into the individual's brain, prompting that person to continually seek out conflict and trauma for excitement. The notion of failure becomes a common theme, especially for those whose disorder went unrecognized in childhood.

Distractibility, hyperactivity, impulsivity, and the frequent inability to learn from past experience have all interfered with the person's skill to accomplish life's important tasks and goals. The repeated image of failure remains a constant theme, and fear that all will not occur as planned for the attention-disordered adult, thus prompting him/her toward avoidance and procrastination. The ADD adult becomes trapped in a terrible bind, cannot finish what he/she cannot even begin, and does not wish to begin what cannot be finished.

Ratey, Hallowell, and Miller (1996) explained that undiagnosed adults come to the attention of professionals because their chronic failure to form healthy intimate relationships due to the physical jumpiness and constant need for intense and/or multiple sources of stimuli, thus making it impossible to sustain the emotional and cognitive contact that intimate relationships demand. The partner of the ADD adult can feel undervalued due to both the distractibility of the ADD and the tendency of that adult to throw existing energy into activities other than the relationship in repeated attempts to achieve order. The ADD adult may develop an attitude toward relationships seeing them as associated with situational demands that the ADD adult finds hard to meet.

A self-fulfilling prophecy is created whereby the individual expects failures in intimacy and becomes defensive, sometimes determining that intimacy is not desired and developing avoidance patterns regarding relationships. Adults face difficulties in being effective in the wider social world and can report a history of antisocial behavior.

The interplay between the constant fears of being bad and falling short of personal and interpersonal expectations and of failing occurs again and again. These feelings of being bad and the inner chaos prompts adults to act out, eliciting negative reinforcement from others and another self-fulfilling prophecy is established. Very often ADD adults go undiagnosed unless exhibiting overt behavior problems due to their intelligence, talents, skills and/or the advantage of a structured environment, allowing them to function and not be noticed as having a problem. They learn to defensively compensate and shield themselves from being noticed as different. This can lead to a sense of shame about oneself and further compensation.

Paradoxically, adults with attention problems cannot tolerate being alone despite their fear and disregard for people or their inability to get along socially. Being alone can be difficult due to the triggering of feelings of emptiness that may cause them to seek or create conflict. These problematic issues become scripts and can be unlearned once an understanding of the disorder has been reached.

Kelley and Ramundo (1993) described the strengths of the ADD adults as active, creative, open-minded, compassionate, having a sense of wonder, curious, enthusiastic, passionate, and a good sense of humor. Weaknesses are that of being impatient, moody, intolerant of noise and chaos, carelessness with details, shaky communication skills, limited capacity of work and stress, easily bored, impulsive, and disorganized. Learning styles can be different and need to be identified as visual vs. auditory vs. tactile kinesthetic learner.

CHAPTER 13

Treatment: Stimulants as the First Line of Defense

Medications: Pharmacological Approach

Unfortunately, there is a paucity of data concerning the impact of medication on the ADD population, and the majority of the research is directed at the ADHD population. It is presumed that this has occurred for a number of reasons: the ADHD population has been easier to define; there is no widely recognized evaluation for ADD; and the ADHD population is consistently more of a behavioral problem and therefore more susceptible to those around them wanting to medication them.

Clinically, it is observed that both subgroups, ADHD and ADD, notice differences on medication, although the ADHD group appears to respond more to the dopamine enhancers and the ADD group to the norepinephrine enhancers. Buitelaar et al. (1995) identified a positive response to methylphenidate (MPH) to be correlated with a high IQ level, a high degree of inattentiveness, young age, less severe disorder, and a lower rate of anxiety.

Catecholaminergic Agonists

The major drugs in this class include L-Dopa, Amantadine, Bromocriptine, Pergolide, Lisuride, and the stimulants.

233

Cholinergic agonists play a role in human memory and cognitive function (McLean et al., 1993). Nootropics refers to a class of drugs known as cognitive activators. Wender (1995) finds that the agonists do not produce euphoria and may appear promising for treatment of ADHD as they directly stimulate the postsynaptic receptors (as compared to the psychostimulants that are indirect agonists increasing release of neurotransmitter substances at the presynaptic site).

Several medications are currently being tested with clinical trials: Pramiracetam, Ganglioside, and Thyrotropin Releasing Hormone.

Levodopa (L-Dopa) has been a classic dopamine agonist with its action occurring presynaptically. It is agonistic at both the D1 and D2 receptor sites. Side effects are numerous, the most frequent being dyskinesias, bradykinetic episodes, psychiatric disturbances, gastrointestinal disturbances, and orthostatic hypotension (Zasler, 1992). Levodopa has both a short duration immediate affect (1 to 4 hours) and long duration slower action of a week or longer, the long duration is thought to be the result of postsynaptic pharmacodynamic changes (Barbato et al., 1997).

Levodopa has been found to have alerting effects in patients with Parkinson's disease, as well as improving attention span in diagnosed ADHD individuals. Research reported cognitive and behavioral improvements specifically in alertness, sustained attention, and concentration. There was more improvement for brain-injured individuals within the first 6 months of injury, as opposed to 1 to 4 years post-injury, raising the potential of spontaneous improvement in the recently head-injured population (Wroblewski and Glenn, 1994).

Amantadine (Symmetrel) has been found to benefit cognitive function and reduce agitation; it is also being utilized for the negative symptoms of schizophrenia (withdrawal, abulia, and bradykinesia) (McLean et al., 1993). Amantadine was also demonstrated to reduce fatigue, control emotional lability and agitation (Elovic, 1996), and improve sustained attention and distractibility in the brain-injured population (Wroblewski and Glenn, 1994). van Reekum et al. (1995) found amantadine useful in treating motivational symptoms following brain injury. More specifically, amantadine was found to have a positive effect on speed of information processing, resistance to distraction, sustained attention, initiation, inhibitory control, and other cognitive self-regulatory abilities (Cowell and Cohen, 1995). The use of amantadine was found to decrease impulsivity and perseveration and to improve executive functioning in a 50-year-old TBI woman with frontal lobe dysfunction. An increased positive response was obtained with the addition of L-dopa/carbidopa. Evidence of improvement was in constructional praxis, divided auditory attention, and cognitive flexibility. This confirmed the benefit of a combination of dopamine agents to remediate the effects of head injury with medical management but without observed side effects and reported maintenance of substantial gains at follow-up (Kraus and Maki, 1997). Methylphenidate and amantadine both produced significant improvement in the TBI population and specifically impacted a measure of distractibility and sustained attention (Allen et al., 1997). Negative symptoms (depression) of dementia subtypes (Alzheimer's Disease and vascular dementia) were responsive to methylphenidate, suggesting that withdrawn, nonagitated patients with moderate degrees of impairment would benefit from stimulant use. A modest improvement in cognitive abilities was evidenced in the vascular, but not the Alzheimer's type of dementia (Galynker et al., 1997). There was a minimal risk of exacerbation of psychosis noted in a study conducted to determine amantadine as a candidate to address symptoms of tardive dyskinesia (TD) in the diagnosed schizophrenic adult. Findings indicated a statistically significant positive impact of amantadine in conjunction with a neuroleptic to address TD symptoms (Angus et al., 1997). Amantadine was found to have a "neuroprotective" effect and improve survival of Parkinson's patients (Utti et al., 1996).

Amantadine hydrochloride has been used clinically as an antiviral agent, as well as an anti-Parkinsonian agent. Its action is not well understood, but it is hypothesized to have a presynaptic action, as well as a possible postsynaptic action. There is speculation that Amantadine may also increase central cholinergic and gabaminergic activity. Side effects include peripheral edema, light-headedness, orthostatic hypotension, hot and dry sin, rash, and liver reticularis (discoloration of the skin). In addition, it may lower the seizure threshold and cause confusion and hallucinations in the geriatric population (Zasler, 1992). This medication was also found to be successful in the treatment of aggression (Cassidy, 1994).

Other dopamine receptor-stimulating agents that have a more direct action are Bromocriptine, Lisuride, and Pergolide. Bromocriptine and Lisuride are antagonistic at the D1 receptor and agonistic at the D2 receptor; Pergolide is agonistic at both the D1 and D2 receptor sites (Zasler, 1992).

As a postsynaptic agonist for dopamine at the striatal and hypothalamic-hypophyseal levels, Bromocriptine (Parlodel) has been used in the head-injured population primarily for speech and language disorders and has also been found beneficial to the hemispatial neglect syndromes and parietal lobe functioning. This medication improved symptoms of apathy and poor initiation, drive, sustained attention, responsiveness, and alertness. Cognitive processing improves and this medication has been found useful to remediate abulia and akinetic mutism. The use of bromocriptine was found to facilitate spatial delayed-memory functions while haloperidol was found to impair these functions thus demonstrating the separate processing mechanism of the *what vs. where* phenomenon apparently operating at both structural and biochemical levels (Luciana and Collins, 1997). Often, however, treatment gains were not preserved on cessation (Elovic, 1996). Like the other dopaminergics, there are side effects of mental disturbances (including agitation, confusion, depression, hallucinations, and nightmares), hypotension, dizziness, drowsiness, and faintness (Wroblewski and Glenn, 1994; Zasler, 1995). Bromocriptine was found to produce a pronounced improvement in motivation at doses at or below 10 mg. Results were maintained subsequent to treatment withdrawal which supported the possibility that just a low dose of this dopamine agonist provided the initial support necessary to help the head-injured individual resume more normalized functioning (Powell et al., 1996).

Pergolide (Permax) is one of the newer dopamine agonist and is approximately ten times more potent than Bromocriptine. There is evidence of its use only with Parkinson's disease. This medication has been useful for nonresponders to Bromocriptine (Wroblewski and Glenn, 1994).

Selegiline (L-Deprenyl) is a selective inhibitor of MAO type B, which is largely located in the brain. Treatment with this medication increases the availability of dopamine (and by selectively inhibiting MAO type B rather than the more widespread Type A), it is not associated with the problematic dietary restrictions or the acute sympathetic effects, such as severe hypertension, tachycardia, headache, and vomiting. It has been noted to improve participation, activation, arousal, attention, mood, and behavior, and to be beneficial in treatment of ADHD adults and Alzheimer's disease (Elovic, 1996; Wroblewski and Glenn, 1994). Deprenyl has been used with positive effects to treat ADHD with Tourette's syndrome. There were no serious side effects over a period of time on the medication and clinically there was meaningful improvement in ADHD symptoms. Deprenyl blocks the metabolism of dopamine to improve dopamine transmission; it is also a potent antioxidant and has a protective effect on the progression of Tourette's syndrome. Excluding occasional reports of nausea, abdominal discomfort, insomnia, and hallucinations, it was remarkably well tolerated and, most importantly, did not exacerbate tics (Jankovic, 1993). In contrast, Feigin et al. (1996) found the effects of Deprenyl to be unclear and warranting further study, indicating beneficial effects for the amelioration of symptoms of Tourette's, but not necessarily of ADHD.

Apomorphine is a dopamine receptor agonist that has been shown in some research studies to have resulted in decreased neglect in rats with cortical and subcortical lesions (Wroblewski and Glenn, 1994).

Stimulants

Stimulants are referred to as catecholamine agonists, meaning that they directly affect these neurotransmitters. The general mechanism has been to directly increase the availability of norepinephrine and dopamine at the receptor sites to provide increased effectiveness of neurotransmission. Stimulants operate on various levels, functioning as inhibitors of monoamine reuptake, as catecholamine agonists, as releasers of monoamines into the synapse and as MAO, preventing catecholamine breakdown within the neuron (monoamine oxidase degrades dopamine). All of these actions result in an initial increase of dopamine, norepinephrine, and 5-HT at their receptor sites.

Amphetamine consists of a simple molecule of only nine carbon atoms with one chiral center and, by its simplicity, it is dwarfed by the structural complexity of most of the other classes of drugs. The most prominent action is that of CNS stimulation, production of euphoria, increased motor activity, and appetite suppression. Reportedly the mechanism by which amphetamine causes catecholamine release is that it reduces intracellular pH gradients of synaptic vesicles, and once the buffering capacity of the vesicle has been exceeded, the decreased proton gradient reduces the driving force for transmitter uptake. Deprotonated catecholamine then may diffuse from the vesicle following its concentration gradient, and this elevated cytosolic monoamine then may be released from the cell by reversal of the uptake carrier. *N*-methyl substitution of amphetamine results in methamphetamine (MPA), which has nearly twice the *in vivo* potency of amphetamine, and the derivative of MPA, MDMA, which was widely abused in the 1980s and 1990s. Amphetamine (AMPH) has been well documented since the 1960s as playing an important role in the extracellular release of dopamine and AMPH, producing a broad spectrum of central and peripheral effects, prompting extraneuronal dopamine release, as well as norepinephrine from peripheral sympathetic norepinephrine nerve terminals (Cho and Segal, 1994).

Carlson and Bunner (1993) reviewed studies examining the effects of psychostimulant medications on learning and achievement in children diagnosed with ADHD. Overall, studies reported considerable effects of medication on daily classroom performance and consistently revealed these effects; however, only on a short-term basis as evidence of achievement in terms of beneficial effects was not sustained over periods of months and years. Thus it remains unclear as to whether stimulants generalize to real-life academic performance. Further, there are wide differences in the response to medications, and variability remains as to whether lower dosages may optimize learning and higher dosages evidence the greatest benefits for behavioral improvement. Horn et al. (1991) found that the effects of a high dose of stimulant medication could be achieved by combining the low dose with a behavioral intervention.

Pelham (1993) found in his review of the literature that the stimulants are the most widely used medication to treat ADHD and the short-term benefits in terms of improved classroom behavior, daily academic productivity, improvement in compliance with teacher commands and teacher rated disruptive behavior, and improvement in peer-directed aggression have all been well documented. Finally, findings indicate that there are individual differences in response to the stimulants and children respond differently with some of the stimulants having more optimal effects than others. Of importance is the finding that use and duration of the use of stimulant medication was not associated with subsequent drug abuse for adolescence and young adulthood. Further, some studies presented data suggesting that a positive response to stimulant medication was associated with a lower probability of drug abuse.

Matochik and associates (1994) examined the effects of chronic stimulant treatment upon cerebral glucose metabolism in adults diagnosed with ADHD. Adults were studied utilizing PET scans prior and subsequent to drug treatment. Findings indicated that stimulant medication did not alter global or whole-brain metabolism, although stimulant medication was associated with significant improvement in behavioral measures with improved ratings for restlessness and ability to maintain attention. Authors conclude that the lack of robust metabolic effects in the measurement of medication effects questions the use of glucose metabolism studies.

Results point to the difficulty with the research in pinpointing the disorder and in measuring changes due to the impact of medication. As stated previously in addressing ADD, measures used do not also measure what they purport to measure and, consequently, findings in this study may also be due to the assessment techniques and diagnostic accuracy. Noncompliance or improper use of psychostimulants in children was seen as the consequence of a number of complex psychosocial factors including the child's passivity and oppositionality, as well as parental concerns and parental reaction (Stine, 1994). Wilens, Spencer, and Biederman (1995) in summarizing research regarding the use of the stimulants found no reports of stimulant abuse for adults, little evidence to support a concern for adverse cardiovascular effects, and mild or no impact of interactions of stimulants with other medicators (excluding co-administration of the sympathomimetics, TCAs, anticonvulsants and MAO inhibitors).

Methylphenidate (Ritalin) is the most popular and most widely used stimulant. Ritalin is clinically suggested as a first line of defense due to its short-acting properties; it tends to take 20 minutes to commence, lasting for approximately 4 hours; and has evidenced positive results for individuals ranging from 2.5 to 76 years. There tend to be few side effects associated with this medication and various research completed over a period of 30 years confirmed the absence of long-term side effects (Weiss, 1996).

There is a short-acting version, which takes 20 minutes to become active and lasts for 4 hours, subject to a high degree of individual variation. The long-acting sustained release takes approximately 45 minutes to 1.5 hours, lasting 6 to 8 hours, again subject to individual variation. At our clinic, we have found excellent results with the combined use of the short- and long-acting version to either combat a rebound or overmetabolizing problem and/or to provide a means of increasing dosage (while maintaining the short-acting dosage at 20 mg). Ritalin is available in dosage strengths of 5, 10, and 20 mg. We have found that the best results occur when:

1. An individual who is fragile or sensitive biologically begins with a low dose and titrates up slowly.
2. There is a dosage cap of 20 mg per dose. Sustained release, present in 20-mg strengths, provides a smooth and consistent means of maintaining continuous coverage and slowing increasing dosage strength.
3. Appetite problems can be combated with continuous eating on a 2-hour interval schedule.
4. Food is taken with each dose and incidents of hypoglycemia are addressed via an eating schedule.
5. Anxiety problems can be addressed by taking calcium (with magnesium) with each dose.

Clinically in the ADD population we observe that anxiety, tension, depression, agitation, hypertension, thought disturbance, and other symptoms that mimic attention disorders are exacerbated by MPH. When individuals do experience problems, it is usually due to the stimulant properties and this medication may tend to "stimulate" underlying disorders. The comorbid symptoms are stimulated by MPH and are not necessarily the consequence of the medication.

Methylphenidate may lower the seizure threshold; however, it may be used in conjunction with seizure medication. Safety has not been established for children under 6 years of age; however, clinical efficacy has been noted for 5-year-olds. There is a rebound effect when the drug wears off. For children, it may be increased symptoms of hyperactivity, and for adolescents and adults, it may evidence as increased moodiness and sensitivity. A rebound fatigue may be more characteristic of ADD than ADHD. Appetite suppression is the most frequent side effect. There may be some difficulty falling asleep. Stomach aches and headaches are complaints at the onset of medication that frequently subside. There may be a significant elevation of the resting heart rate in previously unmedicated children; however, with continued drug treatment only a minor increase is observed. If there is lethargy, the dosage may be too high and if motor tics develop, medication needs to be reduced or discontinued. There are no long-term growth defects, and discontinuation of medication during the summer has no effect either way. Sustained release and/or generic brands have been found to be ineffective. It appears that based on the way the generic brand is formulated the result is an often negative, variable, and unpredictable response, often followed by agitation and behavioral problems after usage for a period of time (Weinberg, 1995). With sustained release, it can be overmetabolized early resulting in overmedication and later undermedication. Stimulant overdoses in non-hyperactive children often have led to hypertension and tachycardia, but generally are not associated with cardiovascular fatality and, therefore, it is not necessary to monitor blood pressure, heart rate or EKG before or during routine treatment unless there are comorbid cardiovascular abnormalities (Copeland, 1991; Fitzpatrick et al., 1992; Safer, 1992; Wender, Wood, and Reimherr, 1991).

A significantly poorer response in subjects with comorbid anxiety when compared to those without anxiety was noted (Pliszka, 1990; Tannock et al., 1995). Similarly DuPaul, Barkley, and McMurray (1994) noted that ADHD children with comorbid internalizing symptoms were poor responders to MPH and suggested that some children may be at a higher risk for adverse medication reaction. Propranolol (a beta adrenergic agent) was found helpful as an augmenter to MPH in ameliorating the rebound effects (Lavenstein and Fore, 1997).

In our clinical practice, we have found that children with internalizing symptoms generally tend to be anxious and sometimes very fragile with symptoms of the overfocused subtype and more often diagnosed as ADD. Stimulant mediation increases the underlying symptoms of anxiety, seizure-like activations, and general fragility, and needs to be addressed to allow the individual to continue to utilize Ritalin and benefit from its use. Concomitant use of nutritional supplements, calcium, Clonidine, anti-anxiety agents, antiseizure medication, and whatever treatment is necessary to address underlying symptoms allows the individual to return to use of MPH with very positive results. Finally, Wilens et al. (1995) noted that adults require more robust dosing to attain a significant benefit from Ritalin.

Wender (1995), in his clinical findings with the adult ADHD population, found that side effects due to excessive doses of the stimulants produced more agitation than euphoria and too large a dose produced sedation and fogginess. Other side effects noted are that of increased systolic and diastolic blood pressure, short-lived appetite suppression, dry mouth, and insomnia (depending on the time of dose). A concern was noted of increased hypertension that could be addressed with additional medication. In patients who became withdrawn, suspicious, and anxious, stimulant use was seen as provoking latent tendencies. In long-term evaluation (1 year), adults diagnosed as ADHD were found to experience positive long-term effects from consistent use of MPH in their personal and professional lives (handling of stress, task completion, organization, and so on). Tolerance to the drug was not evidenced and when tapered, adults re-experienced symptoms with the same degree of severity as premedication status. Gadow et al. (1995) found that MPH did not lead to a worsening of a previously diagnosed tic disorder and ratings indicated some improvement noted with the frequency of motor and vocal tics. It may be possible that MPH reduced stress due to its impact on symptoms of the attentional disorder, which then had a positive impact on the degree of tics observed.

Ritalin is not a "happy pill", and will only serve to increase cognitive or thinking abilities. Thus, the individual should look for results in thinking abilities, whether that is the ability to focus on a task for a longer period of time, process information, and be aware of what is going on around them, not be as distracted, and thinking processes may be faster. The idea is to maximize the dosage within allowable levels until some change in thinking patterns is observed and then to decrease the dose if there are effects from the medication that resemble "speed" effects.

Clinically, we have found via patient report that sustained release used by itself does not produce noticeable effects; however, for those individuals who tend to overmetabolize, whereby the medication is out of their system in approximately 1 to 2 hours as opposed to 4, benefit occurs from the combined use of regular and sustained release. The most effective combination has been to take the regular and sustained-release medications together for the first initial dose, followed by a subsequent dose of the regular after approximately 6 to 7 hours. Generally, this has been a positive combination; however, some individuals have needed to use the combination on a more-frequent basis. Reports from patients as to generic use consistently yielded information that it does not work as well and for adults there appears to be an extremely high degree of agitation and anxiety-like symptoms that accompany its use. Finally, we have found Ritalin to be effective in use with children as young as 2 years of age with no reported problematic effects, and individuals as old as 80 years of age. Mayes et al. (1994) confirmed beneficial effects of MPH for preschool children, as well as children with co-existing neurological disorders.

There is little in the research to suggest the abuse of MPH, although one case was documented presenting intranasal abuse of the medication (Jaffe, 1991; Sarkar and Kornetsky, 1995). Braver and de Wit (1995) evaluated the role of using an animal population and found MAMP (methamphetamine) to significantly lower the threshold for stimulation and have rewarding properties similar to other abused drugs. Dopamine, in either subjective or objective reinforcing effects, pinpointed the impact of amphetamines on humans. Concerns were raised by these animal studies as to the eliciting conditions for abuse. However, overall, results suggested a limited role for dopamine in the subjective effects of D-amphetamine in normal volunteers and effects originally believed to be associated with abuse potential and mediated by the dopamine system were not observed. Dopamine may mediate the reinforcing, but not the euphorigenic effects of stimulants in humans. Finally, the authors warned of the problems of generalizing animal studies to that of humans.

Schubiner et al. (1995) report successful use of MPH with substance abusers, citing the role of the self-medication theory of abuse as explanation for the drug's effectiveness in maintaining abstinence. There were no differences found between boys aged 6 to 16 years diagnosed with ADHD and controls in parameters of the growth-hormone (GH) axis (fasting serum GH levels, GH-binding protein activity, or insulin-like growth factor 1 levels) when treated with MPH. Findings of a study conducted by Toren et al. (1997) provide further confirming evidence that the use of MPH does not have a long-lasting impact upon growth rate. Research indicates that ADHD mediates growth issues, appearing temporarily through midadolescence and resolving itself by late adolescence, unrelated to medical management (Spencer et al., 1996). A report, via questionnaire to physicians (pediatric neurologists and clinic directors) utilizing CNS stimulants in clinical practice, indicated the adverse effects of Ritalin at relatively low percentages although confirmed the ability of this medication to either exacerbate or bring an underlying disorder into existence (personality changes occurred in 7%, tics in 5%, weight loss in 4%, and seizures in less than 1% of the population studied). Ritalin was the most favored (90%) yet Cylert and Dexedrine were equally favored as a second choice. The mean maximum dose was 52 mg (range of 25 to 85 mg) with drug holidays for weekends and vacations recommended by 65% of the physicians. Duration of medical management as treatment was from 1 to 5 years with an average of 3.5 years, resulting in the claim of overuseage remaining unsupported (Millichap, 1997).

To address the issue that is often raised in the general population, Ward et al. (1997) investigated the effects of D-amphetamine on the normal population. Many individuals are diagnosed ADD depending upon the individual's response to medication and if the response is positive and the person displays some of the behavioral symptoms or cognitive complaints associated with this disorder, then the diagnosis is subsequently made. Another issue often raised, is that use of stimulant medication can somehow acquire addictive properties, resulting in overuse and misuse. Findings indicate that the use of D-amphetamine increased performance capacity without stimulant-like effects in *normal* subjects. There were no indications of stimulation, anxiety, or a decrease in sedation.

Redman and Zametkin (1991) found increased levels of brain metabolism with the use of stimulants. Pelham et al. (1992) found that ADHD symptoms improved with administration of MPH. ADHD boys, however, attributed their behavior to effort rather than to the medication. When not on medication, attributions for failure were to the *pill* or to some other person or thing. This tends to be a more classic response of this population and a consequence of the impaired functioning of the frontal processes, whereby they under- or overestimate their behaviors and are subject to continual misattributions. Authors concluded that the ADHD boys needed to have this attributional state to avoid the severe effects on their self-esteem. Overall findings of this study did report large beneficial behavioral effects of the stimulant medication, and the ADHD boys reported themselves happier and liked themselves more on the days when they received the medication as opposed to placebo. Consistent with prior data, recent research by Pelham and Associates (1997) confirms that the pharmacological activity of MPH positively and significantly impacts the self-evaluation and persistence of ADHD children (evidenced as significant in task persistence following failure) and contradicts the idea that this form of treatment is a causal factor in dysfunctional attributions and/or in the production of adverse effects. Children were found to generate internal attributions for success or external attributions for failure irregardless of medication. The concept of medication-mediated success benefiting future performance in ADHD children is proposed. ADHD symptoms were found to be less apparent when the child was engaged in an externally stimulating activity such as television or playing video games, although their behavior was still not within normal limits and symptoms of restlessness, inattentiveness, and being overly, talkative, continued to be observed during these intrinsically stimulating activities. Stimulant medication did produce the expected behavioral improvement, however, had no clear impact upon game performance (Tannock, 1997). Granger, Whalen, and Henker (1993) found overall more positive than negative behaviors when comparing medication to placebo to measure effects of methylphenidate on the interactions of ADHD boys. There was evidence provided of the medication increasing controlled behaviors, compliance, less aggression and disruption. Medication changes were salient enough to attract the attention of adult observers even when not cued by rating scales. MPH has historically produced significantly less hyperactive behavior than use of placebo or antecedent exercise (Barkley, 1993; Silverstein and Allison, 1994). Ritalin was found to increase alertness and cognition demonstrating a significant reduction of hyperactivity and impulsivity. It did not, however, provide significant changes in nonattentional behavioral symptoms (Drak, Johnson, and Clark, 1997). The use of Ritalin revealed increased performance on cognitive measures impacting at least one of the following in a positive direction, verbal learning or memory, and auditory or visual attention (Drak, Johnson, and Clark, 1997). Murphy, Pelham, and Lang (1992) noted a difference in the effects of MPH on observed aggression, citing more positive findings of decreased aggression on direct observation measures versus a laboratory provocation task. MPH effects were less responsive on social information processing measures implicating that social deficits may be due to issues of inattention and impulsivity and not aggression.

Hinshaw, McHale, and Heller (1992) found that methylphenidate resulted in a significant reduction of stealing and property destruction behaviors; however, also served to enhance cheating, which authors attributed to enhancement of task involvement. Although use of medication significantly reduced covert actions of stealing and property destruction, authors speculated as to its long-term impact, given that covert behaviors and delinquency are deeply embedded in cultural and familial networks and as such are not amenable to intervention directed solely to the child. MPH was found to affect the accuracy of processing on a sustained attention task, as well as the speed of processing on focused and divided attention tasks. MPH improved vigilance aspects of sustained attention and enhanced selective search abilities (de Sonneville, Njionktjen, and Hilhorst, 1991). There was some amelioration of symptoms of right-hemisphere dysfunction, left visual-field neglect noted to produce reading difficulties and learning disabilities with the use of MPH (Malone et al., 1994). ADHD boys responded similarly to treatment, regardless of the diagnosis of comorbid conduct disorder. Use of MPH was found to improve focused and sustained attention, vigilance, impulsivity, and the use of feedback as measured on neuropsychological tests and was not found to be effective on conventional psychological tests (de Sonneville, Njionktjen, and Bos, 1994).

Medication has had a significant impact on classroom behavior for the ADHD population. Typically, MPH has been an effective intervention evidencing increased attention span, impulse control, academic performance, and improved peer relationships (DuPaul et al., 1991). MPH increased event-related potential (ERP) waves for parietal functioning and improved selective attention (Verbaten et al., 1994). Pelham et al. (1993) evaluated the effects of MPH on behavior of ADHD boys in a summer treatment program for classroom behavior and academic performance. Findings revealed significant effects for both behavior and learning in the classroom setting and, more importantly, there was relatively small incremental value gained by the higher dose of medication or the addition of behavior modification, compared with the effects of the low dose of MPH. The exact effects of MPH have been unclear. Balthazor, Wagner, and Pelham (1991) attempted to isolate the exact issues that this medication impacts and found that MPH overall has an effect on general aspects of information processing, thus aiding academic learning. MPH was shown to be effective by the middle of the learning curve for nonverbal learning tasks (O'Toole et al., 1996). Rapoport et al. (1994) found MPH positive in normalizing classroom behavior, but not necessarily resulting in the improvement of academic functioning. Improper dosage when corrected indicated improved behavior. The need for supplemental interventions is suggested. This study supports the idea that MPH is not the whole answer and needs to be supplemented by other treatment, development of coping mechanisms, strategies and learning or increasing skills of basic academic functioning. Additionally, the idea of dosage specificity is proposed as being necessary for attentional processes to improve sufficiently enough to attain gains in academic functioning beyond what may be necessary for appropriate classroom behavior. What may be reported as positive effects of medication may in fact still be reflective of underdosing sufficient to improve behavioral functioning, but not cognitive deficits. Stoner et al. (1994) were successful in an initial attempt to develop a curriculum-based measurement of math and reading to evaluate MPH dosage.

Carlson and Bunner (1993) conducted a review of the literature on the effects of MPH on diagnosed ADHD subjects and found that it does result in immediate improvements in various academic tasks. Medication was not found to impact reading performance, and it was suggested that it could not correct extreme deficits and a 24-month lag of acquired abilities. It was proposed that the stimulant medication may impact milder disabilities as opposed to the more severe deficits. Dosage was found to impact accurate completion of work in language arts and mathematics assignments with a linear trend. Sustained release was also found to reveal significant effects on children's independent seatwork. Long-term benefits of medication were not found; however, this may simply illustrate the need for medication in addition to and in combination with other interventions. Finally, there are methodological problems that may have impacted these findings. Klorman et al. (1994) found that the use of methylphenidate and the combination of maturation promoted more efficient strategic skills to cope with symptoms of ADD for children diagnosed with ADD and ADD/aggression/oppositionality. Stimulant treatment overall improved children's behavior at home and in school, impacting the full range of symptoms associated with these subtypes from inattention to hyperactivity, aggression and oppositionality. Stimulant treatment was positive across all ages measured (5.6 to 11.9 years).

Barkley, DuPaul, and McMurray (1991) conducted one of the few studies to compare the response of children diagnosed as ADD vs. those diagnosed as ADHD on methylphenidate. Results indicated decreased errors in a continuous-performance task, improved observed behavior during the performance of an academic task, and improved accuracy during a math task. There were no significant differences of medication response between the two groups.

Pelham (1993), in his review of studies conducted using MPH, found short-term positive effects beyond that of the behavioral treatments similar to other reviews. He also noted that the beneficial effects on peer interaction has contributed to a trend to provide a third daily dose of medication and to medicate on the weekend in order to impact children's behavior when they are with their peers, in organized sports with adults, and activities in general. Irritability, loss of appetite, and insomnia were found to be the most common adverse reactions. Other symptoms such as stomachaches were found to dissipate with repeated administration. A small number of children were found to experience a negative rebound effect in the evening hours or what might be referred to as a return to baseline behavior. Stimulant medication can also cause cognitive overfocusing, blunting, and social withdrawal, and can exacerbate or precipitate motor tics. Other symptoms occurring with less frequency are that of nausea, dizziness, headaches, tachycardia, skin rashes, and drowsiness. Finally, Pelham notes that children's responses to stimulants vary in magnitude and direction across tasks and situations, making it difficult to identify global responders and non-responders based on only a few measures. Evans, Vallano, and Pelham (1994) found that treatment with MPH improved the mother's ability to manage her son's behavior consistently and reduced negative feedback situations.

Solanto and Wender (1989), in studying ADHD children, found an atypical subgroup that became overaroused and exhibited perseveration, which may represent overdosing. Generally, however, there was increased cognitive flexibility and an increase in productivity. Tannock and Schachar (1992) also noted the emergence of symptoms of cognitive perseveration in children and MPH was found to reduce cognitive flexibility temporarily in some ADHD children.

Findings are mixed regarding the effectiveness of methylphenidate in the treatment of closed head-injury individuals on measures of attention, learning and cognitive processing speed, and behavioral correlates (Clark et al., 1990; Speech et al., 1993). MPH was found to increase cognitive function and behavior and to improve arousal in pediatric head injury with ages varying from 3 to 16 years (in one case), from mild to severe in level of severity of injury. Improvement was noted just subsequent to injury as well as up to 50 months post injury, revealing improvements for both the acute and chronic periods following head injury. The most frequently noted side effects were a loss of appetite and sleep disturbance (with this issue being minimized by the last dose occurring in the early afternoon) resulting in MPH being seen as an effective treatment for TBI (Hoynyak, Nelson and Hurvitz, 1997). Tic severity was higher on high-dose dextroamphetamine than on the high-dose methylphenidate (Castellanos et al., 1997). Efficacy of MPH for this population was increased by the addition of behavioral interventions (Johnson et al., 1994). There were adverse side effects of methylphenidate among mentally retarded children with ADHD due to the appearance of motor tics and severe social withdrawal, suggesting that this population is at risk for development of underlying disorders. Higher functioning children had more positive effects than lower functioning mentally retarded children (Aman et al., 1991; Handen et al., 1991). Use of Ritalin was found to have an overall positive effect on independent play and academic functioning in dually diagnosed mental retardation and ADHD (Harden et al., 1995). However, methylphenidate has been found useful to remediate symptoms of ADHD when accompanied by another comorbid disorder such as borderline personality disorder (van Reekum and Links, 1994). Ritalin was found to improve the severe neurobehavioral slowing resulting from cancer and cancer treatment impacting frontal and brain stem regions. Uniform improvement in mood was also noted (Weitzner, Meyers, and Valentine, 1995). Ritalin has been successful for use with the autistic population to address associated comorbid symptoms of attentional problems (Wiznitzer, 1995).

Dexedrine (D-Amphetamine, Dextroamphetamine) is used in approximately 4 to 6% of those on stimulant medication for attention disorders. It has been found to be appropriate for children who utilized MPH as children and now find it no longer effective as adolescents or adults. Dexedrine has traditionally been the only stimulant medication recommended for children aged 3 to 6 years and has been found to improve sustained attention during play and in structured group activity. Dexedrine has both a short- and long-acting version with either rapid onset similar to that of Ritalin (short-acting) or longer-lasting Dexedrine spansules for coverage of up to 6 to 8 hours. There appears to be greater efficacy with the sustained release version of Dexedrine than that found with Ritalin. We have found some addictive properties commensurate with weight loss. Additionally, emotionally fragile individuals may experience a frightening increase in underlying emotions. As with MPH, emotional disorders can be exacerbated with use of Dexedrine. Dexedrine should not be used or used with caution if there is evidence of cardiovascular disease, hypertension, hyperthyroidism, glaucoma, hypersensitivity, and agitation. Gastrointestinal acidifying agents, such as orange juice or gastric juices, decrease the absorption of the amphetamines. Dexedrine may be given after meals to reduce the potential for headaches or stomachaches. There is a rebound similar to that of MPH (Alessandri and Schramm, 1991; Copeland, 1991; Shaywitz and Shaywitz, 1991; Elia and Rapoport, 1991). In its long-acting form, there can be an initial spike experienced as agitation or sedation (Wender, 1995).

D-Amphetamine was compared to the effects of Clonidine and Yohimbine on rates of information processing using normal subjects, and suggests greater effect of speed of the processing of information via facilitation of attentional capacity allocation to specific targets, whereas the norepinephrine medications acted on early stimulus processing (Halliday et al., 1994). Sarbuck,

Bleiberg, and Kay (1995) noted positive aspects in treating attentional deficits in head injury due to D-amphetamine's direct impact on the allocation of resources creating improved efficiency of functioning. The idea of dextro-amphetamine enhancing the response of head-injured and stroke patients' response to rehabilitation suggests the use of this medication as a valuable treatment approach. One mechanism by which it exerts its effect remains nonspecific, but the theory proposed that the enhanced catecholaminergic activity with increased alertness, concentration, initiative, and motor activity enhances learning and retention of compensatory techniques taught in the therapeutic rehabilitation. The amphetamine action was also proposed to augment neuronal plasticity and regeneration (Hornstein et al., 1996). It is suggested that adequate trials of both MPH and Dexedrine occur prior to attempting treatment with nonstimulants. March, Wells, and Conners (1995) suggest a mixed trial of a stimulant medication, Cylert, be implemented prior to implementation of a medication with less benefit for treatment.

Cylert is the newest stimulant available and least favored due to a lack of trial and effectiveness. This, in addition to the side effects of possible liver dysfunction, makes Cylert a third or fourth choice for medication. Cylert has only minimal effects on the autonomic nervous system and operates via stimulation of the dopaminergic mechanism.

Contrary to the above medications, while rapidly absorbed, this is a long-acting medication that lasts from 7 to 8 hours and attains its peak in 2 or 3 hours. Maximum therapeutic effectiveness may take a range of 3 to 8 weeks. Since it does have a build-up, it should be discontinued gradually. Finally, Cylert is not approved for children under 6 years of age and can result in decreased seizure threshold. Best response is administration with a morning and noon dosage, schedule, continued on the weekends. There is no rebound effect, although insomnia and liver damage may occur. Transient side effects are weight loss, insomnia, anorexia, stomach aches and/or nausea (Copeland, 1991; Wender, 1995). Sallee, Stiller, and Perel (1992) found more positive effects for pemoline in that its effect on neuroprocessing was apparent within the first 2 hours after administration, as measured on tasks indicating more efficient memory search and paired-associate learning. A pilot investigation suggests its usefulness in reducing symptoms of conduct disorders for children diagnosed with ADHD/CD and an adjunctive to MPH used solely for MPH non-responders (Shah et al., 1994). Cylert, found to have less addictive properties, was suggested as a medication of choice for substance abusers. This medication was effective in treatment of MS-related fatigue (Elovic, 1996).

Fenfluramine hydrochloride (Ponderal, Pondimin, Ponderax) stimulates the ventromedial nucleus of the hypothalamus and may also impact serotonin metabolism. Fenfluramine is a potent 5-HT-releasing agent *in vitro* and despite the specificity for the serotonergic system, considerable data now indicate that high doses do have effects on the dopaminergic system *in vivo* (Cho and Segal, 1994). Fenfluramine is a halogenated derivative of amphetamine and there is a question as to neurotoxic effects in its depletion of neuronal serotonin. Kapur et al. (1994) report that fenfluramine modulates ongoing neuronal activity with the consequence of a relative increase in metabolism in the prefrontal cortex and relative decrease in occipital temporal regions with reported subjective feelings of activation and euphoria in normal subjects.

Aman et al. (1993) compared the effects of fenfluramine and methylphenidate on mentally impaired children in their performance of tasks of selective and sustained attention visual matching and color matching. Results indicated that fenfluramine is superior to the placebo on the memory task, whereby MPH was more effective on the sustained-attention task. Behavior rating indicated improved performance with other medication on the variables of attention, activity level and mood. Data indicate that fenfluramine may be moderately useful with both mental retardation and ADHD. Findings remain mixed, however, and not nearly as clear, nor as obvious, with the normal population and use of MPH. Methylphenidate, according to the authors, appears to result in arousal both physiologically and attentionally, whereas fenfluramine appears to depress heart rate and blood pressure, and in this study had no impact on vigilance. Finally, MPH tended to reduce response time and fenfluramine resulted in increased reaction time. Fenfluramine has been found successful in controlling panic attacks and depression and has been implicated in the treatment of obesity and obsessive-compulsive disorder (Solyon, 1994; Jenike and Rauch, 1994; Max et al., 1994). It was shown to have some positive effects on cognitive spatial memory tasks (Jansen and Andrews, 1994).

Dextrostat (Dextroamphetamine sulfate), a recently introduced version of Dexedrine, provides cost savings and increased flexibility with 2.5 mg dosage. This form of Dexedrine has been useful in non-responders on other stimulants.

Adderall (mixed salts of a single-entity amphetamine product), removed from sale after being initially well received, has recently received approval for use for treatment of ADD and narcolepsy. We have found Adderall to be an excellent alternative for Ritalin non-responders. Adderall has a therapeutic response to obesity, providing weight loss to those individuals who gained weight on Ritalin and/or are obese. Available in 10 and 20 mg, flexible dosing varies from every 4 to 12 hours, depending on the absorption rate. Common side effects are that of insomnia, loss of appetite, stomach pain, headache, irritability, and weight loss. Side effects similar to that of the other stimulants may disappear after several days and/or deceased dosage. Effects upon the cognitive and behavioral aspects of ADD are similar to that of Ritalin and Dexedrine.

Second Choice Medications: The Antidepressants

The antidepressants, in addition to other medications, are being trialed to address symptoms of ADD when the stimulant medication, for a variety of reasons, is not a viable option. Research is underway to investigate the usefulness of nicotine, decongestant medications, caffeine, and other substances.

The antidepressants can be used to treat attention disorders in addition to comorbid symptoms of bedwetting, migraine headaches, eating disorders, and obsessive-compulsive disorders. Wilens et al. (1995) present findings suggestive of the usefulness of combining stimulant medications and the antidepressants to address comorbid symptoms of ADD for a full-treatment approach. Interestingly, subjects used in their study were identified ADHD and it is proposed that prior problematic results on stimulant medication alone were the result of symptoms related to the disorder of ADD, which was then ameliorated by additional medication. Weiss (1996) indicated a concern regarding the increasing use of polypharmacy with diagnosed ADD children to treat underlying comorbid factors and stressed the need for further rigorous research. A variety of combinations being used with stimulants are that of Clonidine, tricyclics, Risperidome, Guanfacine, and Venlafaxine.

Antidepressants operate by inhibiting the re-uptake of and increasing the concentration of neurotransmitters enabling more efficient transmission. Some block the re-uptake of norepinephrine and some of serotonin, preventing their re-uptake back into the presynaptic neuronal vesicles. Pelham (1993), in his review of medication effects on ADHD, did not foresee antidepressants as useful in long-term treatment. Wilens et al. (1993) noted in their clinical experience that TCAs are useful, specifically desipramine and nortriptyline.

Clinically, we have found the antidepressants to be useful in treatment of vulnerability to distractibility from the internal and external environment, and less behavioral distractibility and tendency to wander from task to task. In the next chapter, the antidepressants commonly used with the attention-disordered population will be discussed further.

CHAPTER 14

Treatment: Antidepressants as the Second Line of Defense to Address Underlying Comorbid Conditions/Other Possible Medical-Management Solutions*

Tricyclic Antidepressants, First Generation

Imipramine (Tofranil) can be used for children 6 years and older and has had a beneficial effect on bedwetting. It blocks the re-uptake of serotonin.

Tofranil requires a build-up for maximum effectiveness. Improvement usually occurs within 2 to 3 days. Children who react to stimulants can benefit from subclinical doses of Tofranil taken at bedtime or in divided doses morning and noon. Tofranil is helpful for those who are anxious, have sleep problems or who have a disturbance of mood or affect with their attention disorder.

Similarly, those described as angry and aggressive have been helped with this medication. There is extreme danger if overdosed and treatment needs to begin with lower doses and increased. There is no rebound effect. Most common side effects in children are nervousness, sleep disturbance, fatigue, and mild gastrointestinal disturbances. It also has the potential to cause neurological, psychiatric, allergic, and endocrine side effects as well. The risks associated with these medications are greater than those of the stimulants. If there is a familial history of tics or seizures, use of imipramine may exacerbate the emergence of motor and vocal tics (Parraga and Cochran, 1992).

---

*The following represents selected medications more commonly used with the stimulants to address underlying comorbid symptoms.

253

Pelham (1993) found in his review of the research and the effect of medication on ADHD symptoms that imipramine benefited some children, but the effects overall were not as positive as with methylphenidate (MPH) and the side effects were a subject of concern. Hunt, Lau, and Ryu (1991) found a slight therapeutic advantage with the stimulants; however, behavioral response to imipramine was nearly equivalent. Imipramine was found to improve ADHD symptoms, insomnia and enuresis in a child with fragile X syndrome (Hilton et al., 1991).

Nortriptyline (Pamelor) appears to be a potent, activating antidepressant thought to inhibit the activity of serotonin and acetylcholine and increase the pressor effect of norepinephrine. This medication was found to have positive effects in ADHD adolescents who had responded poorly to stimulants and teacher reports indicated most significantly a decrease of impulsivity (Hunt et al., 1991).

Wilens et al. (1993) evaluated the potential benefit of Nortriptyline in the treatment of children and adolescent treatment-resistant ADHD individuals; 76% of the subjects were considered to have a moderate to marked improvement in symptoms. There was a linear relationship between the dosage and small increases in heart rate and EKG parameters significant of the onset of asymptotic sinus tachycardia. In treatment of ADHD and chronic tic disorder, Nortriptyline had significantly improved ADHD symptoms without major adverse effects (Spencer et al., 1993).

Heterocyclic Antidepressants, Second Generation

The primary clinical indication for using heterocyclic antidepressants in children and adolescents has been the diagnosis of enuresis and ADHD (Ryan, 1990).

Desipramine (Norapramin) (DMI) acts similar to Tofranil, but with fewer side effects. It blocks the re-uptake of norepinephrine preferentially. Smaller tablets are recommended for adolescents due to potential for overdosage. It is more effective in divided doses morning and later in the day. This medication is effective for those with anxiety and depression co-occurring with the attention disorder. It has not been approved for children under 12 years of age.

Recent information indicates that there are problematic consequences in the use of this medication. Clinically, we have found side effects from consistent use and some impact to CNS functioning. Biederman et al. (1989) identified small, clinically unimportant, but still statistically significant increases in diastolic blood pressure, heart rate, and electrocardiographic conduction, and warned of treatment with children and the need of close clinical supervision. Tingelstad (1991) found significant effects on the cardiovascular system, such as the development of postural hypotension in children diagnosed with ADD. Werry (1995) noted that Desipramine is 2 to 4 times more poisonous than other tricyclic antidepressants.

A response to Desipramine was found in even the most complex cases of ADHD with associated comorbidity, as well as with simple non-comorbid cases of ADHD (Biederman et al., 1993). Desipramine was found to be well tolerated in treatment of children with chronic tic disorder, evidencing significant improvement in both chronic tic and ADHD symptomatology without major adverse side effects over an average follow up period of 16 months (Spencer et al., 1993). Desipramine was found to facilitate cocaine abstinence in an adolescent diagnosed with ADHD (Kaminer, 1992). At a low dose, when used with an adult diagnosed with ADHD, Desipramine resulted in less anxiety, irritability, impulsivity, and mood fluctuation (Magee, Maier, and Reesal, 1992). Wilens et al. (1993) indicated the positive use of this medication for treatment of ADHD in adults. Hunt et al. (1991) concluded in their review of the research that DMI appears to be effective in treating ADHD; however, the lack of change on cognitive tests indicates that DMI's effect may not occur at such a concrete level and, instead, this medication serves to improve task performance by modulating affect and frustration.

In evaluating individuals on this medication we find only the relief of distractibility present and recently in evaluation of a 13-years-old adolescent there was a question of substantial impact to brain functioning after being on this medication for treatment of ADD symptoms over a period of years.

Serotonin Re-uptake Inhibitors, Third Generation

The newer, selective serotonin re-uptake inhibitors operate by blocking the re-uptake of serotonin back into the system and have been found clinically to be very specific and potent, more so than the older antidepressants. Generally, they do not present the anticholinergic side effects. The SSRIs have been found effective in treatment of unipolar and bipolar depression, atypical depression, panic disorder, obsessive compulsive disorder, social phobia, and post-traumatic stress disorder.

There is a serotonin syndrome being reported when other medications are combined with the SSRIs. Specifically, this will occur with such medications as Pondimin, Adipex, Redux, Ultram, Sinemet, Parlodel, Eldepryl, Demerol, and Lithium. The interaction results in the precipitation of the serotonin syndrome by indirectly causing serotonin release on some manner. Elevated serotonin can result in such symptoms as confusion, disorientation, agitation, irritability, anxiety, euphoria, hyper- or hypoglycemia, nausea, flushing, dilated pupils, sinus tachycardia, and other autonomic nervous systems as well as neuromuscular symptoms. In using polypharmacy (and the additional use of the stimulant medications) prescribers need to be alert to the *Serotonin Syndrome*, which refers to a toxic state that occurs with enhanced serotoninergic neurotransmission, evidencing symptoms of changes in mental status and behavior (medications producing at least three of these symptoms are capable of causing this syndrome: agitation, restlessness, myoclonus, hyperreflexia, shivering, tremor, diarrhea, incoordination, fever, and profuse sweating) (Ivanusa, Hécimovic´, and Demarin, 1997). Clinically with the use of stimulants and the SSRIs this has been observed often by the author. Usually this is more of an issue with Dexedrine and/or Adderall than Ritalin. One exception was the individual taking both Ritalin and Serzone, symptoms were resolved with the reduction of the Serzone to very low levels whereby more of the norepinephrine component was triggered, resulting in successful amelioration of symptoms of overfocusing, depression, and anxiety due to continual worrying behavior.

Fluoxetine (Prozac), an SSRI, was initially hailed as the medication that breathed new life into medical management for treatment of depression and obsessive compulsive disorder, without the troubling side effects of the tricyclic and heterocyclic antidepressants. A risk for seizure disorder and the development of mania has been noted. Fluoxetine takes up to 5 weeks to reach a steady state and there is evidence of this medication exacerbating symptomotology of motor restlessness, sleep disturbance, and social disinhibition, also a subjective state of excitability may be present. It is contraindicated for MAO inhibitors with a mandatory 2-week hiatus before commencing medication. Frequent side effects are nausea, nervousness, headache, insomnia, sexual dysfunction (anorgasmia). (Copeland, 1991; Elia and Rapoport, 1991; Venkataraman, Naylor, and King, 1992; Riddle et al., 1991; Weiss and Walkup, 1997).

Gammon and Brown (1993) tested the combination of Fluoxetine and methylphenidate in an effort to find a safe alternative for ADHD children and adolescents whose symptoms had responded inadequately to stimulant medications. All of the subjects (except one) in the study evidenced a positive therapeutic response to the addition of Fluoxetine to MPH. Results indicate that Fluoxetine augmentation can substantially improve symptoms in some MPH-resistant children with ADHD. Bussing and Levin (1993) found that as the symptoms of a child with a history of obsessive-compulsive symptoms subsided with use of Fluoxetine, symptoms of ADHD increased, and as evaluation revealed the presence of the disorder, dextroamphetamine was added. Following increased reports of hyperactivity, medication was changed to methamphetamine with positive results in combination with the Fluoxetine. Fluoxetine evidenced some moderate success when used only in the treatment of ADHD children and adolescents (Barrickman et al., 1995). Wender (1995) had little success with adult ADHD and Fluoxetine when used alone; however, this medication could effectively treat the comorbid disorder of depression when used conjunctively with stimulants.

Common side effects of *Sertraline (Zoloft)* are nausea, headache, diarrhea, insomnia, dry mouth, ejaculatory delay, drowsiness, dizziness, tremor, fatigue, and increased sweating. Clinically, Zoloft works very well for children, adolescents, and the aged as a mild, relatively safe antidepressant. Frankenberg and Kando (1994) found Zoloft successful as an intervention for ADHD and co-morbid Tourette's Syndrome. Clinically, Zoloft works very well for children, adolescents and the aged as a mild, relatively safe antidepressant. Frankenberg and Kando (1994) found Zoloft successful as an intervention for ADHD and comorbid Tourette's syndrome.

Paroxetine (Paxil) does seem to have a slight affinity for the cholinergic receptors and users may experience some anticholinergic effects as a result; however, unless the person is especially sensitive, effects are not observed in the clinical population. It has been found to effectively and quickly relieve depression and symptoms of anxiety (generally within a few days to one week) . Once-daily dosing of 20 mg makes this a comfortable medication to administer. Dosage is titrated upwards to a maximum dose of 50 mg per day. Multiple doses of Paroxetine results in the half-life being extended to 7 to 10 days (Weiss and Walkup, 1997).

Common side effects are nausea, sweating, weakness, sleepiness, nausea, ejaculatory disturbance and other male genital disorders, somnolence, asthma, dizziness, insomnia, tremor, anxiety, cough, sedation, and headache. Bidman, Sherling, and Brunn (1995) found a severe case of development of extrapyramidal side effects (dystonic reaction) to combined treatment of Paxil and Haldol.

There may be a possibility of an interaction with Imitrex and it is recommended when switching from Prozac or Zoloft that this occur in a cautious progression. Paxil was found to provide treatment for generalized social phobia. Relapse rates were high if the medication was discontinued too early. Treatment of approximately six months was effective for abating symptoms of social phobia (Stein et al., 1996).

Buspirone (Buspar)

Buspirone (Buspar) is a novel benzodiazepine anxiolytic that is theorized to work through its serotonergic agonist activity at the 5-HT receptor. This medication is also noted to be presynaptically antagonistic at the D2 dopaminergic receptor. The main side effects are dizziness, headache, nervousness, and light-headedness (Zasler, 1992). This medication was found to have a positive effect in the treatment of aggression (Cassidy, 1994). Buspirone was found to produce significant improvement in impulsivity and hyperactivity, but was not beneficial for cognitive deficits; however, it worked well in combination with MPH for a 6-year-old boy (Mandoki, 1994).

Generally this medication has been found to benefit children and adolescents with generalized anxiety disorder. Buspar has not been found to impair psychomotor or cognitive functioning. There is little or none in the way of an euphoric effect and it is not subject to abuse (Kutcher and Gardner, 1996).

Fourth-Generation Antidepressants

Fluvoxamine maleate (Luvox) is a new antidepressant similar to Venlafaxine that recently became available. Luvox is the newest of the SSRI agents with relatively low incidence of anticholinergic effects. The most commonly adverse reactions are that of somnolence, insomnia, nervousness, nausea, abnormal ejaculation, and asthma. There is a tendency for drowsiness, therefore bedtime administration is suggested. It cannot be used with MAO inhibitors. Heavily trialed overseas, it was brought into the States recently and is showing mixed results, clinically working well when it works. Targeted treatment is that of obsessive-compulsive disorder. However, it has been found to be quite useful for treatment of panic attacks, panic disorder, and generalized anxiety. van Vljiet et al. (1996) found that Luvox leads to a reduction of panic attacks as well as a subsequent reduction of symptoms related to agoraphobia. Symptom relief was similar in effectiveness to that of the MAO inhibitors.

Bupropion (Wellbutrin) weakly blocks the neuronal uptake of serotonin and norepinephrine and may possibly be a weak dopamine agonist. It has been advocated as a means of treatment for ADHD without the abuse potential, producing similar levels of improvement of symptoms equal to that of MPH. Research, however, indicates an absence of behavioral change in the home setting, nor was there any improvement detected in measures of cognitive performance; however, teachers reported significant reduction of classroom hyperactivity. The main side effects consisted of skin rash, tremor, and periodic edema, and thus it appears to be safe, but not effective in prepubertal children. The most important adverse reaction is seizure and activating side effects. When studied with the adolescent population, there was an improvement to a significant degree in behavior and major side effects were mild nausea, stomach discomfort, increased appetite, and vomiting. This suggests that the medication may be useful for treatment of hyperactivity if associated with conduct disorder. Finally, a larger study failed to confirm significant effects on ADD symptoms (Hunt et al., 1991). Recently, further studies are indicating positive effects of this medication, and it is being used in the attention-disordered population. Clinically, we have not found beneficial effects equalizing the stimulants, although some individuals do report feeling better and being less distractible on this medication. Jacobsen, Chappell, and Woolston (1994) described the case of a child who developed repetitive, compulsive behavior, both after the administration of D-amphetamine and the administration of Bupropion for ADHD and casts doubt on the use of this drug for individuals vulnerable to obsessive-compulsive disorder or tics.

Other studies concur that Bupropion is not an appropriate alternative to stimulants in the treatment of ADHD due to exacerbation of tics (Spencer et al., 1993). Wender (1995), in addressing the use of Bupropion from a clinical viewpoint in adults with ADHD, sees this medication as more effective than other antidepressants, although it is not always effective in treatment and symptoms associated with the attentional disorder, and advises the combination with the stimulants if symptoms are not ameliorated. Found effective in treatment of mood and temper, it appeared less effective in its impact on symptoms such as concentration, hyperactivity, disorganization, and impulsivity.

Clinically, we have found *Venlafaxine (Effexor)* highly useful in treating anxiety, depression, and the overfocused subtype of ADD used in conjunction with the stimulants. If tolerated well (and this is variable), this medication serves to specifically impact distractibility, both behavioral and vulnerability to distractibility (being distracted) from the internal and external environment, in addition to resolving symptoms of both depression and anxiety within a relatively short period of time. Effexor is a serotonin and norepinephrine re-uptake inhibitor and weak inhibitor of dopamine re-uptake. It is contraindicated for MAO inhibitors and works within several days to one week in most cases. The most common adverse effects are nausea, somnolence, dry mouth, dizziness, constipation, nervousness, sweating, asthma, abnormal ejaculation/orgasm, and anorexia. In one particular case, Effexor did stimulate seizure activity of the motoric type and this medication, in addition to Serzone does appear to be particularly sensitive to the serotoninergic syndrome. It addresses in a very effective manner symptoms of the overfocused subtype, specifically tendencies to overworry, overfocus, and overreact to emotional stimuli. It can become highly problematic with some cases, requiring immediate cessation due to activating side effects (generally overly fragile, highly emotionally labile patients). Schweitzer et al. (1994) found Effexor to be comparable to the tricyclics without the accompanying side effects. Studies are just beginning to occur with children and reports are favorable. Recent studies indicate that children are metabolizing Effexor more quickly than adolescents or adults. Children with ADHD in these preliminary studies are evidencing improvement behaviorally (even with the more serious problem of conduct disorder). This medication is being seen as a second line of defense for treatment of ADD. The trend for children is the effect on behavioral symptoms to a greater degree than depression (Ferguson, 1995; Pliszka, 1995; Mandoki, 1994). Wilens et al. (1995) see this medication as possibly promising for treatment of adult ADHD.

Similar to Effexor, *Nefazodone HCl (Serzone)* addresses the problem of impotency with little incidence of sexual dysfunction. Patients can experience some adverse side effects similar to Effexor, which occur rather quickly, requiring cessation. Minimal drug-induced anxiety, agitation, and insomnia can occur in addition to asthma, dizziness, and light-headedness. This medication provides effective relief of depression and comorbid panic disorders, anxiety associated with depression, as well as addressing symptoms of the overfocused subtype with tendencies to overreact, overworry and overfocus. Insomnia, fever, and night awakenings are noted. Serzone is related to the other antidepressants with a chemical structure similar to that of Desyrel. It blocks NE reuptake and blocks serotonin postsynaptically and inhibits presynaptic serotonin reuptake. Side effects most often resulting in discontinuation are that of nausea, dizziness, insomnia, weakness, and agitation. Bipolar patients if not treated at the time of taking this medication, may evidence a manic episode. Relief of symptoms of depression may be attained anywhere from 1 to 2 weeks and within 4 weeks of the onset of treatment (Goldberg, 1995). When side effects of dry mouth, sedation, nausea, dizziness, weakness, and agitation can be tolerated, we have found this medication excellent in decreasing obsessive, overfocused, circular thinking.

Monoamine Oxidase Inhibitors

Monoamine oxidase (MAO) inhibitors have great potential benefit for very impulsive ADHD children and adolescents, and have evidenced positive results for symptoms of social phobia, which is more characteristic of ADD. The MAO class of psychiatric medications include phenelyzine (Nardil), isocarboxazid (Marplan), and tranylcypromine (Parnate). The therapeutic effects of MAO inhibitors appear to be linked to their ability to increase the availability of the neurotransmitters norepinephrine, serotonin, and dopamine. The drugs accomplish this by inhibiting the naturally occurring MAO enzyme (monoamine oxidase) that causes the degradation of these neurotransmitters.

A factor weighing against the use of MAO inhibitors is the problem of dietary restrictions that accompany use of the drugs: certain foods, if high in the amino acid tyramine, can interact with the MAO inhibitor to produce increases in blood pressure to the point of critical levels. Taking MAO inhibitors together with SSRIs can result in a potentially fatal metabolic crisis called the serotonin syndrome. Other adverse effects of the MAO inhibitors include danger of hypertensive episodes, insomnia, overstimulation or fatigue, mania, dry mouth, dizziness, constipation, and, on rare occasions, liver toxicity. MAO inhibitors are favorable in the use of panic attacks, and for remediation of intractable anxiety, social phobias, and atypical depressions. A watch-out period of 7 to 14 days is highly encouraged in general when children are placed on this medication.

Hunt, Lau, and Ryu (1991) found MAO inhibitors effective in treatment of ADHD children. Wender, Wood, and Reimherr (1991) found this medication helpful for adults suffering from ADHD–residual type. Wilens et al. (1995) suggest that the MAO inhibitors may have beneficial effects for the treatment of refractory, non-impulsive adult ADHD subjects with comorbid depression and anxiety who are able to comply with the stringent dietary restrictions. Here again, differences in ADHD and ADD present themselves in that in all probability ADHD individuals (defined as being out of control) would not follow such restrictions, nor would they exhibit the anxiety and panic seen with the ADD population who would be in need of MAO inhibitors due to the degree of anxiety exacerbated by the stimulants.

Mirtazapine (Remeron) a Class by Itself

Remeron is a recently released medication which provides a novel noradrenergic and serotonergic pharmacological action. It has been clinically accepted as an excellent medication to address symptoms of the moderately and severely depressed. Due to its unique pharmacology, it remains devoid of anticholinergic, adrenolytic, and serotoninergic side effects. The most frequently reported adverse events are that of transient sedation and weight gain (Burrows and Kremer, 1997). It is designed to provide relief of symptoms of depression and anxiety, similar to that of the MAO inhibitors, with a minimal degree of side effects. The action is to block the 5-HT2 and 5-HT3 receptors, this medication then stimulates the release of norepinephrine and serotonin. It cannot be administered with an MAO inhibitor due to the similarity of action. Clinical improvement with a high dose of Remeron was found to consistently abate symptoms of major depression. Problems occurring with the higher dosage was due to side effects of dizziness and nausea. Better results may occur with a more gradual titration (Rickels et al., 1996).

Antihypertensives

Catapres (Clonidine) has been recently found to be helpful in highly aroused, overactive children who responded poorly to methylphenidate or Dexedrine or have persistent side effects from these medications. This medication has also been found to be beneficial for children who exhibit signs of conduct disorder, oppositional behavior, aggression, and explosiveness. Clinically, it has been found to have little effect on attentional processes (Bauer, 1994).

Overfocused children and adolescents who experience an adverse effect with stimulant use benefit, as well as it tends to reduce side effects of stimulant. Overfocused is defined as that child who is excessively deliberate, has difficulty changing activities, and can be very compulsive and rigid. The use of clonidine resulted in improvement in treatment of ADHD alone and ADHD with tic symptoms and subjects with ADHD and comorbid tic disorders had a more positive behavioral response (Steingard et al., 1993). Clonidine has been helpful for sleep disturbances due to its sedation qualities commonly reported by ADHD children, adolescents and adults (Wilens, Biederman, and Spencer, 1994). Generally, symptoms related to the overfocused subtype of ADD are excessive worry and anxiety, creating a continual restlessness and cyclical emotional process that creates sleep disturbances due to the unrelenting thinking and re-thinking. Deprived sleep only predisposes the individual to a cascade of future problems physically and emotionally. In another study, symptoms of ADHD were treated successfully with Clonidine; however, the individuals continued to experience tics, Clonazepam was added and this addition resulted in the successful reduction of tics as well as sustained behavioral improvement (Steingard et al., 1994).

Clonidine reduces the release of neurotransmission and the intensity of arousal. It inhibits norepinephrine release partially through presynaptic inhibition of locus coeruleus firing and thereby reduces basal brain arousal. This reduced arousal, according to Hunt et.al. (1991), allows background noise to be diminished and reduces the amount of stimuli that must be processed. Clonidine has been found to have an impact on thinking functions and provide support for the role of norepinephrine in attention, the role of the locus coeruleus (LC) in selective attention, inhibiting some activity while alternating another activity (gating mechanism) (Penny, Holder, and Meck, 1996).

It is usually begun in very low doses and gradually increased. The most noticeable side effect is that of drowsiness that occurs 34 to 90 minutes after administration. Sleepiness and fatigue may last for several weeks. If this continues to be problematic medication may require adjustment. Hypotension requires that blood pressure be carefully monitored. Other side effects are transient, including headaches, dizziness, stomachaches, and nausea. Rebound hypertension may occur with sudden withdrawal.

Clonidine and Guanfacine (Tenex), used more often with adults, offer great benefit for disorders involving hyperarousal, such as highly volatile ADHD. While it is not effective in alleviating symptoms of distractibility and inattentiveness, it may be combined with small doses of stimulants. (Copeland, 1991; Elia and Rapoport, 1991). Tenex had beneficial effects (without the sedation of Clonidine) as an alternative to stimulants for treatment of Tourette's and ADHD. Tenex was found to ameliorate attentional deficits and evidence a significant decrease in motor and phonic tics (Chappelle et al., 1995). Hunt et al. (1991) reported clinical effectiveness in aggression and highly aroused ADHD. With individuals with combined hyperarousal and distractibility, Clonidine given with Ritalin is an optimal combination. When administered transdermally (skin patch), this medication allows for a constant and effective blood level for approximately 5 days and is preferred by children who dislike taking pills.

Clonidine is widely used as an augment to the stimulant in the latter part of the day to stabilize behavior in the evening and improve sleeping habits, and clinically it is found that the Clonidine and stimulants have provided a positive treatment approach for the overfocused subtype of the attentional disorder without hyperactivity who is characterized by a great amount of drama, anxiety, and sleep deprivation. Research clearly documents the effectiveness of Clonidine for sleep disturbances associated with both ADHD or ADD. Parents commonly observe less oppositional behavior regarding bedtime; less sleep restlessness; increased number of hours slept; and improved morning awakenings, with fewer ADD symptoms the next day, which parents attributed to improved quality of sleep (Rubenstein, Silver, and Licamele, 1994; Wilens, Biederman, and Spencer, 1994).

Propranolol (Inderol) is a nonselective antihypertensive beta adrenergic blocking agent impacting the central and peripheral nervous system. It is utilized in the treatment of vascular hypertension. In a preliminary study, Inderol was found useful either by itself or as an adjunctive medication for treatment of aggressive, explosive rage, and self-injurious behavior with both children and adolescents (Simeon, 1997).

Desmopressin acetate nasal spray (DDAVP) has been designed to treat primary nocturnal enuresis, based on the theory that abnormally low nocturnal secretion of plasma vasopressin (AVP) or antidiuretic hormone (ADH) may play an etiologic role. DDAVP is a nasal spray provided as an aqueous solution of desmopressin acetate with cholorobutanol, sodium chloride, and hydrochloric acid for intranasal administration. Reported improvement ranged from 10 to 65% fewer wet nights compared to placebo or pretreatment. Short- and long-term effectiveness was assessed and found to positively ameliorate a statistically significant or number of prior non-responders. Individuals may see a reduction in bed wetting as early as 1 to 3 nights posttreatment. Treatment initially lasts 2 months followed by gradual tapering of the spray for long-term abstinence, which can be longer than 3 months and less than 12 months. Adverse side effects are nasal congestion, rhinitis, flushing, and mild abdominal cramps, and individuals can use the spray for at least 12 months without adverse effect (Miller, Goldberg, and Atkin, 1989; Phône-Poulenc Rorer Pharmaceuticals, 1995).

The most recent development is that of DDAVP nasal spray/rhinal tube (desmopressin acetate) which is a synthetic analogue of 8-arginine vasopressin. This formulation has been found to be helpful for the treatment of primary nocturnal enuresis (PNE), as well as central diabetes insipidus (CDI). ADD children have commonly been found to have problems with enuresis and, less commonly with encopresis. Eisenberg et al. (1994) examined the hypothesis that vasopressin derivatives would facilitate learning and memory in ADD and/or learning-disabled children. There were clear findings of improvement following administration of the medication in learning task and a measure of logical memory. In addition, there was a non-significant trend for the more-impaired children to benefit less from DDAVP as compared to placebo than children with less baseline impairment. Stemberg and Lackgren (1993) concluded that oral desmopressin was comparable to the nasal spray evidencing a positive, long-term effect in adolescents with primary nocturnal enuresis.

Neuroleptics

In some cases of ADHD that do not benefit from the stimulants, Haloperidol and Thioridazine have been found to be useful alternatives. However, side effects are of great concern and the risk of developing tardive dyskinesia remains high. Generally, neuroleptics are found to have a limited role in treatment of ADHD; however, individuals likely to benefit would be those diagnosed with an underlying thought disorder (Hunt et al., 1991). Clinically, neuroleptics and stimulants have been found useful in individuals with underlying thought disorder and we find this to be correlated more with an attentional disorder without hyperactivity. Non-responders to the neuroleptics have been found to benefit from Ritalin alone or in addition to the prescribed neuroleptic (Pine et al., 1993).

Clozapine (Clozaril) is a fairly recent antipsychotic agent whose mechanism is that of a dopamine blockade operating more actively at the limbic area, rather than the nigrostriatal sites. Although less likely to result in the common extrapyramidal side effects, there are many risks to this medication requiring constant maintenance and the consequence of it not being the hopeful answer that initially was thought when it first became available.

Risperdal (Risperidone) has been very effective in the treatment of psychosis and is tolerated well with MPH if a comorbid ADD disorder exists. Risperdal appears to block serotonin via a modulatory effect of dopamine activated in the frontal cortex and basal ganglia area, while blocking dopamine receptors in the limbic system. It is not associated with as many of the side effects of the other neuroleptics. Risperdal treats the outward symptoms or positive symptoms of schizophrenia, such as delusional thinking, hostility, hallucinations, feelings of persecution, disorganized thinking, incoherence or excitement. It also treats the negative and more hidden symptoms of emotional withdrawal or isolation, apathy, social withdrawal, lack of emotion or display of inappropriate emotion, as well as an inability to follow the flow of the conversation. Treatment is based upon the lowest and most effective dose for that individual. Certain antihistamines may have an additive effect upon the severity of some of the side effects. When used with medications such as Sinemet, Levadopa, and Tegretol, this medication may become less effective. Predominant side effects are that of dizziness, agitation, anxiety, sleep disorders, weight gain, headache, constipation, upset stomach nausea, drowsiness, tiredness, sun-sensitivity, and sexual dysfunction. There is now an oral form of this medication, *Oral Solution Risperdal*. Cosgrove (1994) found positive effects in the use of Risperdal for dual diagnoses of ADHD and schizophrenia. The use of low dosages of Risperdal with behaviorally disturbed children may be a possibility yet remains in question (Weiss, 1996). Risperdal was, however, found to be effective in the treatment of acute mania associated with psychotic features (Tohen et al., 1996).

Olanzapine (Zyprexa) is a recent medication once daily dosing designed to address symptoms of psychosis. Generally well tolerated in clinical trials, this medication revealed excellent control of both the positive symptoms (delusions, hallucinations, and disordered thinking) and negative symptoms (emotional withdrawal, flat affect, and inability to enjoy things) of psychosis. It is reported to target symptoms of those early diagnosed patients with chronic illness and/or those with intolerance to other antipsychotic medication. Diminished side effects are noted with a low incidence of extrapyramidal symptoms. Tamminga, Kane, and Lahti (1996) report that properties of this medication resemble that of Clozapine. Zyprexa impacts all dopamine receptors as an antagonist, operates at many of the serotonin receptors as an antagonist as well as at the noradrenergic cholinergic (muscarinic) and histaminergic receptors. The regionally selective impact upon only dopaminergic neurons impacting limbic and frontal cortex is also similar to that of Clozapine. Olanzapine was found to have significantly fewer adverse reactions, incidence of extrapyramidal side effects, hyperprolactinemia, and sexual dysfunction, as compared to risperidone; response can be maintained at 28 weeks (Tran et al., 1997).

Serentil (Serlect) is a medication designed to treat psychotic symptoms. It is more specific than either the Clozapine or Zyprexa, interacting predominantly with the dopamine D2 family of receptors. Side effects are diminished in that it does not attach to receptors that produce the sedative and anticholinergic effects. The action of this medication is similar to that of Haldol in the treatment of psychosis (Tamminga, Kane, and Lahti, 1996). Serentil has the longest half-life for once daily dosing and is, therefore, effective for both positive and negative symptoms. To bring symptoms under immediate control, an increase of 4 mg every other day was found to be a safe method of titration as opposed to a daily increase. Schizophrenic patients tolerated this medication quite well, demonstrating efficacy for treatment while maintaining extrapyramidal symptoms similar to that of placebo. The most frequent side effects noted were dry mouth, tachycardia, headache, decreased ejaculatory volume, mild weight gain, mild nasal congestion and nausea. Targeting of negative symptoms was greatest for olanzapine and serentil (Jibson and Tandon, 1996; Sramek et al., 1997).

Quetiapine is another new neuroleptic with the absence of muscarinic M_1 receptor activity to avoid the commonly seen anticholinergic side effects. Studies show improvement of both positive and negative symptoms of schizophrenia (less potent for negative symptoms) common side effects of somnolence, agitation, constipation, dry mouth, weight gain, postural hypotension, dizziness and mildly increased alanine aminotransferase (ALT) and aspartate aminotransferase (AST). Its strength lies in the low incidence of extrapyramidal side effects, diminished occurrence of autonomic side effects, and efficacy for treatment of schizophrenia (Jibson and Tandom, 1996). *Ziprasidone,* another new antipsychotic was found to be effective in the treatment of positive symptoms and lowering extrapyramidal effects. It has commonly reported side effects of somnolence, dizziness, nausea, postural hypotension, and lightheadedness (Jibson and Tandon, 1996).

Amino Acid Supplementation

Amino acids are the precursors to the catecholamines and indolamines. as precursors to the neurotransmitters, serotonin, norepinephrine, and dopamine, they have been hypothesized for treatment. Phenylalanine, tryptophan, and tyrosine in increased amounts could lead to increased levels of neurotransmitters and theoretically be an alternative treatment. However, the use of amino acids generally has not shown great effectiveness in treatment of an attentional disorder, excluding tryptophan, which is no longer available (Hunt et al., 1991). Issues of toxicity, development of tolerance, and the overall question of therapeutic effects has minimized amino acids as effective alternatives (Wender, 1995).

Phenylethylamine (PEA), an endogenous neuroamine, has been found to be structurally related to the amphetamines, producing similar effects on energy and attention in addition to mood enhancement. The PEA precursor phenylalanine, in combination with the dopamine agonist, selegiline, was found useful in treatment for depression (Sabelli et al., 1996).

Antiseizure

Gabapentin (Neurotonin) is a relatively new antiseizure medication, originally introduced to augment the major antiseizure medications available. Recent studies, however, are showing that it can be used by itself in the treatment of partial or complex partial seizures. There are less side effects than the older antiseizure medications. Side effects are that of dizziness, ataxia, fatigue, nystagmus, and somnolence; however, it is usually well tolerated (Chadwick, 1995).

As an adjunctive treatment for partial seizures (simple, complex, and secondarily generalized), Gabapentin's (Neurotonin) low inherent toxicity and lack of drug interaction provides an excellent additional treatment for partial epilepsy that is not being completely remediated by a first line of defense antiseizure medication. The use of Gabapentin provided positive results with almost complete remediation of symptoms for up to 6 months in treatment of Restless Legs Syndrome (Adler, 1997).

Divalproex/sodium (Depakote) is currently being introduced as a first line of defense for mania symptoms, operates as a mood stabilizer, is highly effective and well tolerated (Papatheodorou, 1996; Keck et al., 1992). Adverse effects primarily are vomiting, followed by nausea, somnolence, tremor, weight gain, transient hair loss, and dizziness. Patients need to be closely monitored due to the susceptibility of hepatotoxicity and it is not to be used during pregnancy. Clinically, Depakote has been helpful as an adjunct to Ritalin for highly agitated, anxious, explosive personalities, in addition to adolescent mania. Recommended use is not for children under 3 years of age. Depakote has been demonstrated as one of the first-line monotherapy treatments to address symptoms of partial-onset seizures (Beydoun, Sackellares, and Shu, 1997). Primarily released for use with absence seizures, this medication has also been found to be effective for myoclonic and tonic-clonic seizures, partial and generalized seizures as well as an adjunctive medication (Bourgeois, 1995). We have found Depakote evidencing positive effects on ameliorating the seizure-like activation noted by aggressive outbursts and complementing the impact of the stimulants on symptoms of the attentional disorder.

Lamotrigine (Lamictal) is a rather new medication that originally targeted the adult population. Studies, however, are showing use for children and the elderly. It's potential for use with the elderly is a chewable tablet form. Side effects are that of rash headache, nervousness, asthenia, ataxia, diplopia, nausea, blurred vision, dizziness, vomiting and somnolence. Similar to that of phenytoin and carbamazepine in action, it has demonstrated efficacy for children, adolescents and adults for partial and secondary, generalized seizures (Leach and Brodie, 1995; Leach, Lees, and Riddall, 1995).

Phenytoin (Dilantin) has been utilized as an antiseizure medication, yet also has a long history of use for medical management of aggression, evidencing secondary gains in improved social behaviors and feelings of well being. Research has been controversial with mixed results regarding the relief of impulsive behavior and aggressive acts. Recent studies, employing very careful design as well as accurate definition and measurement of aggression, reports unequivocally reduced impulsive aggressive acts (that are not premeditated) to a significant degree (Barratt et al., 1997). Phenytoin has been the most commonly used antiepileptic medication for treatment of simple and complex partial seizures as well as generalized tonic and tonic-clonic seizures. It is well tolerated by both children and adults; dose-related dysfunction of ocular and cerebellovestibular systems can exist (Wilder, 1995).

Carbamazepine (Tegretol) was approved for treatment of complex partial or partial seizures and generalized tonic-clonic seizures and is another widely used antiepileptic medication with less toxicity effects than either phenytoin or phenobarbital. It was demonstrated for efficacy for both children and adults, this medication has been utilized singly or in combination with other antiepileptics (Loiseau and Duché, 1995). *Tegretol-XR* is a newly released sustained version. Side effects are that of aplastic anemia, agranulocytosis, thrombocytopenia, dizziness, vertigo, drowsiness, fatigue, ataxia, and a worsening of symptoms, as well as the aggravation of coronary artery disease. Post et al. (1997) has found improvements over that of lithium for treatment of bipolar disorder.

Topiramate, a rather new medication, has also been found to be an effective treatment for partial-onset seizures in children (Elterman, 1997). *Felbamate* was found to have a high risk for hematologic and hepatic toxicity. It was, however, the first new antiepileptic medication to be approved with such structural differences from the other medications, offering a broader spectrum for efficacy for treatment of generalized as well as localized epilepsies. Suggested for cautious use, this medication is approved for children and adults (Theodore, Jensen, and Kwan, 1995).

Benzodiazepines

Clonazepam (Klonopin) has been utilized for a variety of disorders, panic attacks, generalized anxiety, depression, obsessive-compulsive disorder, and pain control. Klonopin, together with Clonidine, was found effective in treating tic disorder and comorbid ADHD (Leonard et al., 1994); the addition of Kloropin has ameliorated the tics (Steingard et al., 1994). Davidson et al. (1993) found successful results in the use of Klonopin for treatment of social phobia.

Alprazolan (Xanax) has been widely prescribed for panic attack symptoms, generalized anxiety, and sleeping problems. Side effects include sedation, withdrawal symptoms, and disinhibition, and it is contraindicated for patients with substance-abuse problems. One positive aspect is its rapid onset and immediate relief of symptoms. Clinically, this medication has worked well with the alcoholic and marijuana addicted population for relief of the overwhelming anxiety that has not been addressed by either antianxiety or antidepressant medication, and when cravings remain intense and unremediated by a medication such as ReVia.

Naltpexone (ReVia) is being used for alcohol treatment similar to that of Antabuse, to prevent relapse by blocking the brain's reinforcing effects and cravings. This medication has evidenced some gains in behavior and social communication with autistic children and may become useful in the treatment of Autism. ReVia is classified as an opioid blocker and alcohol detoxification. It is designed to decrease the cravings and the overall general consumption of alcohol. It may also operate to block the development of physical dependence to opioid-based narcotics such as Heroin, Morphine, Methadone, and Codeine. It may induce withdrawal in individuals dependent upon opiate substances. Major side effects associated with the detoxification process are that of nausea, headache, fatigue, and nervousness. Individuals withdrawing from alcohol report symptoms of insomnia, anxiety, abdominal cramping, vomiting, and joint and muscle pain, however these side effects may occur as a result of alcohol withdrawal and not necessarily this medication. Roth, Ostroff, and Hoffman (1996) found positive effects in decreasing repetitive self-injurious behavior.

Overall, clinically to treat ADD, we have found the best results occur with the use of the stimulant medications as the first line of defense, followed by additional medications to treat the comorbid symptomology. Underlying disorders do need to be addressed with medical management prior to commencing with stimulant use when it is clearly apparent that the stimulant medication will exacerbate that condition. The seriousness of the underlying condition will determine which disorder is addressed first.

CHAPTER 15

Evaluation of
Attention Deficit Disorder

Oshman (1992) discussed the need for and absence of standardized tests or procedures to use for diagnosis of ADD–RT (adult deficit disorder, residual type). Consequently, for assessment he recommended a clinical interview (a process whereby the individual is questioned about the problems he/she is experiencing and the extent to which functional capacity is impaired). Questions should be asked about the core symptoms of the disorder and how it is affecting the person's life. Because ADD–RT usually has a comorbidity disorder, this is questioned as well. It is important to distinguish ADD from depression and manic depression, its look-alikes as well as personality disorders. Finally, in order to diagnose ADD–RT, childhood has to be discussed and an attempt to determine presence or absence of the disorder during that time of life.

Shibagaki, Yamanaka, and Furuya (1993) identified the method of measuring electrodermal activity during passive and active listening tasks with children diagnosed with ADHD. Their findings indicate that ADHD children tended to exhibit a lower arousal as indicated by a decrease in the amplitude of the skin conductance response. Thus, they concluded that hyperactive school children evidence less electrodermal responsiveness to stimuli than normal children and this correlates with the common findings of short attention spans in these identified children.

Clinical tests for attention and concentration as well as measures of the frontal lobe functions have been well documented in the neuropsychology

271

literature. Tests utilized are validated to measure symptoms of attention and concentration as well as functioning of the frontal area (specifically the prefrontal area, involved in planning and control, use of feedback, shifting and maintaining a set, sequencing, divided and alternating attention), and parietal area (information processing, cognitive processing speed).

Wherry et al. (1993) examined the validity of the Gordon Diagnostic System and results failed to demonstrate the validity of this measure to discriminate ADHD individuals from normal individuals. Authors suggested the use of multiple behavior ratings as an alternative to clinical evaluation.

Shun, McFarland, and Bain (1990) examined the processes involved in different attention measures. A motor component specified by visually tracking particular stimulus features, complex scanning and tracking aspects of attention, was found for the Letter Cancellation Test, Digit Symbol, Trail Making Test and Symbol Digit Modalities Test. The second component of attention, the ability to select and manipulate particular stimulus and response features while growing others, sustain ongoing mental processes, and select features for processing, was found for Serial 7s and 13s and the Stroop Color Word Test. This component is similar to a definition of concentration. The third component defined by an immediate attention span was the Digit Span Test and Knox Cube Test and represents simple mental tracking. A final note by the authors was that the Serial 7s and 13s was subject to patient anxiety, and thus the Stroop represented a better measure of sustained selective processing.

Screening measures for children with ADD involved the measurement of frontal lobe functions. Barkley et al. (1992) examined a battery composed of the Continuous Performance Test by Gordon, Grooved Pegboard Test, Controlled Word Association Test, Hand Movements Scale, Porteus Mazes, Rey–Osterrieth Complex Figure, Stroop Color Word Test, Trail Making Test and Wisconsin Card Sorting Test for validity. Barkley's group also summarized that the Continuous Performance Test, Stroop (interference score) Hand Movements, and Go-No-Go tests have some reliability in determining differences between ADHD and normals. The Wisconsin Card Sorting Test may have some validity for differentiating ADHD and normals for 6 to 11 year olds.

Boucugnani and Jones (1989) evaluated subjects of the Wisconsin Card Sorting Test and Trail Making Test, and Stroop findings point to significant differences between ADHD and normals on test variables measuring perseveration, self-directed attention, and inhibitory capacity. Gorenstein, Mammato, and Sandy (1989) found that an inattentive–overactive group of children as compared to matched normals performed in the direction of a prefrontal deficit on three measures, The Wisconsin Card Sorting Test (WCST), errors on the Sequential Matching Memory Test, and Necker Cube Reversals. The Trail Making Test, Stroop Color Word and Sequential Memory Tasks also exhibited deficits for the inattentive-overactive group. Shue and Douglas (1989) found ADHD children to perform greater than normal for perseverence errors as well as the Trail Making Test Parts A and B for errors and time. A test of everyday attention was designed to measure everyday attentional activities comprised of a range of tests addressing such issues as searching maps, looking through telephone directories, listening to lottery number broadcasts, and predicting recovery of function 6 month subsequent to a stroke. The above categories were found to correlate with performance on known attentional measures such as the Stroop, Trails B, PASAT, WCST, and Digit Span Backwards (Robertson et al., 1996).

Neuropsychological evaluation revealed poorer performance on measures of distractibility (A Cancellation Auditory and Visual Test) verbal fluency (Verbal Fluency Test) a measure of whole brain functioning (Digit Symbol) novel learning task (WCST) and measure of sequencing ability (Picture Arrangement). The ADHD group evidenced visuomotor difficulties as well as problems with sequences and it was hypothesized that this disorder is related to visuomotor, sequential and temporal symptoms of an executive dysfunction disorder (Pineda et al., 1997). The types of tasks that Pineda denotes as symptoms of an executive dysfunction, however, can be attributed to spatial dysfunctioning (inability to view the whole). In our research, typically children with this type of deficit demonstrate poor performance on the above tasks for this reason. This demonstrates how the tests themselves are subject to differential interpretation and become misleading. Typically children and adults evidence a lower Performance IQ as a consequence of the impact of time and spatial dysfunctioning (impacting all of the five measures comprising this index in some capacity). There were more perseverative errors on the WCST delineating the ADHD group in Pineda's study. What may appear as perseveration, however, which may actually be information processing deficits the loss of information which result in the repetition of an answer already identified as incorrect. Similar findings were obtained with children ages 10 to 12 years, whereby neurological soft signs contributed to predict a variable FSIQ, the PIQ as well as scholastic achievement (whether a cause or effect of the executive dysfunction) was lower (Pineda et al., 1997).

Seidman et al. (1997) examined individuals 9 to 22 years on several neuropsychological measures to determine the enduring quality of ADHD.

The ADHD group was found to be significantly more impaired on measures of attention and executive function, impairment was significant across the age span (in comparing the younger, less than 15 years, to the older population). This study supports findings of underlying neuropsychological issues associated with the attentional disorders, and although authors implicate the frontal attentional network, measures may have been subject to the impact of the posterior attentional network. The three measures reaching significance in this study, was the Stroop, WCST, and the Rey-Osterrieth Complex Figures, which the authors used as confirmation of the frontal attentional network. The Rey-Osterrieth figures revealed a problem with copy organization which may have been related to spatial issues. Analysis of the Stroop indicates an overall lower raw word score, significant of slow reading. As noted in our research, however, the discrepancy between the word and color-word scores (interference task) still provides clear evidence of the difficulty gating out and focusing in, to read the color of the ink, providing assessment of distractibility. Differences for the WCST were significant in the number of categories obtained as well as errors (perseverative and nonperseverative) although there were actually more nonperseverative errors. In using the Stroop and the WCST in our clinical practice, we find that both measures although utilizing logic in their performance, are primarily measuring issues of distractibility (Stroop) and information processing (WCST) with variables of distractibility and sustained attention having additional impact on the WCST (this would support the finding of greater nonperseverative errors as confirmation of a problem of missing information as opposed to frontal processes).

Reitan and Wolfson address the issue of frontal-lobe functions in a number of their writings and conclude in general that when a measure purports to be measuring frontal lobe deficits, this may not in fact be the case. They concur with Costa (1988), who summarized the conflict by stating: "It is easy to find tests that are sensitive to frontal lobe dysfunction, and very difficult to find tests that are specific for it." The idea is that perhaps the discrepancies in the above-mentioned literature may be due to the fact that we are attempting to measure a specific entity that cannot be measured. The idea that frontal-lobe functioning is not a discrete entity unto itself, but rather an integrative process; what one measures is a combination of processes that subserve frontal functions and there is no ability to measure discrete frontal functions as a result. Bigler (1988) indicates that tests purported to measure frontal-lobe functioning, such as the WCST and the Category test, are not specific to frontal-lobe damage. The same is true for Part B of the Trail

Making Test in that research of Reitan and Wolfson (unpublished) concludes that this measure fails to demonstrate significant differences between identified frontal vs. nonfrontal brain dysfunctioning. Thus, these measures are more sensitive to cerebral damage and perhaps frontal processes (encompassing the frontal areas and areas that subserve the frontal areas) than specifically frontal cerebral cortex. Axelrod and associates (1993) summarized with the idea that neurocognitive measures are factorially complex.

This issue is again addressed in the studies using positron emission tomography (PET) measurements of regional cerebral blood flow (CBF). Comparisons of CBF changes using paired image subtraction provides the opportunity to isolate cerebral areas participating in the use of the processes that differentiate task performance. Results of Sergent et al. (1992) indicate that an attempt to interpret patterns of activation is confronted by difficulties of automatic and uncontrolled processing of stimuli, resulting in a tendency for errors of interpretation. Not all areas of component operation that differentiate two tasks produce significant CBF changes due to this uncontrolled activation. Thus, there are many difficulties inherent in using PET experiments to identify anatomical functional relations of higher-order cognitive processes. Designing a task that specifically taps a restricted set of subprocesses does not guarantee that other operations are not conjointly performed during its performance. This potential for error suggests the need for converging evidence to ensure valid anatomical functional correlations. Authors suggest the idea of several task comparisons within a study as an alternative way of achieving a comprehensive account of the pattern of cerebral activation by providing converging information about anatomical–functional correlation.

van Zomeren and Brouwer (1994) view attention as a term applied to a broad class of phenomena that cannot be obtained or contained in a single definition and thus cannot be tested with a single unitary measure nor would a single condition test provide a sufficient measure due to the presence of other limiting factors necessitating other separate assessment to rule them out as variables. Recommended are measures that encompass all of the aspects of attention:

▪ General observation of the individual's attention in daily life
▪ Mental control
▪ Alertness
▪ Hemineglect
▪ Focused attention

- Divided attention
- Sustained attention
- Supervisory control

The purpose of neuropsychological evaluation is to address the problems frequently found in using self-report measures alone. In using self-report measures and structured interviews, Sherman, McGue, and Iacono (1997) noted a high degree of variance between self-reporting practices of parents and teachers. Teachers more frequently endorsed ADHD items as well as a variety of other behavioral problems and mothers appeared to under-report the information. Misdiagnosis of ADD tends to be rather prevalent, occurring as a consequence of the absence of sufficient data with which to arrive at an informed conclusion.

The battery of tests that have been utilized at our clinic for the past 10 years address the above attentional issues; neuropsychological tests allow for the direct measure of brain functioning while factoring out such extraneous variables as race, educational level, culture, and prior learning. This battery has been extremely effective in differentiating the two subtypes of this disorder, specifically revealing the same pattern of results (the degree remains highly variable) implicating specific symptoms on a continual basis and demonstrating this pattern across all of the developmental ages from 5 to 76 years. In an evaluation of the aged population (ages 75 to 99 years) patterns still emerge (especially if the brain remains somewhat intact) which can be suggestive of a pre-morbid attentional disorder. The use of neuropsychological tests allows for issues of brain dysfunctioning to be ruled in or out depending upon the severity of results and/or evidence of distortion errors. In utilizing several different measures to address each of the symptoms of this disorder, checks and balances are inherent in the battery to provide a very accurate and consistent diagnostic process. Research to date has provided converging evidence for specific subprocesses loading on certain test measures. These patterns have been consistently identified, as well as specific means of responding, depending on the nature of the disorder, and the individual's specific characteristics. Thus, dependent measures and test performance are impacted in clearly definable patterns due to the impact of independent variables of severity of the disorder, type of disorder, intellectual potential, degree of compensation, motivation, and personality type. Patterns have been specifically replicated on a continual basis allowing clear-cut diagnosis, ruling in and ruling out of other intervening variables.

A concern that has been raised is the validity of evaluation in regard to the impact of substance abuse, especially those substances that remain in the system for long periods of time. Drugs that have immediate effects and/or are relatively easy to detect would be apparent at the time of evaluation thus obviously negating the examination (which would subsequently not occur). However, marijuana, known to remain in the system for long periods of time, would remain undetected and may have an impact upon the evaluation process. Neuropsychological evaluations were administered to adult subjects (ages 27 to 42 years) who were given doses of ethanol, marijuana, amphetamine, hydromorphone, and pentobarbital at different dosage levels over a period of 5 weeks. Marijuana had a significant impact on only 1 of the 14 measures administered. Research indicates that of the measures in the evaluation process for marijuana, only the PASAT evidenced a decline of abilities due to a slowed reaction time, however there was not an impact upon the number of errors obtained. Ethanol and phenobarbital produced impaired performance on the WCST (computer administration) which was evident at lower doses and became more apparent as the task increased in its cognitive demands. Amphetamine had little effect upon any of the measures administered. Hydromorphone had a small, although significant effect, evidencing a decrease of 10% in the number of correct responses on a search task (Pickworth, Rohrer, and Fant, 1997). Sher et al. (1997) evaluated alcohol-use disorders and neuropsychological functioning in college students and identified deficits in visuospatial and motor speed that varied with increased dependence upon alcohol. They specifically noted the deficits with the block design subtest of the WAIS-R and the visual reproduction subtest on a memory measure. Those alcohol abusers who were alcohol dependent revealed more impairment on Part B of the Trail Making Test.

In evaluating the attention-disordered population over the past 10 years, we have isolated the effects of low blood sugar or hypoglycemia as having an impact on those measures demanding greater amounts of complex thinking and/or highly affected by psychomotor speed, such as the PASAT, SDMT, WCST, Stroop, and Parts A and B of the Trailmaking Test. Those who suffer from this condition frequently report feeling confused, foggy, dizzy, lightheaded, distractible and having diminished energy. When levels of blood sugar fall below normal ranges, the CNS faces a condition of hypoglycemic. Research indicates that during this state, healthy adult subjects (mean age range 26 years) have delayed reactions on measures of selective attention and motor response selection which evidences recovery when normal blood sugar is restored (Smid et al., 1997).

Descriptions of Individual Measures

The following battery was selected based on the research and identification of these tests as measures of identified symptoms of ADD. Tests are reported in the literature as measurements of the frontal and parietal areas of the brain. They are as follows:

Trail Making Test, Parts A and B have generally been seen as a measure of frontal lobe functioning.

The Trail Making Test is identified as a test for speed of visual search, attention, mental flexibility, and motor function. The test was originally part of the Army Individual Test Battery (1944) and was added by Reitan to the Halstead Battery. There are two parts: Part A requires the connection of making pencil lines and keeping the pencil on the paper between 25 encircled numbers randomly arranged on a page in proper order; Part B is comprised of 25 encircled numbers and letters to be completed in alternating order. The adult form is used from 15 years of age and older. Approximate time for administration is 5 to 10 minutes. Scoring is in the form of seconds or time and number of errors.

The Trail Making Test has been found to be loaded on both a rapid visual search and visuospatial sequencing. It has been found to be highly sensitive to brain damage, including closed head injury and alcoholism. Young adult learning-disabled subjects differed from normals only on Part B, but not on Part A. Part B has been found to require some information-processing ability, Part A does not. Part B has clearly been found to be the more sensitive of the two measures, requiring the ability of shifting course during an ongoing activity and the ability to deal with more than one stimulus at a time. Part B, requiring the alternation between numbers and letters is said to be particularly sensitive to frontal-lobe damage and prefrontal lesions in particular (Golden, 1981; Pontius, 1973; Reitan and Wolfson, 1985, 1994, 1995; Stuss et al., 1992; des Rosiers and Kavanagh, 1987; Dodrill, 1978; O'Donnell, 1983; Pontius and Yudowitz, 1980; Eson et al., 1978). Mesulam (1985) views the measure as addressing the issues of response inhibition and vulnerability to interference with performance being influenced by both age and intelligence.

This measure has also been used extensively with the ADD population as it is seen as a measure of frontal-lobe functioning. There have been mixed results in some studies clearly finding ADHD children to have impairments, usually more so on Part B (Gorenstine et al., 1989). Shue and Dagras (1989) found more errors on Part B in ADHD when compared to normals. Boucaghani and Jones (1989) found ADHD children deficient only on time measures of Part B. In Johnson's (1981) study of ADD adolescents, teens performed more slowly on Part B than ADHD teens.

Holdnack et al. (1995) evaluated adults diagnosed with residual ADD and found that trail and performance were considerably slower than that of normals exhibiting overall slow psychomotor speed and integration. There was no psychomotor speed problem evidenced on Trails B, which authors felt might reflect some accommodation in performance as Part B was no longer novel having been preceded by Part A. Authors felt that intact functioning on Part B was significant of intact cognitive flexibility and intact executive functioning processes. Adults utilized in the study were well-educated, successful individuals who clearly fit the prototype of ADD—hence, the absence of frontal functioning deficits and characteristic deficit of slow cognitive speed. This is an excellent example of the controversy surrounding the use of these measures and the need to approach performance from a qualitative rather than quantitative approach.

Recently, Reitan and Wolfson (1994, 1995) found no significant differences between frontal and non-frontal brain damaged patients, indicating that the Trail Making Test Part B is not necessarily a measure of the frontal cerebral cortex, but rather functions subserved by the entire cerebrum. Arnold et al. (1994) found that the Trail Making Test was not impacted by the effect of acculturation. van Zomeren and Brouwer (1994) see the Trails B measure as a measurement of processing speed. Clinically, we have found that there can be the tendency to perform excellently on this measure without mistakes, only to receive a poor score due to time. Thus, we have found it important to first distinguish the type of errors (confusion and/or capacity problem, resulting in a loss of place vs. inability to perform the task). Thus, an individual (generally with ADD) could perform quite well on this measure; however, it takes them an extensive amount of time, characteristic of what appears as impairment, but is merely the speed component.

The Progressive Figures Test and Color Shape Test are versions of the Trail Making Test for the ages of 5 to 8 years.

The WCST (Grant and Berg, 1948) assesses the ability to form abstract concepts and shift and maintain a set. It was originally developed by Berg and Grant to assess abstraction ability. Heaton (1981) points out that there has been increasing interest in this measure, as it is quite versatile in providing information on several aspects of problem-solving behavior beyond the basic indices of task success or failure. Scoring methods include the number of perseverative responses, the number of perseverative errors, the failure to maintain a set, and number of categories achieved.

The WCST typically has been found to be especially sensitive to lesions of the frontal lobe. Ozonoff (1995) found the WCST to be a very reliable instrument for autistic and LD children and adolescents utilizing executive functioning properties and a level of solid awareness, suggesting its ability to assess multiple dimensions of cognition and behavior. Holdnack et al. (1995) in administering the WCST to a group of residual ADD adults found no evidence of problematic performance when compared to normal counterparts. This study again points to the need to qualitatively assess these measures in identifying ADD and its subtypes. It remains difficult to identify ADD, relying on executive functions and skills of logic to operate as well as they do. Further, it is important when using neuropsychological measures to be aware of the problems of using the comparison of "normal" as being acceptable when the individual's potential may be well above the average.

Heaton (1981) standardized the test instructions and scoring procedures for the long version and formally published it as a clinical instrument. The test consists of four stimulus cards placed in front of the subject who is then given two packs of cards (each containing 64 response cards) that have designs similar to the stimulus cards. The subject is instructed to match each of the cards in the decks to one of the four key cards. The subject is provided with immediate feedback as to whether the response is correct or incorrect.

Milner (1963) found clear differences between patients with dorsolateral frontal lesions and those with orbitofrontal and posterior lesions. Patients with dorsolateral lesions revealed an inability to shift from one sorting principle to another, apparently due to perseverative influence from the previous response. As such the WCST exposes the fragility of the interrelationships that usually connect many cognitive components. It has been found that patients cannot easily shift strategies for selecting cards when the rules for the correct response is changed. Perseveration as well as lack of initiative are common problematic behaviors observed. Milner (1963) and Taylor (1979) suggested that the test is sensitive to problems of the dorsolateral areas of the frontal lobe, the left more than the right. Researchers generally agree that the WCST is a good measure of frontal-lobe function, but have found perseveration to be associated with right rather than left frontal damage (Bornstein, 1986; Hermann et al., 1994). Bondi et al. (1993) found non-demented Parkinson's disease patients to evidence selective deficits pointing to the use of this measure as an indicator of striato-frontal outflow operations. Cuesta et al. (1995) suggested that the

WCST may not specifically be a measure of frontal-lobe functions and poor performance appears to provide evidence of a more global cerebral impairment. By approximately the age of 10, children perform similar to adults and there is not a significant decline in performance until after age of 80 years (Heaton, 1981).

However, Axelrod, Jiron, and Henry (1993) found in examining healthy adults, from the ages of 20 to 90 years, that there are significant linear trends for age, and demonstrated decreased competence on variables of accuracy and perseverance. Age of subjects (young adult 18 to 38 years vs older adult 60 to 86 years) resulted in decreased feedback usage, speed of processing and memory processes impacting performance in a negative direction on the computer-administrated version of this measure (Fristoe, Salthouse, and Woodard, 1997). Stratta and associates (1993) found educational attainment to have an impact on performance with both the schizophrenic and control population.

Williams et al. (1994), in evaluating the effect of wavelength on the performance of attention-disordered children on the WCST, were attempting to determine the involvement of the dorsal neural stream, believed to mediate key attentional operations. Children diagnosed as ADHD were administered this measure and compared with the performance of matched controls. First, findings confirmed prior research in that ADHD children differed from normal children in the number of perseverative responses, errors, percentage of perseverative errors, total errors, and percentage of conceptual responses. Second, the wavelength manipulation affected attentional processing and on all measures there were significant effects for color with the short wavelength (blue) enhancing performance. This was found to be consistent with prior research that the short wavelength stimuli increased the speed and magnitude of M channel response and enhanced reading performance. In the case of the ADHD population, performance improved to the degree that it approached the normal range. On all WCST measures affected by color, short wavelength stimuli brought the performance of the attention-impaired group into the same range of performance that the normal group showed in the control condition, which was clear. Thus, short wavelength materials or overlays may compensate for the attentional impairment in the ADHD population.

Patients with prefrontal lesions have been found to commit more errors than normal on non-frontal lesioned patients (Milner, 1963). Children with a physician's diagnosis of ADD have been found to have more perseverative errors than controls (Chelune et al., 1986). In comparing the ADHD population with matched controls, only the WCST perseverative errors and responses provided significant discrimination and designated the impact of the attentional disorder (Pineda et al., 1997). The WCST tends to be used in the majority of ADD studies and emerged as a highly viable measure of the disorder. Significant deficits were found in most of the studies for ADHD children when compared with normals. There is some question as to its ability to differentiate ADD as the child matures, and for adolescents, studies become more inconsistent with their results (Barkley, Grodzinsky, and DuPaul 1992).

McBurnett et al. (1993) found no significant interaction between aggression and hyperactivity on WCST performance. Axelrod and associates (1994) addressed this issue in finding that WCST performance can result from deficiencies in many different cognitive processes than just the frontal cerebral cortex. The WCST failed to differentiate the dysexecutive from the nondysexecutive subjects. Performance on this measure is not linked to a single neuroanatomical area of functioning which confirms its validity as a measurement of a multicomponent executive system (Axelrod et al., 1996; Baddeley et al., 1997). Similar to findings of Reitan and Wolfson (1994, 1995), there was no differential performance on the WCST among the schizophrenic, mood-disordered, and traumatically brain-injured populations. Results suggest that this measure may be multifaceted with regard to its functional specificity and that impaired performance may point to the frontal processes comprised of the frontal cortex and the subcortical regions that subserve it as well as those regions with frontal interconnections. The WCST was found to involve a number of regions in task performance, specifically that of the left or bilateral, dorsolateral prefrontal cortex, parietal association cortex (bilateral inferior parietal lobes) left occipital cortex, and cerebellum and striate cortex (Nagahama et al., 1996). This confirms the problem of evaluation with the WCST and assumptions regarding specific brain areas in use, such as that of the SPECT scans. Further, finds provide confirmation of why some individuals are able to perform well on this measure utilizing frontal processes, however may also experience a problem in performance due to deficits in other areas of function (such as the IPL) despite intact logic processes. The idea of information processing being a component to thus is also confirmed. Westerveld et al. (1996) presented findings of research conducted with ADHD and ADD citing both similar and different performance problems. ADD children had greater problems with failure to maintain a set, suggestive of a sustained attention disorder consistent with findings observed in our clinical setting. Also noted was poorer performance for girls.

The Bender Gestalt measure asks the individual to copy all of nine designs just as they are seen from a total of nine cards on one piece of paper.

The task of copying all nine designs on one page is an excellent means for enabling the examiner to observe whether and how well the individual plans the layout of their drawings on the page.

Frequently noted in the ADD population has been a consistent spatial problem, whether spatial neglect of the page and/or difficulty with spatial orientation and placement of the designs. More often than not, the designs are intact from a visual spatial point of view; however, it is the spatial component that seems to be more of the problem which evidences a specific pattern of responding. At times there is a neglect of one side of the design. Drawings are characteristic of the "hemineglect syndrome" defined by Heilman and colleagues (1985, 1994), whereby there is the failure to attend to the whole of the page, and thus the neglect of one-half of space that is commonly found in lesions in the right hemisphere.

Sergent and associates (1992) noted that the spatial discrimination of letters and their mirror images mainly engaged the inferior parietal lobule of both hemispheres on PET scan studies. In examining the mildly demented population using PET studies of regional cerebral metabolic rates for glucose, the posterior parietal cortex was implicated, identifying aspects of location-based selective attention that is impaired in the early stages of the development of Alzheimer's disease. The idea that superior parietal lobe damage indicates deficits in the disengagement of spatially directed attention and the view that the right posterior parietal lobe has a dominant role in the control of spatially directed attention (Parasuraman and Nestor, 1993). Resta and Eliot (1994) found significantly more errors for ADHD children on the Bender. Both groups, ADD and ADHD, performed poorly on measures of written language, evidencing writing, copying, and composition.

Thus, research tends to confirm the clinical findings consistently observed in that when an individual demonstrates a spatial problem on this measure, he/she also may or may not evidence the following to a greater or lesser degree:

1. They tend to evidence problems with reading, as identified by a problem of sight vocabulary and ability to know the word, but not to pronounce it correctly on seeing it and reading it. Individuals with this problem also consistently report losing their place as they read down the page and additionally, not being able to find things or sentences embedded within a page. The first word of a line or a whole line may be skipped.
2. This function also tends to subserve mathematical computations that need to be completed within one's head and/or geometric design.

3. Further, spelling and writing skills are impacted as well to a greater or lesser degree, whether that be the inability to see from sight that the word is spelled incorrectly (not being able to see the whole of the word) or letters than run into each other or down the page. Adults tend to adopt use of capital letters, made quite small, to hide the inconsistencies of the written letters as a consequence of this spatial problem.

4. There are time management problems and an inability to accurately judge how long a project will take.

5. Finally, there is a clumsiness that results in the tendency to bump into things, trip over objects apparently "not seen" and difficulty with specific dance routines within a set portion of space due to right–left confusion.

The Stroop Color Word Test measures the ease with which an individual can shift his or her perceptual set to conform to changing demands and suppress a habitual response in favor of an unusual one. This measure of cognitive flexibility was originally developed by Stroop in 1935 and has since been modified by Golden in 1976. The subject is now asked to read randomized color names (red, green, blue, and yellow) printed ink black type. The subject is then asked to read a second sheet and name the colors of x's printed in green, blue, yellow, and red. Finally, the subject is asked to complete the interference task (primary measure of scoring) and name the color of the ink in which the names are printed and disregard the verbal content. Stroop reported that normal people can read colored words printed in colored ink as fast as words printed in black ink. The time increases significantly when the subject is asked to name the color of the ink rather than to read the word aloud. This decrease in color naming speed is called the "color word interference effect".

Mesulam (1985) views the Stroop as a measure of the susceptibility to interference and a measurement of the inability to inhibit immediate and inappropriate response tendencies. Posner and Synder (1975) maintain that many complex habitual mental processes can operate automatically and be strategy independent. Many cognitive tasks may be viewed as continuing automatic activation and conscious strategies. An example of processing without intention occurs with the Stroop effect whereby the individual cannot avoid processing aspects of an input item that he or she decides to ignore. The magnitude of the Stroop interference effect increased for the older (as opposed to younger) population, pointing to the susceptibility of the anterior attentional system to the effects of age. Younger subjects (age range of 18 to 28 years) evidenced significantly less activation as measured by continuous EEG record-ings over the medial and lateral frontal and parietal areas when compared to older subjects (age range of 62 to 78 years) (West and Bell, 1997).

Rafal and Henik (1994), in researching the biological aspects of the Stroop effect, concluded that this "effect" reflects dysfunction in the fronto-striatal circuit, which normally modulates automatic cognitive operations. Thus, it impacts the anterior attentional system that is necessary for the maintenance of focused attention on selected information, while at the same time sup-pressing other information to allow that planned behavior to be carried out, thus utilizing the inhibitory properties of the frontal lobe and its connections. Lavoie and Charlebois (1994) found significantly lower scores for the atten-tion-disordered population and more hesitations when compared to controls and disruptive boys without ADD.

The Stroop has been studied in psychiatric and brain damaged-patients and has been found fairly effective in distinguishing normals from these groups. It appears to be related to that left frontal area. It has been considered a measure of focused attention (Shiffrin and Schneider, 1977). Henik (1996) finds the Stroop to be a reliable and robust measure of the attentional processes. Other researchers have found the measure an important assessment of the frontal lobe and its capacity to inhibit interfering stimuli and adapting behavior to unusual situations. Deficits in sensory gating have been commonly reported in researching the schizophrenic population and related to dysfunctioning of the limbic circuits (Skinner and Garcia-Rill, 1994). The Stroop has been used to investigate attentional bias in a woman who has delusions, the hypothesis being that someone with delusional beliefs would have a decreased perfor-mance on this interference task measuring gait problems. Evidence provided confirmation of selective process deficits from stimuli salient to one's specific belief system, in this instance a delusional one (Leafhead, Young, and Szulecks, 1996). George et al. (1994), using PET scans with normal volunteers, found that the left mid-cingulate region was highly activated, activity in different regions of the cingulate/gyrus correlated with performance speed, and overall findings implicated the left mid-cingulate region as part of the neural network activated for overriding one response over another. Parasuraman and Nestor (1994), in addressing the impact of Alzheimer's disease, found that this was one measure sensitive to mild and early stages of dementia. The Stroop is one measure that was also indicated as being very sensitive to medical manage-ment. TBI subjects improved substantially on this measure when administered medical management with the stimulant medications, methylphenidate and amantadine (Allen et al., 1997).

The Stroop has been used extensively in ADD research and found to be quite successful in delineating the disorder. The majority of researchers found ADHD children to be more impaired than their normal counterparts and this measure appears to be particularly sensitive to the attentional disorders. In our research we find that typically, on a consistent basis, the individual (irregardless of age or gender or intellectual level) is unable to attain a score in the interference task (reading the color of the word) equivalent to that of the word score (reading the name of the color) and usually the interference score will be one-half to two-thirds less than that of the word score. We have found that individuals who are very adept utilizing logic as a compensatory mechanism, will strategize their performance by internally using self-talk, saying the world *color,* to themselves to successfully increase their score. The Cancellation task, provides further information regarding a vulnerability to being distracted, evidenced by increased errors (demonstrating an inability to gate out some stimuli and focus on other stimuli, similar to that of the Stroop effect) and/or increased time to complete the task successfully.

The Pasat (Paced Auditory Serial Addition Task) is a serial addition task used to assess the rate of information processing and sustained attention. The test was originally designed by Gronwall and associates (Gronwall, 1977). Gronwall and coworkers (Gronwall and Sampson, 1974; Gronwall and Wrightson, 1974) provided estimates of information processing on the amount of information that can be handled at one time. The individual is required to comprehend the auditory input, respond verbally, inhibit encoding of one's own response while attending to the next stimulus in a series and perform at an externally determined pace.

This measure was adapted for use with children in 1988 in England and re-evaluated in 1991 with more specific norms. The adult version has proven to be a clear indicator of information processing and a useful clinical tool to explain the tendency of adults to miss small bits of information from their environment and as a result, miscommunicate, not understand directions and instructions, and can present itself as an auditory verbal comprehension problem. Not surprisingly, this has resulted in negative social consequences for the individual.

The PASAT is thought to measure some central information-processing capacity similar to that seen on reaction time and divided-attention tasks. It can be a very demanding and frustrating task. Deary et al. (1994), using PET analysis on insulin-treated diabetics, found decreased activation in the right anterior and left posterior cingulate areas previously implicated by prior research as activated and increased. Authors question the impact of anxiety and the possibility of emotional changes being a causal factor in the findings. This study points to the problem of assessing neuropsychological measures and the brain areas implicated as well as the impact of other intervening factors and the difficulty of using animal research to predict human performance.

Thompson and Gottesman (1994) found no significant differences between individuals with the diagnosis of post-traumatic stress disorder and normals on performance of the PASAT, which serves to firmly establish this measure as related to brain functioning. Use of reaction time and the PASAT appear to have a degree of predictive ability for return to work after head injury. Subjects suffering from a mild concussive injury did not differ in performance on this measure post injury, substantiating this measure as an accurate predictor of substantial impact to brain functioning (Maddocks and Saling, 1996). The PASAT was used to measure significant and stable gains as a consequence of various attentional training programs (van Zomeren and Bouwer, 1994). Age and IQ impact performance and norms were revised (Brittain et al., 1991; Roman et al., 1991).

The PASAT and CHIPASAT are notoriously indicated by the ADD population to be the most difficult measure comprising the battery. Performance provides clear evidence of the impact of additional variables of sustained attention deficits and distractibility, in addition to that of information processing difficulty. When performance is significant of extensive severity, impact to brain functioning becomes a question. It is primarily this measure that results in individuals giving up and quitting either after several unsuccessful trials and/or immediately upon experiencing difficulty, providing a measure or index of frustration tolerance and also the psychological response to avoid and procrastinate any failure that may occur.

The *CHIPASAT* (Children's Paced Auditory Serial Addition Task) was developed based on the adult test of attention (PASAT) to assess the capacity and rate of information processing in children in 1988 (Johnson, Roethig-Johnson, and Middleton, 1988). The child's general intellectual ability and sex were found to be unrelated to CHIPASAT performance. Age and, to a lesser extent, arithmetic ability had a significant impact on performance, making this a reliable measure of information processing.

Dyche and Johnson (1991) provided more thorough norms for the CHIPASAT. Analysis suggested that normal children can maintain a relatively uniform information processing rate, even when the presentation rate has increased in speed and even doubled.

The Visual Search and Attention Test (VSAT) (Trenerry et al., 1990) has been standardized and validated for use with adults aged 18 years and older.

This addresses the individual's ability to scan accurately and sustain attention on each of four different visual cancellation tasks. Reliable administration requires that individuals possess adequate color discrimination and have the necessary vision for normal reading. It consists four visual cancellation tasks and provides a measurement of sustained attentional effort. Trials are timed and scored based on number correct and we have found in our clinical experience that this measure serves as an identification of slow cognitive speed characteristic of an attentional disorder without hyperactivity.

The Cancellation Test was originally developed by Mesulam and Weintraub (Mesulam, 1985) to evaluate the motor aspects of hemispatial neglect and specifically to assess visuospatial attention capabilities, visuo-scanning and the efficiency of attentional allocation (Geldmacher and Hills, 1996; Mesulam, 1985). The four test forms consist of random and structured arrays of verbal and nonverbal stimuli. The individual is asked to circle of the targets and normally under the age of 50 years can complete all four forms under two minutes. No errors are expected; however, over the age of 50 years, one error per field would still be considered normal and over the age of 80 years, 4 errors per field would still be considered normal. Normally individuals conduct a systematic search beginning on the left and proceeding to the right in horizontal or vertical rows, even in the random arrays. The examiner interrupts after the individual completes ten targets and provides the individual with another pencil to measure the interference and if the individual loses his/her place. Schwartz et al. (1997) evaluated subjects on the cancellation test, noting a common left to right tendency (probably related to a common reading and/or scanning bias) and the influence of both the sensory attentional and motor intentional systems. This measure is useful in the detection of spatial abnormalities in the distribution of visual attention to the individual's overall signal detection capacity (Cohen and Salloway, 1997). In our clinical assessment with this measure, those individuals with more severe spatial difficulties will reveal a difference in their performance, evidencing greater difficulty on the nonverbal portion, discriminating the stimulus to be circled.

Zelko and Brill (1996), in presenting their research with diagnosed ADHD and LD children on tests of visuographic motor-free perceptual, simple motor coordination and search skills, found that specifically ADHD performed worse on the visuographic and search tasks with search deficiencies due to errors in commission. Simple motor coordination and motor-free perception evidenced no differences between the groups. Although the authors indicated the above findings as providing support of frontal processes in the diagnosis of ADHD, in our clinical assessment we find the difference between the two groups to be both the patterning used to complete the task as well as the time taken for successful completion. This allows us to discriminate between the two subtypes for accurate diagnosis of ADD as well as addressing issues of distractibility and the ability to gate out some stimuli while focusing in on other stimuli.

A normal-aged population was studied by Geldmacher, Doty, and Heilman (1994), who located a pattern of results, demonstrating biases towards distant and leftward portions of visual stimuli. Results demonstrated the impact of normal aging on the spatial aspects of visual processing and established the validity of this measure to assess attentional or intentional performance in two areas of space concurrently. These tests have proved useful in determining the spatial allocation of attention. Damage to the left hemisphere results in left-sided neglect, however the right-hemisphere damage results in mild nonlateralized inattention on the cancellation tasks (Geldmacher and Hills, 1996; Marshall and Halligan, 1996).

Clinically, we have used this measure to distinguish hyperactivity from the predominantly inattentive individual without hyperactivity. This measure has been very informative in use with the attention-disordered population, whereby patterns distinct of responding have been observed clinically in ADHD children and adults, evidencing one of the specific subtypes. Generally, for both ADHD and ADD, the individual who is more distractible will have a greater number of errors and/or take a longer time to complete the task, providing evidence of a vulnerability to being distracted. The time taken to complete the task increases from the structured to the unstructured (and more chaotic) environment; time increases and is exacerbated with the compulsive, perfectionistic individual.

The Speech Sounds Perception Test and the Seashore Rhythm Test are designed to measure basic attention and concentration to allow input or information to get into the brain. The Speech Sounds Perception Test consists of 60 spoken nonsense words, which are variants of the "ee" sound and the subject responds by underlining one of the four alternatives printed for each item on the test form. This measure requires the ability to pay close and continued attention to the stimulus material. Very few errors are expected. Clinically, we have observed that attention-disordered individuals may experience problems on this measure as opposed to the Seashore Rhythm Test due to how slow and boring it is, and thus they tend to lose their focus. The Seashore Rhythmn Test is a subtest of the Seashore Measures of Musical Talent, whereby the individual is asked to differentiate between 30 pairs of rhyming beats. This measure requires alertness to non-verbal auditory stimuli, sustained attention to the task and the ability to perceive and compare different rhythmic sequences. In our clinical experience, when an attention-disordered individual has a difficult time on this measure, it indicates that as things become more complex and fast paced, there is more difficulty with taking in information or with input into the brain (Reitan and Wolfson, 1993).

The Symbol Digit Modalities Test (SDMT) was introduced by Smith (1976) based on the results of 10 years of data. The measure is based on neuropsychological principles and administered to both adults and children. Children are normed for both age and gender. There is a written and oral form to address those individuals with handicaps as well as provide a different modality with different variables impacting the functioning. The written form provides a useful measure of the status of the cerebral and peripheral sensorimotor mechanisms involved in written symbol substitutions and the sensitivity of this measure to the presence or absence of brain dysfunctioning has been well confirmed. This measure operates as a screening device to measure the general integrity and functioning of the brain. Clinically, we have found that this can be an accurate measure of the individual's potential when that potential cannot be measured due to the impact of the disorder on the individual's functioning. Finally, there is a trend that has been observed in that, when individuals have a problem of distractibility, they will have more errors and a poorer score in the oral section whereby there is less control and structure (Smith, 1976).

This measure is also seen as being impacted by the attentional processes. Cohen and Salloway (1997) view the SDMT as a measure of focused attention, requiring rapid processing of symbolic information, and the ability to code symbol-number pairs that are unfamiliar. The oral version of this measure appears to measure information processing capability and has also been used to predict driving capability. Performance has also provided indications of rehabilitation success on various attentional training programs (van Zomeren and Brouwer, 1994). Beatty et al. (1995) found that MS patients produced fewer correct responses than controls and found this to be a measure of speeded novel information processing.

Digit Span, Subtest of the Wechsler Scales

The Digit-Span subtest requires attentional focus and controlled effort. Cohen and Salloway (1997) cited the average number of digits that adults can normally repeat as ranging from 5 to 7, and the discrepancy between the forward and backward version should not exceed two digits. At our clinic, in evaluating ADD we have found a consistent pattern of greater than two points between the recall of digits forward vs backward for the Digit Span task of the Wechsler intelligence scales, with the gap ranging from 3 to 7 points. This pattern is correlated with the severity of the spatial issue and the difficulty that the ADD population experiences subsequent to their diminished ability to view the whole in a mental visual set for short-term recall. Franzen, Lovell, and Smith (1997), in researching the head-injured population, found that the degree of severity of performance for the backward recall on this measure was significantly correlated with the severity of the head injury.

Time as a Measure

van Zomeren and Brouwer (1994) suggest that reaction time and mental slowness is one of the various aspects of attention that can be assessed with standardized tests using adequate age-adjusted norms and will provide valuable information. Characteristic of the brain-damaged population, the mentally retarded, and the ADD is this mental slowness that can range from increased time problems as the task becomes more complex to time problems when the task is heavily speeded and the individual cannot compensate with complex operations of logical analysis and reasoning.

Self-Report Measures

Child Behavior Checklist (CBC) is a self-report measure completed by the parents for the age range of 4 to 18 years, revised as of 1991. According to the authors, parents (and parental surrogates) are among the most important source of data regarding a child's competencies and problems, presenting the most knowledgeable data about the child's behavior across time and situations. The CBC is a total of 118 problem items designed to address behavioral and emotional problems of children, yielding a multi-axial empirically based assessment to provide diagnosis and severity of symptoms in addition to a competency section addressing the quality of the child's participation in sports, hobbies, games, activities, jobs, and chores. Each of the 118 specific problem items and 2 open-ended problem items are scored on a three-step response scale. Syndromes identified encompass the following categories: withdrawn, somatic complaints, anxious/depressed, social problems, thought problems, attention problems, sex problems, delinquent behavior, and aggressive behavior (Achenbach, 1991).

Chen et al. (1994) examined the accuracy of he CBC scales for ADHD and found this measure to have the highest discriminating power for ADHD (when compared with other measures) and suggests that this measure is valid as a rapid screening instrument to identify ADHD (Biederman et al., 1993).

The Attention Deficit Disorders Evaluation Scale Home Version (ADDES) (McCarney, 1989) was designed to be a relevant measure of attention deficit disorders for the home environment and relies on the reporting of the parents or significant caregiver. The 46 items were developed according to the recommendations of diagnosticians professionally involved in measuring ADD and normed on a total of 1,754 students from 12 states and provides norms from ages 4 to 20 years. The three subscales were that of inattentivenes, impulsivity, and hyperactivity. Clinically, in our research this measure has been found to be quite accurate in reporting symptoms of the disorder. Adesman (1991) reviewed the measure and found that both the home and school version were helpful in measuring behavior over time; however, there are no studies to support its use in the measurement of interval change or response to treatment intervention.

The ADD–H Comprehensive Teacher's Rating Scale (ACTeRS) (Ullmann, Sleator, and Sprague (1991) includes 24 items relevant to classroom behavior to factor into the categories of inattention, hyperactivity, social skills, and oppositional behavior. This measure is completed by the teachers on observing behavior of the child in the classroom. Authors found this to be a useful measure in differentiating learning-disabled from attention-disordered children. Clinically, we have found this to be a relatively accurate measure, although anxiety can easily load on the factor of hyperactivity and mistakenly diagnose ADHD.

Other self-report measures include a developmental history for children or adults, and children and adolescent problems checklist to determine historical information and to rule in or rule out additional emotional problems. The Adolescent Behavior Checklist, a 44-item checklist completed by the adolescent, and utilized to provide indications of emotional issues evidenced through recent evaluation, was determined to be a fairly stable and significant measure of ADHD and its associated symptoms. Analysis of responses revealed consistent acknowledgment of conduct problems, impulsivity/hyperactivity, poor work habits, inattentiveness, emotional lability, and social problems (Adams, Kelley and McCarthy, 1997). Finally, measures are utilized from Barkley (1991) to assess functioning in both the home and school environment in terms of behavior and cognitive skills. The only problem we have experienced clinically with these measures is that due to the way they are normed and evaluated there is the tendency for misdiagnosis of ADHD based on the anxiety so prevalent in the ADD population.

CHAPTER 16

Other Treatment Methods

Research generally supports a step-by-step procedure of treatment for ADD, beginning with accurate diagnosis and initial remediation with medication, followed by intervention in the school setting and, finally, specific interventions for the home environment. The more specific the diagnosis, the more one is able to rule in or out other confounding issues, the better the treatment prognosis (Aust, 1994; Varley, 1984; Woodrum, Anderson, and Unger, 1994). An individual's physical, chemical, emotional, attitudinal, and motivational state impacts the use of mental strategies available to him, external aids in the physical environment (i.e., computer, planners, electronic schedulers, watches with alarms) and social interaction skills to receive help from community resources (Hermann and Parente, 1994). Virtual reality is a new addition to the computer that will enhance interest and allow increased generalization of learning. The use of computers to generate virtual environments (Virtual Reality) has been successful in helping the head-injured child to generalize training to their real-life environment. Training using Virtual Reality (VR) forces the child to address consequences of their responses and adapt their mental processing and behavior accordingly. The environmental interaction becomes contingent upon the response repertoire that the child has, thus providing a situation that is specifically commensurate with the child's sensory and motor capabilities, specifically targeting these areas and allowing them to benefit from training at any level of disability (Rose, Johnson, and Attree, 1997). By appealing to all sensory modalities, virtual reality will specifically help remediate spatial issues characteristic of an inattention to the whole that subserves basic language-skill development by adding a dimensional component to task completion. Failure to address all of these issues and their reciprocity will most certainly lead to treatment failure.

In considering ADD as a disorder of higher-level cognitive thinking processes, this population would benefit from methods of rehabilitation designed to address specific neuropsychological issues. Research indicates that, cognitively, there is much to be gained with specific rehabilitation of identified problem areas, developing specific coping mechanisms to address deficit issues, building skill levels and targeting problem areas with specific training to strengthen neural connections.

Remediation or rehabilitation is dependent on adaptive and remedial approaches. Adaptive approaches operate from the idea that intact brain functions can be increased in utilization as a compensatory mechanism. Adaptive retraining provides substitute methods to attain the goal of functioning subserved by deficit areas. Remediate treatment targets recovery or reorganization of brain function, teaching intact cells to take over the role of deficit cells. Environmental stimulation influences these processes. The idea of working specific areas of brain functioning (such as perceptual and sensorimotor exercises) to address visual processing deficits (Raymond et al., 1996).

Parents of ADHD children were found to view this disorder as neurobiological in etiology, with the positive or negative behavior of their child being subject to internally driven forces and not subject to any action they or their child might undertake towards remediation (Johnston and Freeman, 1997). This would automatically negate any type of intervention program that a professional attempted to implement. Both parents and children need to fully comprehend the duality of this disorder: although etiologically genetic in origin, changes can occur with significant impact to brain functioning as a result of the continual interplay occurring between internal and external forces. The lament of the ADD-without-hyperactivity population is that often their emotional reaction and, subsequent, failure to learn stretch their resources and maximize their potential. This can be far worse than the symptoms of the disorder itself. Our research over the last 10 years has revealed the overwhelming impact on academic skill development, specifically that of reading and math. As a result of the failure to develop spatial areas of function, it can become further compromised because the efforts to utilize compensatory mechanisms to address symptoms of the attentional disorder result in the maximizing of logical reasoning areas instead. By the time we see a child at the age of 5 years (our minimum for diagnosis due to the normative data available) the spatial problem evidenced is due to the failure to utilize that area and is no longer amenable to treatment by stimulant medication, all that is left is to retrain and utilize this unused area of functioning. The brighter the individual, the more compulsive they become, the more they dislike failure, and the greater the gap between logical reasoning skills (developed to superior levels) and spatial functioning (often within below average ranges).

Sturm et al. (1997) found efficacy for the development of game-type computer programs designed to address each of the specific aspects of attention, alertness, vigilance, selective and divided attention in patients with localized vascular lesions. Findings support a hierarchical attentional organization. Significant improvement was obtained only with specific training. Training for alertness and selective attention was necessary prior to divided attention training, and training in alertness was a necessary prerequisite for selective attention training to occur.

Rehabilitation of Specific Deficits Identified in the Diagnostic Process

van Zomeren and Brouwer (1994) suggested a compensation model for impaired driving skills describing traffic behavior as a hierarchy of subtasks that occur at strategic, tactical, and operational levels. *Strategic* is defined as choices and decisions concerning route, time of day, and general operations decisions. These decisions are usually made without the pressure of time and before actual driving occurs. The tactical level involves preparatory actions that need to be taken while driving, such as slowing down or braking at an intersection, and there is a slight degree of time pressure at this level. The operational level demands the most in terms of thinking processes and actions that involve the continual issues that arise while driving and analysis of driving (indicating that time pressure exists more so at this operational level). Higher-level decisions designed to offset the possibility of a problem, such as not driving during a certain time of day, can provide a means of compensation.

Sohlberg, Mateer, and Stuss (1993) provided an outline for developing problem-solving by using the following:

1. Generation of goal-directed ideas, brainstorming, and using a variety of alternatives for a given consequence or program.

2. Training in the systematic and careful comparison of information and the framework of looking at each idea and seeing if it is valuable.
3. Use of multiple pieces of information processes simultaneously by examining each idea, seeing what will work, prioritizing which to try first.
4. Finally, trying ideas as solutions, getting feedback, and preparing to try another new idea if this does not work.

Treatment for social skills and inattentiveness has involved specific training and the most successful has been training to the point of automatization, whereby individuals are trained to automatically perceive social cues (van Zomeren and Brouwer, 1994). Cicerone and Giacino (1992) describe *remediation of executive function deficits* after head injury as self-prediction for treatment of anticipatory deficits, self-instructional training for planning deficits and self-monitoring training.

Rehabilitation *for hemi-inattention or unilateral neglect* has typically attempted to remind the individual to pay attention to the unattended side or field of vision. Training for visual scanning was found to have a positive effect on reading ability; however, improvement was generally limited to the trained tasks and evidenced little generalization. Found to be helpful and longer lasting in effects were training strategies that were cue-specific (meaning that training was tied to specific cues), were likely to be present in the individual's everyday life, and by using specific cues, these cues generalized to the ability to perform a number of tasks related to the cues, that were previously problematic (van Zomeren and Brouwer, 1994).

Stimulation Therapy for Attentional Deficits

The major premise behind the stimulation model was that attentional impairments could be alleviated by means of direct stimulation of brain structures assumed to be involved in attentional processes. Treatment was based on having individuals utilize repetitive exercises and providing them with feedback and was found to have substantial success by Ben Yishay and his associates. Some of the training effects were visible however (for the most part) these effects did not generalize beyond the trained tasks and the effects on daily life were not significant to support this theoretical idea (van Zomeren and Brouwer, 1994).

Strategy Substitution Methods for Attentional Training

This model was originally based on the idea that individuals could be helped with compensatory strategies in the form of external aids or internal self-instruction and self-mediation. This method has been found to have the greatest efficacy and support of van Zomeren and Brouwer. Strategy training involves instructions and general guidelines that should be adjusted for each individual and related to specific tasks based on known deficits. The following considerations are suggested:

1. *Task analysis:* Specific analysis of such issues as time pressure, interruptions, degree of structure necessary to complete the task, subtasks subserving the task, kinds of information to be processed, requirement of a particular skill set, and so on.
2. *Analysis of impairments:* Knowledge of specific impairment areas to be able to predict performance problems and thus provide compensation. Knowledge of particular stress areas and prediction of when the individual will be the most impaired and/or stressed.
3. *Analysis of compensatory potential:* This correlates with the analysis of impairments, in that the strengths and weaknesses are assessed specifically to plan available resources and allocations of that resource using the greatest deficit as necessitating the greatest compensatory strategy.
4. *Adaptation to the task and/or the environment:* Using all of the above information to provide adjustment to the task. Interruptions need to be minimized, reduction of number of subtasks involved in the job, sequential checklists made, and supervision and feedback provided.
5. *Elimination of risk of non-optimal risk performance:* The cost of errors need to be estimated and whether there is a question of risk that is beyond the person's abilities needs to be addressed. Emotional issues need to be addressed at this point and the cost effectiveness of the task performance.

Mateer, Sohlberg, and Youngman (1990) suggest specific training strategies for specific types of attention. For selective attention, it is recommended that training involve the incorporation of distracting or irrelevant stimuli during task performance. Training of alternating attentional deficits require flexible redirection and reallocation of attention. Multifaceted approaches are critical and need to include direct training through practice and education to increase awareness, cognitive behavioral treatment to address feelings and attitudes, and structured generalization for both the home and the workplace. To develop effective remediation strategies it is important to take into consideration the effortful demands such strategies will place on an already depleted system. External aids provide a means of ensuring that the individual does not rely solely on mnemonic devices that place heavy demands on cognitive processing (Schmitter and Edgecombe, 1996; Mateer and Mapou, 1996). Sohlberg and Raskin (1996) provide principles to ensure generalization of learning.

1. The idea of actively planning from the onset for generalization to occur
2. Identification of suitable reinforcers present in the natural environment
3. Stimuli utilized are conducive to both the training and the home environment
4. Use of enough examples when teaching new ideas for increased understanding; there is a need to minimize errors
5. Selection of a method to determine measurement of generalization

Divided Attention: ADD Training

Training for divided attention involve the use of tasks in which multiple kinds of information must be attended to simultaneously or the simultaneous use of two or more tasks. Sohlberg and Mateer (1987) designed an Attention Process Training program combined with selective computer programs. They based administration of hierarchically organized treatment tasks on a five level model of attention: focused, sustained, selective, alternating, and divided attention. More than 60 exercises corresponding to the specific components of attention were used to provide repeated exercises of attention in a gradual and progressively more demanding sequence. Treatment was individualized and varied from 4 to 8 weeks with each patient receiving seven to nine sessions per week. Positive results were noted.

Weber (1990) suggests ways to work with capacity and control deficit issues by reducing the capacity required by a task, by training control strategies to the point where they become relatively automatic, by providing awareness of the problem and increase of confidence in the ability to improve attentional functioning. *Feedback* is important and the development of compensatory strategies to apply to everyday life. Training is thought of as a three-tier process involving the identification of the problem, the special training tasks used for compensation and the transfer of this knowledge to everyday life activities.

Parente, Stapleton, and Wheatley (1991) suggest that due to the distractibility and feelings of overload experienced by the attention-disordered individual, others may get them started on particular tasks and remind them to stay on task until it is completed. When left to their own devices, individuals can lose track of what they are doing, saying, or thinking, and outside sources can help to put them back into focus. Training is suggested using task-specific routines, specific attention-process training with the use of computer programs, use of metacognitive self-instruction, and asking questions during task execution that becomes helpful for organization and error monitoring. Error monitoring has been found to mobilize the use of feedback. Social inclusion is an important issue that if not addressed will impact motivation. Social inclusion is defined as being involved in all of the activities that make up the life of the family (Ried et al., 1995).

Addressing ADD Specifically

In the school setting, Burnley (1993) provided a four-step follow-up plan for working with the attention-disordered population (ADHD specifically) in the school setting. Step 1 involved preliminary assessment using observations and self-report measures from both home and the school setting. Step 2 is the follow-up meeting to address the needs of the ADHD child and, based on a positive finding of the disorder, suggestions are made for parent training, specific knowledge of ADHD, and educational training and medication. Step 3 is that of developing strategies to address the symptoms of the disorder comprising the learning of rules, structure, minimizing distractions in the class setting, use of cues to teach the child to stop and think prior to acting, use of immediate and variable contingencies as reinforcers, method of monitoring classroom behavior, and written contracts with notations for keeping expectations both reasonable and consistent. Finally, step 4 is that of follow-up on the progress of the ADHD child. A team approach is strongly recommended to provide services to the child and support for the teacher.

Webster-Stratton (1993), in addressing the conduct-disordered and oppositional-defiant population, reports that the early school and pre-school grades are the optimum and strategic time for early identification, intervention, and prevention programs to facilitate children's social competence and conflict resolution skills. In reviewing the research, Stratton found that there are two basic types of child skill training approaches: the attempt to train the child in specific target social behaviors based on the hypothesized social skill deficit, and the reliance on cognitive-behavioral methods and focus on training children in the cognitive process. In training to correct social behaviors, program focus is on coaching children in positive social skills such as play skills, friendship, and conversational skills. In training on the cognitive processes, focus is on problem-solving, self-control, and self-statements, as well as empathy training and perspective taking. The method used by both of these approaches usually includes verbal instructions and discussion opportunities to practice the skill with peers, role-playing, games, stories, and feedback and reinforcement. Parent training programs comprise the largest research and have presented the most effective and promising results; however, programs do not encompass all that is needed for change to generalize and remain constant. Suggested is that training programs incorporate multiple settings and multiple individuals with the idea that this is not a "quick fix" type of intervention.

Classwide peer tutoring procedures involving the use of frequent and immediate feedback revealed its effectiveness in a singular case study involving one-on-one interaction with an ADHD child. Peer tutoring was described in-depth. It was the role of the teacher to monitor the behavior of the tutoring pairs in the classroom and to provide assistance as necessary. In peer tutoring, the tutor is provided with a "script" of academic material related to the current content of instruction occurring in the classroom. Items are given to the ADHD child by the tutor one at a time and the child responds orally. Points are awarded by the tutor for each correct initial response and in case of error the tutor provides the correct answer and opportunity to practice and learn the correct response. The child then can earn rewards after practicing the correct response a number of times (DuPaul and Henningson, 1993).

Abikoff (1991) addresses the need of multimodal treatment for ADD. Interventions in addition to medication involve the learning of social skills, academic skills, specific cognitive remediation strategies, psychotherapy are hypothesized as necessary for total treatment of the disorder. Abikoff and Klein (1992) suggest the consideration of comorbid disorders in treatment approaches to further implement changes specifically targeted to treat problem areas when dealing with the combination of ADHD and Conduct Disorder.

In the Home

Parent training programs have shown success in remediation of ADHD. The idea is to address the disorder from a family systems perspective to understand the very powerful reciprocal impact of the parent–child interaction (Bernier and Siegel, 1994). Families of ADHD children often have characteristic instability (both familial and marital), conflicted parent-child interactions, high levels of parental stress, and maternal depression. Families face specific challenges around borders and boundaries (underdeveloped homeostasis, difficulty with transition and change), and feedback (continual miscommunication). Accurate diagnosis, training, and education as well as referral to community resources are suggested to cope with this multifaceted disorder.

The majority of the research, unfortunately, has focused on ADHD and studies generally have not addressed the issues of the ADD child. Strayhorn and Weidman (1989) experimented with a preventative mental health intervention program with low income ADHD parent–child dyads. Improvement was seen with specific parent training programs both in terms of parent's ratings of their child's behavior and observed interactions between child and parent. Authors suggest that the aspects of the treatment that was most helpful in reduction of attention deficit symptoms was the practice and reinforcement for longer and longer periods of time in listening to stories, conversing with parents, and participating in the dramatic play that helped the child improve in attending to verbal information and that a protective factor against development of ADHD symptoms was learned competence in sustaining attention to verbally encoded information.

Pisterman and associates (1989) introduced a parent training program aimed at improving child compliance with ADHD preschoolers. Positive treatment effect was obtained on measures of compliance, parental style of interaction and management skills with improvements being sustained and maintained at a three-month follow-up. However, evaluation of treatment effects indicated an absence of generalization and there were no treatment effects for non-targeted behaviors. Improved management skills were evidenced in the parent's more consistent reinforcement of their child's compliance and parents learned a set of skills that resulted in overall improved compliance in their children. The program consisted of providing information about the etiology, course, and treatment of ADHD in addition to addressing practical issues regarding the home setting and finally, sessions were skill oriented (utilizing modeling, role-playing and didactic material) to teach strategies of how to give differential attention to appropriate behavior, how to issue appropriate commands and how to use time-outs for noncompliance.

Anastopoulos et al. (1993) found significant post-treatment gains in both parent and child functioning on completion of a behavioral parent training program specifically designed for school-aged children diagnosed with ADHD. Gains were maintained 2 months subsequent to treatment and there were reductions found in parenting stress and increases in parenting self-esteem. The nine week program included an overview of ADHD, child management principles, teaching of positive reinforcement skills, the use of positive attending and ignoring skills, punishment strategies and ways to modify strategies to generalized settings.

Behavior Management Programs

Lochman and Klimes-Dougan (1993) provided a conceptual model to provide universal interventions and a specific school based anger coping program for aggressive children. The anger coping program consisted of 18 weekly group sessions (comprised of 4 to 6 children) and group sessions included discussion, activities, role playing, video taping, and goal setting. Topics addressed in these groups were perspective taking, awareness of the physiological arousal (introduced with anger outbursts), use of self-instruction to inhibit impulsive responding and evoke social problem solving.

Barkley et al. (1992) provided 12 to 18 year olds diagnosed adolescents with ADHD with 8 to 10 sessions of child behavior management training or problem solving and communication training as compared with structural family therapy. All three treatment approaches produced significant improvements in parent-adolescent communication, number of conflicts and anger intensity during conflict resolution as well as less depression and significant improvement in parent reported school adjustment. All improvements were maintained at a three month follow up.

Whalen and Henker (1991), in their review of the research of therapies for ADHD children, found the need for multimodal approaches encompassing medication and behavioral programs. Social skills is a deficit area for both ADHD and ADD and most studies have found that social skills training alone is not enough. Training in appropriate social behavior in addition to exposure to real life social situations helps to substantiate the learning and provide later generalizability.

The above research findings point to a generalizability of the different programs utilized with the ADHD population whether it be directed at anger, behavioral constraints, or cognitive training. Programs that are successful generally employ sessions over a period of several weeks, incorporate sort of feedback mechanisms and follow-up, address parental issues of how to manage and discipline the child, address the child learning coping skills and finally education and understanding of the disorder itself to allow for specific remediation. One final note is that specific targeting of the problem area, whether it is cognitive deficits and/or behavioral issues is critical to address exactly what needs to be done and it appears that the more specific the identification of the problem the more long lasting the treatment effects. Treatment also needs to address the emotional issues of the ADHD and the ADD child and the impact of symptomatology that produces emotional consequences that will become a variable to contend with in any treatment intervention.

Physiological Approaches

There has been a great amount of controversy regarding the use of biofeedback for treatment of ADHD and results remain inconclusive (Barkley, 1993; Lubar, 1995).

Williams et al. (1994), in evaluating the effects of wavelength on the performance of attention-disordered children on the WCST found that the *wavelength manipulation* affected attentional processing and on all measures there were significant effects for color with the short wavelength (blue) enhancing performance. This was found to be consistent with prior research that the short wavelength stimuli increased the speed and magnitude of M channel response and enhanced reading performance. If the dorsal (attentional) system is an extension of the M channel, the enhancement found with short wavelength stimuli suggests that the use of such stimuli may increase the speed and magnitude of the dorsal system response, resulting in enhanced attentional performance. Studies indicate that contrast reduction may provide a second mechanism for enhancing attentional processing. Further, the efficacy of color intervention is not specific to attention-impaired groups and short wavelength stimuli was found to enhance attentional performance in both ADHD and the normal population. In the case of the ADHD population, performance improved to the degree that it approached the normal range. On all WCST measures affected by color, short wavelength stimuli brought the performance of the attention impaired group into the same range of performance that the normal group showed in the control condition which was clear. Thus short wavelength materials or overlays may compensate for the attentional impairment in the ADHD population. This intervention will require further confirmation and research to be considered as a viable means of remediation.

Adult ADD and Treatment Findings

Weinstein (1994) substantiated the need for a multimodal approach to adult ADHD including medication, psychotherapy and cognitive remediation strategies to enhance functioning by enhancing attention, memory and problem-solving skills. Remediation was found to be effective when both the cognitive and emotional aspects of the disorder were addressed.

Ratey (1993) offered a number of "tips" on the management of adult ADD breaking down the treatment of ADD into five basic areas:

1. Diagnosis
2. Education
3. Structure, support, and coaching
4. Various forms of psychotherapy
5. Medication

In the area of insight and education, he suggested that the individual be sure of the correct diagnosis, separating the disorder from its various look-alikes. Coaching and encouragement, educating others, listening to feedback from others, joining a support group, letting go of the negativity and allowing others to help all are critical variables for successful management of ADD. In the area of performance management, it is important to have an external structure, operate with color coding, acknowledge and anticipate consequences of behavior, use deadlines, break large tasks down, prioritize, notepads in the car and working both to the strengths and the weaknesses. In the area of mood management, he recommended structured time to let go, recharging of batteries, exercise and helpful addictions, understanding of the mood changes, anticipation of problems in social situations, and generally working with the disorder and its emotional issues. Finally, in the area of interpersonal life, the idea is to learn to laugh about mistakes, schedule activities with friends and set social deadlines.

Ratey and Hallowell (1993) went on to suggest management tips for ADD adult within the family system. He again suggested the issue of making an accurate diagnosis and education regarding the disorder and it symptomology.

He proposed understanding of the disorder as it relates to the family system and to have the family negotiate and plan for behavior and consequences. Family therapists are helpful and generally provide a means to disengage from the idea of struggles. Finally there are ideas of family brainstorming, targeting of problem areas, setting of borders and boundaries and making use of feedback.

Ratey, Hallowell, and Miller (1996) talked about the need for education and the undoing of the negative cycle the ADD adult tends to fall into. A common complaint of the ADD adult is that of an immature, childlike behavior and a lagging behind of peers in terms of achievement of life goals. They suggested that a practical and immediate means of augmenting the process of relearning for the ADD adult is to offer support and assistance to help the person structure and bring order to the chaos of everyday life. Planning and organizational tools are essential to provide an external sense of control.

Parker (1993) provided ideas on the management of ADD in couples. Again he indicated the need for an accurate diagnosis and education. He discussed setting up a time for talking and communication with one's partner. Writing down complaints, making a treatment plan, making lists and use of bulletin boards are all help management techniques. Partners should write down what they want from their ADD spouse, avoiding the patterns of one person compensating for the ADD spouse in some way (thus leading to low self-esteem in the ADD adult). Generally, watching out for the tendency towards dominance and submission with someone being in control. Working with the moodiness, providing encouragement and not using ADD as an excuse, are all important in management of this disorder.

Kelly and Ramundo (1993) provided excellent and easy ideas to employ for the different areas of the adult ADD individual. General tips are offered to watch and listen, observe distractibility typical of the ADD person, work on reading skills and use of feedback on an habitual basis. In the area of communication, he suggested getting used to the rhythm of the language in the environment, synchronizing to its flow and thus knowing when and where and how much to contribute, realization of both verbal and nonverbal communication and the idea that communication is an interplay of both words and body language. He cited the difficulty of the ADD adult in their ability to read body language and interpret this correctly.

Getting along on the job, Kelly and Ramundo (1993) indicated that the ADD adult must make sense of the rules, procedures and policies that run the office. ADD adults need to be aware of the unwritten rules, procedures, and policies as well in an attempt to get inside the inner circle in the office situation.

Suggestions such as watching impassivity, stopping and thinking, spacing of children, planning in advance of financial resources, creating a positive living space, establishing borders and boundaries, rest and relaxation, teaching communication skills to family members, not arguing at dinner and use of family meetings and family fun are quite helpful in addressing concomitant emotional factors. Organization is critical and can be attained by putting limits on problem areas, prioritizing lists, establishing a personal work space, use of plenty of cabinets, planners and paperwork completed in the same place and handled at the same time each day.

Addressing Specific Issues Related to Comorbid Symptoms and Disorders with Nutritional Supplements

The diagnosis of ADD appears to preclude the individual for risk, physiologically, genetically, biochemically, and psychologically. The comorbidity identified in this population substantiates a biochemical vulnerability. Physiologically as a group, there is higher evidence of stress and stress-related disorders, possible increased risk to environmental toxins associated with cancer and emotional ability that exacerbates stress.

Specifically, for the late adolescent, young adult, and especially for the aged population, nutrition becomes an essential part of the treatment program. Research is indicating the efficacy of the botanicals as a means of addressing emotional concerns. Blanel (1995) stressed the role of nutritional factors helping to regulate neuronal function and action of the neurotransmitters. Nutritional status is seen as influencing all phases of the nervous system. Treatment is confirming prevention, control, and treatment of various disorders with nutritional substances. Mounting scientific evidence is pointing to the free radicals (molecules or atoms that have increased chemical reactivity due to at least one unpaired electron) that then react with other molecules to cause cell damage or DNA mutation. A condition of oxidative stress (enzymes produced by the body working to repair free radical damage) appears to contribute to cardiovascular disease and cancer. There are implications of essential trace elements in endocrinological processes impacting specific problematic conditions related to thyroid function, use of insulin, adrenal system and gonadal function and correctable with adequate supplementation (Capwell, 1993; Diplock, 1991; Halliwell, 1994; Janzen et al., 1995; Mertz, 1993; Neve, 1992).

Biofeedback

Lubar (1995) developed EEG biofeedback techniques for treatment of ADHD and an ERP event-related potential assessment. He has been researching the efficacy of this treatment for approximately 15 years following diagnosed ADHD children into adulthood. Treatment sessions are integrated with academic work and planned out gradually. Janzen et al. (1995) confirmed the data of Lubar, the ratio of theta to beta discriminated ADD children and finally the most significant differences with treatment for the parietal area. This would confirm the idea that the majority of diagnosed ADHD are actually ADD and thus the targeting of the parietal area. Lubar et al. (1995) found significant effects of neurofeedback training on both objective intellectual measures and attentional subjective reports demonstrating neurofeedback training as a viable treatment for ADHD. Reduction of theta activity was seen as the key factor associated with improvement in ADD. Lubar et al. conclude that there is a necessity for further research with natural control groups. Unfortunately this method of rehabilitation for attentional deficits remains controversial and will require further documentation as an adjunctive treatment technique.

References

Abi-Dargham, M. D., Larulle, M., Aghajanian, G. K. (1997) The role of serotonin in the pathophysiology and treatment of schizophrenia, *The Journal of Neuropsychiatry and Clinical Neurosciences, 9(1),* 1–17.

Abikoff, H. and Klein, R. G. (1992). Attention-deficit hyperactivity and conduct disorder: Comorbidity and implications for treatment. *Journal of Consulting and Clinical Psychology, 60,* 881–892.

Accardo, P. J., Blondis, T. A., and Whitman, B. Y. (Eds.) (1991). *Attention Deficit Disorders and Hyperactivity in Children.* New York: Marcel Dekker.

Acharya, J. N., Wyllie, E., Lüders, H. O., Kotagal, P., Lancman, M., and Coelho, M. (1997). Seizure symptomatology in infants with localization-related epilepsy, *Neurology, (48)* 189–196.

Achenbach, T. M. (1991). *Manual for the Child Behavior Checklist/4-18 and 1991 Profile.* Burlington, VT: University of Vermont Department of Psychiatry.

Acherman, P. T., Dykman, R. A., Oglesby, D. M., and Newton, J. E. O. (1994). EEG power spectra of children with dyslexia, slow learners, and normally reading children with ADD during verbal processing. *Journal of Learning Disabilities, 27(10),* 619–630.

Adams, C. D., Kelley, M. L., and McCarthy, M. (1997). The adolescent behavior checklist: Development and initial psychometric properties of a self-report measure for adolescents with ADHD, *Journal of Clinical Child Psychology,* 26(1), 77–86.

Adesman, A. R. (1991). The attention deficit disorders evaluation scale. *Journal of Developmental and Behavioral Pediatrics, 12(1),* 65–66.

Adler, C. H. (1997). Treatment of restless legs syndrome with gabapentin, *Clinical Neuropharmacology,* 20(2), 148–151.

Adrian, C. and Hammen, C. (1993). Stress exposure and stress generation in children of depressed mothers. *Journal of Consulting and Clinical Psychology, 61,* 354–359.

Aglioti, S., Beltramello, A., Girardi, F., and Fabbro, F. (1996). Neurolinguistic and follow-up study of an unusual pattern of recovery from bilingual subcortical asphasia, *Brain,* 119, 1551–1564.

311

Aharon-Peretz, J., Brenner, B., Amyel-Zvi, E., Metz, L., and Hemli, J. A. (1996). Neurocognitive dysfunction in the antiphospholipid antibody syndrome. *Neuropsychiatry, Neuropsychology, and Behavioral Neurology, 9,* 123–126.

Alberts-Corush, J., Firestone, P., and Goodman, J. T. (1986). Attention and Impusivity Characteristics of the Biological and Adoptive Parents of Hyperactive and Normal Control Children. *American Journal of Orthopsychiatry, 56,* 413–423.

Alessandri, S. M. and Schramm, K. (1991). Effects of dextroamphetamine on the cognitive and social play of a preschooler with ADHD. *Journal of the American Academy of Child and Adolescent Psychiatry, 30,* 768–772.

Alexander-Roberts, C. (1994). The ADHD Parenting Handbook: Practical Advice for Parents from Parents. Dallas, TX: Taylor Publishing Company.

Alexrod, B. N., Goldman, R. S., Heaton, R. K., Curtiss, G., Thompson, L. L., Chelune, G., and Kay, G. G. (1996). Diuscriminability of the wisconsin card sorting test using the standardization sample, *Journal of Clinical and Experimental Neuropsychology, 18,* 338–342.

Allen, J., Brennan, P., Garrett, R., and Moore, R. (1997). A comparative study of methylphenidate and amantadine with traumatic brain injury, ANPA Abstracts *Journal of Neuropsychiatry and Clinical Neurosciences, 9*(1) 156, P90, *American Journal of Psychiatry,* 154(8) 1101–1106.

Allison, M. (1993). Exploring the link between violence and brain injury. *Headlines, March/April,* 12–15.

Aloia, M. S., Gourovitch, D. R., Weinberger, D. R., and Goldberg, T. E. (1996). An investigation of semantic space in patients with schizophrenia, *Journal of the International Neuropsychological Society,* (2), 267–273.

Aman, M. G., Marks, R. E., Turbott, S. H., Wilksher, C. P., and Merry, S. N. (1991). Methylphenidate and thioridazine in the treatment of intellectually subaverage children. Effects on cognitive motor performance. *Journal of the American Academy of Child and Adolescent Psychiatry, 30,* 816–824.

Aman, M. G., Kern, R. A., McGhee, D. E., and Arnold, L. E. (1993). Fenfluoramine and Methylphenidate in children with mental retardation and attention deficit hyperactivity disorder: Laboratory effects. *Journal of Autism and Developmental Disorders, 23*(3), 497–506.

Aman, M. G., Kern, R. A., McGhee, D. E., and Arnold, L. E. (1993). Fenfluoramine and Methylphenidate in children with mental retardation and attention deficit hyperactivity disorder: Clinical and side effects. *Journal of the American Academy, 32*(4), 851–859.

Aman, M. G., Marks, R. E., Turbott, S. H. and Wilksher, C. P. (1991). Clinical effects of methylphenidate and thioridazine in intellectually subaverage children.

Ambrosini, P. J. (1993). Antidepressant treatments in children and adolescents: II. Anxiety, physical, and behavioral disorders. *Journal of the American Academy of Child and Adolescent Psychiatry, 32,* 483–493.

Amen, D. G. (1996). (1994–95) Windows Into the A.D.D. Mind: *MindWorks Press,* 1996.

Amen, D. G. (1993). Windows Into the A.D.D. Mind: Understanding and Treating Attention Deficit Disorders in the Everyday Lives of Children, Teenagers and Adults. Fairfield, CA: Daniel G. Amen.

Amen, D. G., Paldi, J. H., and Thisted, R. A. (1993). Brain SPECT imaging. *Journal of the American Academy.* 32(5), 1080–1081, Ann. NY. Academy of Science, 270, 45–55.

Amin, K., Douglas, V. I., Mendelson, M. J., and Dufresne, J. (1993). Separable/integral classification by hyperactive and normal children. *Development and Psychopathology, 5,* 415–431.

Ammerman, R. T. and Patz, R. J. (1996). Determinants of child abuse potential: Contribution of parent and child factors, *Journal of Clinical Child Psychology,* 25(3), 300–307.

Anastopoulos, A. D., Shelton, T. L., DuPaul, G. J., and Guevremont, D. C. (1993). Parent training for attention-deficit hyperactivity disorder: Its impact on parent functioning. *Journal of Abnormal Child Psychology, 21(5),* 581–596.

Anderson, B. (1996). A mathematical model of line bisection behavior in neglect, *Brain,* 119, 841–850.

Anderson, C. A. and Hammen, C. L. (1993). Psychosocial outcomes of children of unipolar depressed, bipolar, medically ill, and normal women: A longitudinal study. *Journal of Consulting and Clinical Psychology, 61,* 448–454.

Anderson, C. A., Hinshaw, S. P., and Simmel, C. (1994). Mother–child interactions an ADHD and comparison boys: Relationships with overt and covert externalizing behavior. *Journal of Abnormal Child Psychology, 22(2).*

Anderson, C. V. and Bigler, E. D. (1994). The role of caudate nucleus and corpus callosum atrophy in trauma-induced anterior horn dilation. *Brain Injury, 8,* 565–569.

Anderson, R. A., Polansky, M. M., Bryden, N. A., and Canary, J. J. (1991). Supplemental-chromium effects on glucose, insulin, glucagon, and urinary chromium losses in subjects consuming controlled low-chromium diets. *American Journal of Clinical Nutrition, 32,* 173–185.

Anderson, V., Bond, L., Catroppa, C., Grimwood, K., Keir, E., and Nolan, T. (1997). *Journal of the International Neuropsychological Society, 3,* 147–158.

Angold, A. and Costello, E. J. (1993). Depressive comorbidity in children and adolescents: Empirical, theoretical, and methodological issues. *American Journal of Psychiatry, 150,* 1779–1791.

Angus, S., Sugars, J., Boltezar, R., Kosewich, S., and Schneider, N. M., (1997). A controlled trial of amantadine hydrochloride and neuroleptics in the treatment of tardive dyskinesia, *Journal of Clinical Psychopharmacology,* 17(5), 88–91.

Anon. Child Psychopharmacology, Alternatives sought for Ritalin. *Psychopharmacology Update, 7,* 1–2.

Anthony, J. C., Warner, L. A., and Kessler, R. C. (1994). Comparative epidemiology of dependence on tobacco, alcohol, controlled substances, and inhalants: Basic findings from the National Comorbidity Survey. *Experimental and Clinical Psychopharmacology, 2,* 244–268.

Arcia, E. and Gualtier, C. T. (1994). Neurobehavioral performance of adults with closed-head injury, Adults with attention, deficit, and controls. Brain Injury 8(5) 395–404.

Ardila, A., Rosselli, M., Arvizu, L., and Kuljis, R. O. (1996). Alexia and agraphia in posterior cortical atrophy. Neuropsyschiatry, Neuropsychology, and Behavioral Neurology, 10(1), 52–59.

Arnold, B. R., Montgomery, G. T., Castaneda, I., and Longoria, R. (1994). Acculturation and performance of Hispanics on selected Halstead-Reitan Neuropsychological tests. Assessment, 1(3), 239–248.

Arnold, E., Harvey, O'Leary, S. G., and Edwards, G. H. (1997). Father involvement and self-reported parenting of children with attention deficit-hyperactivity disorder, Journal of Consulting and Clinical Psychology, 65(2), 337–342.

Aronowitz, B. R., Hollander, E., DeCaria, C., Cohen, L., Saoud, J. B., Stein, D., Liebowitz, M. R., and Rosen, W. G. (1994). Neuropsychology of obsessive compulsive disorder: Preliminary findings. Neuropsychiatry, Neuropsychology, and Behavioral Neurology, 7, 81–86.

Asikainen, M., Kaste, and Sarna (1996). Patient with traumatic brain injury referred to a rehabilitation and re-employment programme: social and professional outcome for 508 finnish patients 5 or more years after injury Brain Injury, 10 (pp. 883–899).

Attention deficit hyperactivity disorder: ADHD Task Force report (1993, May). Michigan Department of Education.

Auerbach, S. H. (1986). "Neuroanatomical Correlates of Attention and Memory Disorders in Traumatic Brain Injury: An Application of Neurobehavioral Subtypes", Journal of Head Trauma Rehabilitation, 1(3), 1–12.

August, G. J. and Garfinkel, B. D. (1989). Behavioral and cognitive subtypes of ADHD. Journal of the American Academy of Child and Adolescent Psychiatry, 28, 739–748.

August G. J. and Garfinkel, B. D. (1990). Comorbidity of ADHD and reading disability among clinic-referred children. Journal of Abnormal Child Psychology, 18(1), 29–45.

August, G. J. and Garfinkel, B. D. (1993). The nosology of attention-deficit hyperactivity disorder. Journal of the American Academy of Child and Adolescent Psychiatry, 32, 155–165.

Aust, P. H. (1994). When the problem is not the problem: Understanding attention deficit disorder with and without hyperactivity. Child Welfare, 73(3), 215–227.

Avissar, S., Nechamkin, Y., Roitman, G., and Schreiber, G. (1997). Reduced G protein functions and immunoreactive levels in mononuclear leukocytes of patients with depression, American Journal of Psychiatry, 154(2) 211–217.

Axelrod, B. N., Jiron, C. C., and Henry, R. R. (1993). Performance of adults ages 20 to 90 on the Abbreviated Wisconsin Card Sorting Test. The Clinical Neuropsychologist, 7(2), 205–209.

Axelrod, B. N., Goldman, R. S., Tompkins, L. M., and Jiron, C. C. (1994). Poor differential performance on the Wisconsin Card Sorting Test in schizophrenia, mood disorder, and traumatic brain injury. Neuropsychiatry, Neuropsychology, and Behavioral Neurology, 7(1), 20–24.

Baddeley, A. D. and Hitch, G. J. (1994). Developments in the concept of working memory. *Neuropsychology, 8,* 485–493.

Baddeley, A., Sala, S. D., Papagno, C., and Spinnler, H. (1997). Dual-task performance in dysexecutive and nondysexecutive patients with a frontal lesion, *Neuropsychology,* 11(2) 187–194.

Baker, G. B., Bornstein, R. A., Rouget, A. C., and Ashton, S. E. (1991). Phenylethylaminergic mechanisms in attention-deficit disorder. *Biological Psychiatry, 19(1),* 15–22.

Baldwin, K., Brown, R. T., and Milan, M. A. (1995). Predictors of stress in caregivers of attention deficit hyperactivity disordered children. *American Journal of Family Therapy, 23(2),* 149–160.

Ball, S. A., Carroll, K. M., and Rounsaville, B. J. (1994). Sensation seeking, substance abuse, and psychopathology in treatment-seeking and community cocaine abusers. *Journal of Consulting and Clinical Psychology, 62,* 1053–1057.

Balthazor, M. J., Wagner, R. K., and Pelham, W. E. (1991). The specificity of the effects of stimulant medication on classroom learning-related measures of cognitive processing for attention deficit disorder children. *Journal of Abnormal Child Psychology, 19(1),* 35–52.

Banich, M. T. and Shenker, J. T. (1994). Investigations of interhemispheric processing: Methodological considerations. *Neuropsychology, 8,* 263–277.

Banks, S. R., Guyer, B. P., and Guyer, K. E. (1995). A study of medical students and physicians referred for learning disabilities. *Annals of Dyslexia, 45,* 233–245.

Barbato, L., Stocchi, F., Monge, A., Vacca, L., Ruggieri, S., Nordera, G., and Marsen, D. (1997). The long-duration action of levendopa may be use to a postsynaptic effect, *Clinical Neuropharmacology,* 20(5), 394–401.

Barber, B. L. and Eccles, J. S. (1992). Long-term influence of divorce and single parenting on adolescent family- and work-related values, behaviors, and aspirations. *Psychological Bulletin, 111(1),* 108–126.

Barkley, R. A. (1990). *Attention deficit hyperactivity disorder: A handbook for diagnosis and treatment.* New York: The Guilford Press.

Barkley, R. A. (1991). The ecological validity of laboratory and analogue assessment methods of ADHD symptoms. *Journal of Abnormal Child Psychology, 19(2),* 149–179.

Barkley, R. A. (1993). Eight principles to guide ADHD children. *The ADHD Report, 1(2),* 1–5.

Barkley, R. A. (1993, June). Continuing concerns about EEG biofeedback/neurofeedback. *ADHD Report, 1(3),* 1–3.

Barkley, R. A. (1993, December). Pseudoscience in treatments for ADHD. *ADHD Report, 1(6),* 1–3.

Barkley, R. A. (1994, February). Can neuropsychological tests help diagnose ADD/ADHD? *ADHD Report, 2(1),* 1–3.

Barkley, R. A. (1994, April). More on the new theory of ADHD. *ADHD Report, 2(2),* 1–4.

Barkley, R. A. (1995, June). A closer look at the DSM-IV criteria for ADHD: Sopme unresolved issues. *ADHD Report, 3(3),* 1–5.

Barkley, R. A. (1997). Behavioral Inhibition, Sustained Attention and Executive Functions: Constructing a unifying theory of ADHD, *Psychological Bulletin,* 1, 65–94.

Barkley, R. A., DuPaul, G. J., and McMurray, M. B. (1991). Attention deficit disorders with and without hyperactivity: Clinical response to three dose levels of methylphenidate. *Pediatrics, 87,* 519–531.

Barkley, R. A., Grodzinsky, G., and DuPaul, G. J. (1992). Frontal lobe functions in attention deficit disorder with and without hyperactivity: A review and research report. *Journal of Abnormal Child Psychology, 20(2),* 163–185.

Barkley, R. A., Guevremont, D. C., Anastopoulos, A. D., and Fletcher, K. E. (1992). A comparison of three family therapy programs for treating family conflicts in adolescents with attention-deficit hyperactivity disorder. *Journal of Consulting and Clinical Psychology, 60,* 450–462.

Barkley, R., Koplowitz, S., Anderson, T., and McMurray, M. B. (1997). Sense of time in children with ADHD: Effects of duration, distraction, and stimulant medication, *Journal of the International Neuropsychological Society,* 3, 359–369.

Barnhill, J. L. and Horrigan, J. P. (1997). Tourette's syndrome in patients with developmental disorders. ANPA Abstracts *Journal of Neuropsychiatry and Clinical Neurosciences, 9(1),* 139, P30.

Barns, S., Kappenberg, R., McKenna, A., and Wood C. (1994). Brain injury; personality, psychopathology and neuropsychology. *Brain Injury, 8(5),* 8(5), 413–427.

Baron-Cohen, S. and Hammer, J. (1997). Parents of children with asperger syndrome: what is the cognitive phenotype? *Journal of Cognitive Neuroscience,* 9(4) 548–554.

Barratt, E. S., Stanford, M. S., Feltlhous, A. R., and Kent, T. A. (1997). The effects of phenytoin on impulsive and premediated aggression: A controlled study, *Journal of Clinical Psychopharmacology,* 17(5), 3451–349.

Barry, C. A., Shaywitz, S. E., and Shaywitz, B. A. (1985). Girls with attention deficit disorder: A silent minority? A report on behavioral and cognitive characteristics, *Pediatrics,* 76, 801–809.

Barta et al. (1997). Planum temporale asymmetry reversal in schizophrenia: Replication and relationship to gray matter abnormalities, *American Journal of Psychiatry,* 154(5) 661–667.

Barrickman, L., Noyes, R., Kuperman, S., Schumacher, E., and Verda, M. (1991). Treatment of ADHD with fluoxetine: A preliminary trial. *Journal of the American Academy of Child and Adolescent Psychiatry,* 30, 762–767.

Barrickman, L. L., Perry, P. J., Allen, A. J., Kuperman, S., et al. (1995). Bupropion versus methylphenidate in the treatment of attention-deficit hyperactivity disorder. *Journal of the American Academy of Child and Adolescent Psychiatry, 34(5),* 649–657.

Bassetti, C., Aldrich, M. S., Chervin, R. D., and Quint, D. (1996). Sleep apnea in patients with transient ischemic attack and stroke: A prospective study of 59 patients. *Neurology,* 47, 1167–1173.

Bauer, K. E. (1994). *A Primary Care Physician's Desk Reference to the Medical and Medication Management of Attention Deficit Hyperactivity Disorder.* Milwaukee, WI: PER Publications.

Baumgardner, T. L., Singer, H. S., Denckla, M. B., Rubin, M. A., Abrams, M. T., Colli, M. J., and Reiss, A. L. (1996). Corpus callosum morphology in children with tourette syndrome and attention deficit hyperactivity disorder. *Neurology, 47,* 477–482.

Bear, D. M. (1995). Psychiatric presentations of epilepsy, In *Neurology of Behavior and Cognition,* Seminar held at the Knickerbocker Hotel, Chicago, Illinois, December 12–16, 1995.

Beatty, W. W., Hames, K. A., Bianco, C. R., Paul, R. H., and Wilbanks, S. L. (1995). Verbal abstraction deficit in multiple sclerosis. *Neuropsychology, 9(2),* 198–205.

Beatty, W. W. and Monson, N. (1996). Problem solving by patients with multiple sclerosis: Comparison of performance on the Wisconsin and California Card Sorting Tests. *Journal of the International Neuropsychological Society, 2,* 134–140.

Becker, M. E. and Vakil, E. (1993). Behavioural psychotherapy of the frontal-lobe-injured patient in an outpatient setting. *Brain Injury, 7,* 515–523.

Beers, S. R. (1992). Cognitive effects of mild head injury in children and adolescents. *Neuropsychology Review, 3,* 281–320.

Beers, S. R., Morrow, L., Ryan, C. M., Wasko, M. C., Rarie, J., and Manzi, S. (1996). The use of information processing measures to detect cognitive deficits on systemic lupus erythematosus (SLE). *Journal of the International Neuropsychological Society, 2(1),* 15.

Begley, S. (1994, February 7). One pill makes you larger, one pill makes you small. *Newsweek,* 37–40.

Beidel, D. C., Christ, M. A. G., and Long, P. J. (1991). Somatic complaints in anxious children. *Journal of Abnormal Child Psychology, 19,* 659–670.

Bellak, L. (1994). The schizophrenic syndrome and attention deficit disorder: Thesis, antithesis, and synthesis? *101st Annual Convention of the American Psychological Association. American Psychologist, 49(1),* 25–29.

Benes, F. M., Sorensen, I., Vincent, S. L., Bird, E. D., and Sathi, M. (1992). Increased density of glutamate-immunoreactive vertical processes in superficial laminae in cingulate cortex of schizophrenic brain. *Cerebral Cortex, 2,* 503–512.

Bennett, K. M. B., Waterman, C., Scarpa, M., and Castiello, U. (1995). Covert Visualspatial attentional mechanisms in Parkinson's disease. *Brain,* 118, 153–166

Benton, A. L. (1969). Disorders of spatial orientation, In P. O. J. Winken & G. W. Bruyn (Eds). Handbook of Clinical Neurology (Vol. 3). Amsterdam: North Holland.

Benton, A. L., Sivan, A. B., Hamsher, K. deS., Varney, N. R., and Spreen, O. (1994). *Contributions to Neuropsychological Assessment: A Clinical Manual* (Second ed.). Oxford: Oxford University Press.

Berg, A. T. and Shinnar, S. (1966). Unprovoked seizures in children with febrile seizures: Short-term outcome. *Neurology, 47,* 562–568.

Berk, L. E. and Landau, S. (1993). Private speech of learning disabled and normally achieving children in classroom academic and laboratory contexts. *Child Development, 64,* 556–571.

Bernat, J. L. and Vincent, F. M. (1987). *Neurology: Problems in Primary Care.* Oradell, NJ: Medical Economics Books.

Bernier, J. C. and Siegel, D. H. (1994). Attention-deficit hyperactivity disorder: A family and ecological systems perspective. *Families in Society: Journal of Contemporary Human Services,* 142–150.

Berthier, M. L., Campos, V. M., and Kulisevsky, J. (1996). Echopraxia and Self-Injurious Behavior in Tourette's Syndrome A Case Report. *Neuropsychiatry, Neuropsychology, and Behavioral Neurology, 9,* 280–283.

Berthier, M. L., Kulisevsky, J., Gironell, A., and Heras, J. A. (1996). Obsessive-compulsive disorder associated with brain lesions: clinical phenomenology, cognitive function, and anatomic correlates. *Neurology, 47,* 353–361.

Berti, A., Làdavas, E., and Corte, M. D. (1996). Anosognosia for hemiplegia, neglect dyslexia, and drawing neglect: Clinical findings and theoretical considerations, *Journal of the International Neuropsychological Society,* (2), 426–440.

Bertolino, A., Nawroz, S., Mattay, V. S., Barnett, A. S., Duyn, J. H., Moonen, C. T. W., Frank, J. A., Tedeschi, G., and Weinberger, D. R. (1996). Regionally specific Pattern of Neurochemical Pathology in Schizophrenia as Assessed by Multislice Proton Magnetic Resonance Spectroscopic Imaging. *American Journal of Psychiatry, 153,* 1554–1563.

Beydoun, A., Sackellares, J. C., Shu, V., and the Depakote Monotherapy for Partial Seizures Study Group (1997). Safety and efficacy of divalproex sodium monotherapy in partial epilepsy: A double blind, concentration-response design clinical trial, *Neurology, 48,* 182–188.

Bezirganian, S., Cohen, P., and Brook, J. S. (1993). The impact of mother–child interaction on the development of borderline personality disorder. *American Journal of Psychiatry, 150,* 1836–1842.

Bhatara, V. S., Kummer, M., McMillin, J. M., and Bandettini, F. (1994). Thyroid function and attention-deficit hyperactivity disorder: Comment. *Journal of the American Academy of Child and Adolescent Psychiatry, 33(7),* 1057–1058.

Bidman, C. L., Sherling, M., and Bruun, R. D. (1995). Combined pharmacotherapy risk. *Journal of American Academy of Child and Adolescent Psychiatry, 34(3),* 263–264.

Biederman, J., Baldessarini, R. J., Wright, V., Knee, D., Harmatz, J. S., and Goldblatt, A. (1989). A double-blind placebo controlled study of desipramine in the treatment of ADD: II. Serum drug levels and cardiovascular findings. *Journal of the American Academy of Child and Adolescent Psychiatry, 28,* 903–911.

Biederman, J., Baldessarini, R. J., Wright, V., and Keenan, K. (1993a). A double-blind placebo controlled study of desipramine in the treatment of ADD: III. Lack of impact of comorbidity and family history factors on clinical response. *Journal of the American Academy of Child and Adolescent Psychiatry, 32,* 199–204.

Biederman, J., Faraone, S. V., Doyle, A., Lehman, B. K., Kraus, I., Perrin, J., and Tsuang, M. T. (1993b). Convergence of the Child Behavior Checklist with structured interview-based psychiatric diagnoses of ADHD children with and without comorbidity. *Journal of Child Psychology and Psychiatry, 34,* 1241–1251.

Biederman, J., Faraone, S. V., Spencer, T., Wilens, T., Norman, D., Lapey, K. A., Mick, E., Lehman, B. K., and Doyle, A. (1993c). Patterns of psychiatric comorbidity, cognition, and psychosocial functioning in adults with attention deficit hyperactivity disorder. *American Journal of Psychiatry, 150,* 1792–1797.

Biederman, J., Milberger, S., Faraone, S. V., Guite, J., and Warburton, R. (1994). Associations between childhood asthma and ADHD: Issues of psychiatric comorbidity and familiality. *Journal of the American Academy of Child and Adolescent Psychiatry, 33(6),* 842–848.

Biederman, J., Milberger, S., Faraone, S. V., Lapey, K. A., et al. (1995a). No confirmation of Geschwind's hypothesis of associations between reading disability, immune disorders, and motor preference in ADHD. *Journal of Abnormal Child Psychology, 23(5),* 545–552.

Biederman, J., Munir, K., Knee, D., Habelow, W., Amentano, M., Autor, S., Hoge, S.K., and Watermaux, C. (1986). A family study of patients with attention deficit disorder and normal controls. *Journal of Psychiatric Research,* 20, 263–273.

Biederman, J., Wilens, T., Mick, E., Milberger, S., et al. (1995b). Psychoactive substance use disorders in adults with attention deficit hyperactivity disorder (ADHD): Effects of ADHD and psychiatric comorbidity. *American Journal of Psychiatry, 152(11),* 1652–1658.

Bigler, E. D. (1988). *Diagnostic, Clinical Neuropsychology, Austin, TX: Pro-Ed.*

Black, D. W., Noyes, R., Pfohl, B., Goldstein, R. B., and Blum, N. (1993). Personality disorder in obsessive–compulsive volunteers, well comparison subjects, and their first-degree relatives. *American Journal of Psychiatry, 150,* 1226–1231.

Black, L. M. (1996). Affect processing problems of preschool-aged language disordered children. *Journal of the International Neuropsychological Society, 2(4),* 378.

Bland, J. S. (1995). Psychoneuro-nutritional medicine: An advancing paradigm. *Alternative Therapies, 1(2),* 22–27.

Bohnen, N., Van Zutphen, W., Twijnstra, A., Wijnen, G., Bongers, J., and Jolles, J. (1994). Late outcome of mild head injury: Results from a controlled postal survey. *Brain Injury, 8,* 701–708.

Bohnen, N. I., Jolles, J., Twijnstra, A., Mellink, R., and Wijnen, G. (1995). Late neurobehavioural symptoms after mild head injury. *Brain Injury, 9,* 27–33.

Bondi, M. W., Kaszniak, A. W., Bayles, K. A., and Vance, K. T. (1993). Contributions of frontal system dysfunction to memory and perceptual abilities in Parkinson's disease. *Neuropsychology, 7(1),* 89–102.

Borchardt, C. M. and Bernstein, G. A. (1995). Comorbid disorders in hospitalized bipolar adolescents compared with unipolar depressed adolescents. *Child Psychiatry and Human Development, 26(1),* 11–18.

Borcherding, B., Thompson, K., Krusei, M., Bartko, J., Rapoport, J. L., and Weingartner, H. (1988). Automatic and effortful processing in attention deficit/hyperactivity disorder, *Journal of Abnormal Child Psychology,* 16, 333–345.

Bornstein, R. A. (1986). Classification rates obtained with "standard" cut-off scores on selected neuropsychological measures. *Journal of Clinical and Experimental Psychology,* 8, 413–420.

Boucugoani, L. L. and Jones, R. W. (1989). Behaviors analogous to frontal lobe dysfunction in children with attention deficit hyperactivity disorder. *Archives of Clinical Neuropsychology,* 1, 161–173.

Bouma, P., Bovenkerk, A. C., Westendorp, G. J., and Brouwer, O. F. (1997). The course of benign partial epilepsy of childhood with centrotemporal spikes: A meta-analysis, *Neurology*, 48, 430–437.

Bouma, P. A. D., Westendorp, R. G. J., Van Dijk, J. G., Peters, A. C. B., and Brouwer, O. F. (1996). The outcome of absence epilepsy: A meta-analysis. *Neurology*, 47, 802–808.

Bourgeois, B. (1995). Valproic Acid, Clinical Use, In *Antiepileptic Drugs, Fourth Edition*, Eds., Levy, R. H., Mattson, R. H., and Meldrum, B. S., Raven Press, Ltd., New York, 633–640.

Bowen, J. D., Malter, A. D., Sheppard, L., Kukull, W. A., McCormick, W. C., Teri, L., and Larson, E. B. (1996) Predictors of mortality in patients diagnosed with probable Alzeheimer's disease. *Neurology*, 47, 433–439.

Boyle, M. H., Offord, D. R., Racine, Y. A., and Szatmari, P. (1992). Predicting substance use in late adolescence: Results from the Ontario Child Health Study follow-up. *American Journal of Psychiatry*, 149, 761–767.

Boyle, M. H., Offord, D. R., Racine, Y., Fleming, J. E., Szatmari, P., and Sanford, M. (1993). Evaluation of the revised Ontario Child Health Study scales. *Journal of Child Psychology and Psychiatry*, 34, 189–213.

Braaten, E. B. and Rosén, L. A. (1997). Emotional reactions in adults with symptoms of attention deficit hyperactivity disorder, *Personality and Individual Differences*, 22(3), 355–361.

Brady, E. U. and Kendall, P. C. (1992). Comorbidity of anxiety and depression in children and adolescents. *Psychological Bulletin*, 111, 244–255.

Brady, K. D. and Gerring, J. P. (1997). Cognitive recovery following pediatric closed head injury: role of age at injury and lesion location, ANPA Abstracts, *Journal of Neuropsychiatry and Clinical Neurosciences*, 9(1) 135.

Branch, W. B., Cohen, M. J., and Hynd, G. W. (1995). Academic achievement and attention-deficit/hyperactivity disorder in children with left- or right-hemisphere dysfunction. *Journal of Learning Disabilities*, 28(1), 35–43.

Braun, A. R., Varga, M., Stager, S., Schulz, G., Selbie, S., Maisog, J. M., Carson, R. E., and Ludlow, C. L. (1997). Altered patterns of cerebral activity during speech and language production in developmental stuttering: An H(15 O positron emission tomography study, *Brain*, 120, 761–784.

Brawman-Mintzer, O., Lydiard, R. B., Emmanuel, N., Payeur, R., Johnson, M., Roberts, J., Jarrell, M. P., and Ballenger, J. C. (1993). Psychiatric comorbidity in patients with generalized anxiety disorder. *American Journal of Psychiatry*, 150, 1216–1225.

Bray, G. A. (1988). Sympathetic nervous system and a nutrient balance model of food intake, In Morley, J. E., Sterman, M. B., and Walsh, J. H., Eds., Nutritional Modulation of Neural Function, San Diego, Academic Press Inc., 87–94.

Breier, J. I., Plenger, P. M., Castillo, R., Fuchs, K., Wheless, J. W., Thomas, A. B., Brookshire, B. L., Willmore, L. J., and Papnicolaou, A. (1996). Effects of temporal lobe epilepsy on spatial and figural aspects of memory for a complex geometric figure. *Journal of the International Neuropsychological Society, 2*, 535–540.

Bremer, D. A. and Stern, J. A. (1976). Attention and distractibility during reading in hyperactive boys, *Journal of Abnormal Child Psychology,* 4, 381–387.

Bremner, J. D., Southwick, S. M., Darnell, A., and Charney, D. S. (1996). Chronic PTSD in Vietnam combat veterans: Course of illness and substance abuse. *American Journal of Psychiatry, 153,* 369–375.

Brent, G. A. (1994). The molecular basis of thyroid hormone action. *New England Journal of Medicine, 331,* 847–853.

Brittian, J., LaMarche, J., Reeder, K., Roth, D., and Ball, T. (1991). Effects of age and IQ on Paced Auditory Serial Addition Task (PASAT) performance. *The Clinical Neuropsychologist,* 5, 163–175.

Broadbent, D. E. (1958). *Perception and Communication.* New York-Pergamon Press.

Brook, J. S., Whiteman, M. M., and Finch, S. (1991). Childhood aggression, adolescent delinquency, and drug use: A longitudinal study. *Journal of Genetic Psychology, 153(4),* 369–383.

Brown, A. (1995, Winter). ADD through the eyes of a child: A first person account. *Attention!, 1(3),* 32–38.

Brown, A. S., Mallinger, A. G., and Renbaum, L. C. (1993). Elevated platelet membrane phosphatidylinositol-4,5-bisphosphate in bipolar mania. *American Journal of Psychiatry, 150,* 1252–1254.

Brown, D. (1993, May/June). Job accommodation ideas for people with learning disabilities. *LDA Newsbriefs,* p. 7.

Brown, R. T. and Wynne, M. E. (1992). Correlates of teacher ratings, sustained attention, and impulsivity in hyperactive and normal boys. *Journal of Clinical Child Psychology, 11,* 262–267.

Brown, T. E. (1994, Fall). The many faces of ADD: Comorbidity. *Attention!, 1(2),* 29–36.

Brown, W. S., Marsh, J. T., and La Rue, A. (1982). Expotential electrophysiological aging: P3 latency: *Electroencephalography and Clinical Neurophysiology, 55,* 277–285.

Brumback, R. A. (1992). The primary disorder of vigilance. *Challenge,* 6(3), 1–2.

Budman, C. L., Sherling, M., and Bruun, R. D. (1995) Combined pharmacotherapy risk. *Journal of the American Academy of Child and Adolescent Psychiatry, 34(3),* 263–264.

Buchanan, R. W., Strauss, M. E., Breier, A., Kirkpatrick, B., and Carpenter, W. T. (1997). Attentional impairments in deficit and nondeficit forms of schizophrenia, *American Journal of Psychiatry,* 154(3) 363–370.

Buchsbaum, M. S., Someya, T., Teng, C. Y., Abel, L., Chin, S., Najafi, A., Haier, R. J., Wu, J., and Bunney, W. E. (1996). PET and MRI of the thalamus in never-medicated patients with schizophrenia. *American Journal of Psychiatry, 153,* 191–199.

Buck, B. H., Black, S. E., Behrmann, M., Caldwell, C., and Bronskill, M. J. (1997). Spatial- and object-based attentional deficits in Alzheimer's disease: relationship to HMPAO-SPECT measures of parietal perfusion, *Brain,* 120, 1229–1244.

Buitelaar, J. K., Van der Gaag, R. J., Swaab-Barneveld, H., and Kuiper, M. (1995). Prediction of clinical response to methylphenidate in children with attention-deficit hyperactivity disorder. *Journal of the American Academy of Child and Adolescent Psychiatry, 43(8),* 1025–1032.

Burke, M. S., Josephson, A., and Lightsey, A. (1995). Combined methylphenidate and imipramine complication. *Journal of the American Academy of Child and Adolescent Psychiatry, 34(4)*, 403–404.

Burnley, G. D. (1993). A team approach for identification of an attention deficit hyperactivity disorder child. *School Counselor, 40(3)*, 228–230.

Burns, D. D., Sayers, S. L., and Mora, K. (1994). Intimate relationships and depression: Is there a causal connection? *Journal of Consulting and Clinical Psychology, 62*, 1033–1043.

Burrows, G. D. and Kremer, C. (1997). Mirtazapine: Clinical advantages in the treatment of depression, *Journal of Clinical Psychopharmacology, 17(2)*, (Suppl. 1), 34S–39S.

Bussing, R. and Levin, G. M. (1993). Methamphetamine and fluoxetine treatment of a child with attention deficit disorder and obsessive-compulsive disorder. *Journal of Child and Adolescent Psychopharmacology, 3(1)*, 53–58.

Bustillo, J. R., Thaker, G., Buchanan, R. W., Moran, M., Kirkpatrick, B., and Carpenter, W. T. (1997). Visual information processing impairments in deficit and nondeficit schizophrenia. *American Journal of Psychiatry, 154(5)*, 647–654.

Cabeza, R. and Nyberg, L. (1997). Imaging condition: An empirical review of PET studies with normal subjects. *Journal of Cognitive Neuroscience, 9(1)*, 1–26.

Cadoret, R. J. and Stewart, M. A. (1991). An adoption study of attention deficit/hyperactivity/aggression and their relationship to adult antisocial personality. *Comprehensive Psychiatry, 32(1)*, 73–82.

Caffara, P., Riggio, L., Malvezi, L., Scaglioni, A., and Freedman, M. (1997). Orienting of visual attention in alzeheimer's disease: Its implication in favor of the inter-hemispheric balance. *Neuropsychiatry, Neuropsychology, and Behavioral Neurology, 10(2)*, 90–95.

Cahn, D. A., Malloy, P. F., Salloway, S., Rogg, J., Gillard, E., Kohn, R., Tung, G., Richardson, E. D., and Westlake, R. (1996). Subcortical Hyperintensities on MRI and Activities of Daily Living in Geriatric Depression. *Journal of Neuropsychiatry, 8*, 404–411.

Cahn, D. A. and Marcotte, A. C. (1996). Recall and rate of forgetting in attention deficit hyperactivity disorder. *Journal of the International Neuropsychological Society, 2(1)*, 58.

Calhoun, G., Fees, C. K., and Bolton, J. A. (1994). Attention-deficit hyperactivity disorder: Alternatives for psychotherapy? *Perceptual and Motor Skills, 79(1, Pt 2)*, 657–658.

Campbell, J. M. (1992). Attention Disorders (ADD and ADHD): Their Identification and Implications. Lapeer, MI: JAM Publications.

Campbell, S. (1993). Some issues in identifying problem behaviors in very young children. *The ADHD Report, 1(2)*, 5–7.

Canter, L. and Canter, M. (1987). *Homework Without Tears*. Santa Monica, CA: Canter and Associates, Inc.

Capwell, M. (1993). Chromium and longevity? *Prevention, 45(3)*, 33.

Cardon, L. R., Smith, S. D., Fulker, D. W., Kimberling, W. J., et al. (1995). Reading disability, attention-deficit hyperactivity disorder, and the immune system: Response. *Science, 268(5212)*, 787–788.

Carlson, C. L. and Bunner, M. R. (1993). Effects of methylphenidate on the academic performance of children with attention-deficit hyperactivity disorder and learning disabilities. *School Psychology Review, 22,* 184–196.

Carlson, E. A. (1995). A developmental investigation of inattentiveness and hyperactivity. *Child Development, 66(1),* 37–54.

Carroll, K. M. and Rounsaville, B. L. (1993). History and significance of childhood attention of deficit disorder in treatment-seeking cocaine abusers. *Comprehensive Psychiatry, 34,* 75–82.

Carter, S. C., Robertson, L. C., and Nordahl, T. E. (1992). Abnormal processing of irrelevant information in chronic schizophrenia: Selective enhancement of Stroop facilitation. *Psychiatry Res., 41,* 137–146.

Casey, B. J., Castellanos, F. X., Giedd, J., and Marsh, W. L. (1997). Implication of right frontostriatal circuitry in response inhibition and attention-deficit hyperactivity disorder. *Journal of the American Academy of Child and Adolescent Psychiatry, 36(3),* 374–383.

Cassidy, J. W. (1994). Neuropharmacological management of destructive behavior after traumatic brain injury. *Journal of Head Trauma Rehabilitation, 9(3),* 43–60.

Castellanos, F. X., Elia, J., Kruesi, M. J., Gulotta, C. S., et al. (1994). Cerebrospinal fluid monoamine metabolites in boys with attention-deficit hyperactivity disorder. *Psychiatry Research, 52(3),* 305–316.

Castellanos, F. X., Giedd, J. N., Eckburg, P., March, W. L., Vaituzis, C., Kaysen, D., Hamburger, S. D., and Rapaport, J. L. (1994). Quantative morphology of the caudate nucleus in attention deficit hyperactivity disorder. *American Journal of Psychiatry, 151(12),* 1791–1796.

Castellanos, F. X., Giedd, J. N., Hamburger, S. D., Marsh, W. L., and Rapoport, J. L. (1996). Brain morphometry in Tourette's syndrome: the influence of comorbid attention-deficit/hyperactivity disorder. *Neurology, 47,* 1581–1583.

Castellanos, F. X. et al. (1997). Controlled stimulant treatment of ADHD and comorbid Tourette's syndrome: Effects of stimulant and dose, *Journal of American Academy Child and Adolescent Psychiatry, 36,* 589–96, Referenced in *Journal Watch for Psychiatry, 3(7),* 54.

Ceffen, G. M., Butterworth, P., Forrester, G. M., and Ceffen, L. B. (1994). Auditory verbal learning test components as measures of the severity of closed-head injury.

Cerella, J. and Hale, S. (1994). The rise and fall in the information-processing rates over the life span. *Acta-Psychologica, 86(2–3),* 109–197.

Cerella, J., Rybash, J., Hoyer, W., and Commons, M. L. (Eds.) (1993). *Adult Information Processing: Limits on Loss.* New York: Academic Press.

Chadwick, D. (1995). Gabapentin, clinical use, In *Antiepileptic Drugs, Fourth Edition,* Eds., Levy, R. H., Mattson, R. H., and Meldrum, B. S., Raven Press, Ltd., New York, 851–856.

Chang, K., Neeper, R., Jenkins, M., Penn, J., Bollivar, L., Israeli, L., Malloy, P., and Salloway, S. (1995). Clinical profile of patients referred for evaluation of adult attention-deficit hyperactivity disorder. ANPA Abstracts, *The Journal of Neuropsychiatry and Clinical Neurosciences, 7(3),* 401.

Chapman, S. B., Levin, H. S., Matejka, J., Harward, H., and Kufera, J. A. (1995). Discourse ability in children with brain injury: Correlations with psychosocial, linguistic, and cognitive factors. *Journal of Head Trauma Rehabilitation, 10(5),* 36–54.

Chappelle, P. B., Riddle, M. A., Scahill, L., Lynch, K. A., et al. (1995). Guanfacine treatment of comorbid attention deficit hyperactivity disorder and Tourette's syndrome: Preliminary clinical experience. *Journal of the American Academy of Child and Adolescent Psychiatry, 34,* 1140–1146.

Chaskelson, M. (1991). Identification of hidden cognitive deficits with attention deficit disorders. *Chadder Box, Jan.*

Chassin, L., Pillow, D. R., Curran, P. J., Molina, B. S. G., and Barrera, M., Jr. (1993). Relation of parental alcoholism to early adolescent substance use: A test of three mediating mechanisms. *Journal of Abnormal Psychology, 102,* 3–19.

Chatterjee, A., Mennemeier, M., Vezey, E., and Rapcsak, S. Z. (1996). Neglect within and across regions of space. *Neurology, 46(2, Suppl.),* A156.

Cheluene, G. J., Ferguson, W., Koon, R., and Dickey, T. O. (1986). Frontal lobe disinhibition in attention deficit disorder. *Child Psychiatry and Human Development, 16,* 221–234.

Chen, W. J., Faraone, S. V., Biederman, J., and Tsuang, M. T. (1994). Diagnostic accuracy of the Child Behavior Checklist scales for attention-deficit hyperactivity disorder: A receiver-operating characteristic analysis. *Journal of Consulting and Clinical Psychology, 62,* 1017–1025.

Chervin, R. D., Dillon, J. E., and Bassetti, C. (1996). Symptoms of sleep-related breathing disorders and hyperactivity in a child psychiatry clinic. *Neurology, 46(2, Suppl.),* A486.

Chieffi, S. (1996). Effects of stimulus asymmetry on line bisection. *Neurology, 47,* 1004–1008.

Children with Attention Deficit Disorders, American Academy of Child and Adolescent Psychiatry (1991, Fall/Winter). Medical Management of Children with Attention Deficit Disorders: Commonly asked questions. *Ch.A.D.D.er,* 17–19.

Chiron, C., Jambaque, I., Nabbout, R., Lounes, R., Syrota, A., and Dulac, O. (1997). The right brain hemisphere is dominant in human infants, *Brain, 120,* 1057–1065.

Cho, A. K. and Segal, D. S. (Eds.) (1994). *Amphetamine and its Analogs: Psychopharmacology, Toxicology, and Abuse.* New York: Academic Press.

Ciaranello, R. D. (1993). Attention deficit-hyperactivity disorder and resistance to thyroid hormone: A new idea? *New England Journal of Medicine, 328,* 1038–1039.

Cicerone, K. D. (1996). Attention deficits and dual task demands after mild traumatic brain injury. *Brain Injury, 10(2),* 79–89.

Cicerone, K. D. and Giacino, J. T. (1992). Remediation of executive function deficits after traumatic brain injury. *Neuro Rehabilitation, 2(3),* 12–22.

Cicerone, K. D. and Kalmar, K. (1997). Does premorbid depression influence post-concussive symptoms and neuropsychological functioning? *Brain Injury, 11(9),* 643–648.

Clark, D. A., Beck, A. T., and Beck, J. S. (1994). Symptom differences in major depression, dysthymia, panic disorder, and generalized anxiety disorder. *American Journal of Psychiatry, 151,* 205–220.

Clark, E., Baker, B. K., Gardner, M. K., and Pompa, J. L. (1990). Effectiveness of stimulant drug treatment for attention problems: A look at head-injured children. *School Psychology International, 11(3),* 227–234.

Clark, V. P., Parasuraman, R., Keil, K., Kulansky, R., Fannon, S., Maisog, J. Ma., Ungerleider, L. G., and Haxby, J. V. (1997). Selective attention to face identity and color studied with fMRI, *Human Brain Mapping, 5,* 293–297.

Clarkin, J. F. and Kendall, P. C. (1992). Comorbidity and treatment planning: Summary and future directions. *Journal of Consulting and Clinical Psychology, 60,* 904–908.

Cockerell, O. C., Rothwell, J., Thompson, P. D., Marsden, C. D., and Shorvon, S. D. (1996). Clinical and physiological features of epilepsia partialis continua. *Brain, 119,* 393–407.

Cohen, D. J. and Leckman, J. F. (1994). Developmental psychopathology and neurobiology of Tourette's syndrome. *Journal of American Academy of Child Adolescent Psychiatry, 33(1),* 2–13.

Cohen, J. (1994). On the differential diagnosis of reading, attentional and depressive disorders. *Annals of Dyslexia, 44,* 165–184.

Cohen, M. D. (1993a, October). Opportunities and obstacles in educating children with ADD. *Chadder Box,* 8–9.

Cohen, M. D. (1993b, November). Section 504 v. IDEA eligibility or when is a little better than a lot? *Chadder Box,* 8–9.

Cohen, M. D. (1995, January/February). Are gifted children with ADD entitled to special education and related services? It depends. *Chadder Box,* 6–7.

Cohen, M. L. (1996, March). Controversy, comorbidity attend the child with ADHD. *Psychiatric Times,* 54–56.

Cohen, P., Cohen, J., and Brook, J. (1993). An epidemiological study of disorders in late childhood and adolescence: II. Persistence of disorders. *Journal of Child Psychology and Psychiatry, 34,* 869–877.

Cohen, P., Cohen, J., Kasen, S., Velez, C. N., Hartmark, C., Johnson, J., Rojas, M., Brook, J., and Struening, E. L. (1993). An epidemiological study of disorders in late childhood and adolescence: I. Age- and gender-specific prevalence. *Journal of Child Psychology and Psychiatry, 34,* 851–867.

Cohen, R. A. (1993). Response selection and the executive control of attention. In R. A. Cohen, (Ed.). *The Neuropsychology of Attention.* New York: Plenum Press.

Cohen, R. A. and Sparling-Cohen, Y. A. (1993). Response selection and the executive control of attention. In R. A. Cohen, (Ed.). *The Neuropsychology of Attention.* New York: Plenum Press.

Cole, P. M. and Putnam, F. W. (1992). Effect of incest on self and social functioning: A developmental psychopathology perspective. *Journal of Consulting and Clinical Psychology, 60,* 174–184.

Coleman, W. (1994, November/December). Medication: Your questions answered. *Challenge, 8(6),* 1–4.

Colquhoun, I. D. (1994). Attention-deficit/hyperactive disorder: A dietary/nutritional approach. *Therapeutic Care and Education, 3(2),* 159–172.

Coltheart, M. and Coltheart, V. (1997). Reading comprehension is not exclusively reliant upon phonological representation. *Cognitive Neuropsychology, 14(1),* 167–175.

Comings, D. E. (1995). The role of genetic factors in conduct disorder based on studies of Tourette's syndrome and attention-deficit hyperactivity disorder probands and their relatives. *Journal of Developmental and Behavioral Pediatrics, 16(3),* 142–157.

Commissaris, K., Verhey, F. R. J., and Jolles, J. (1996). A Controlled Study Into the Effects of Psychoeducation for Patients With Cognitive Disturbances. *Journal of Neuropsychiatry, 8,* 429–435.

Controversial treatments for children with ADD (1993). *Ch.A.D.D. Facts.*

Cope, D. and Nathan, M.D. (1986). The pharmacology of attention and memory. *Journal of Head Trauma Rehabilitation, 11(3),* 34-42.

Copeland, E. (1995, January/February). Social, emotional, and behavioral disorders. *Challenge, 9(1),* 4–6.

Copeland, E. D. (1991a). *A Parenting Odyssey: Attention Deficit Disorders (ADHD/ADD).* Atlanta, GA: Southeastern Psychological Institute.

Copeland, E. D. (1991b). *Medications for Attention Disorders (ADHD/ADD) and Related Problems: A Comprehensive Handbook.* Atlanta, GA: SPI Press.

Copeland, E. D. (1994, November/December). Why children don't succeed in school: Part II. Learning disabilities. *Challenge, 8(6),* 6–9.

Copeland, E. D. and Love, V. L. (1991). *Attention, Please!: A Comprehensive Guide for Successfully Parenting Children with Attention Disorders and Hyperactivity (ADHD/ADD).* Atlanta, GA: SPI Press.

Corballis, M. C. (1994). Neuropsychology of Perceptual Functions. In Dahlea, W. Zaidel, (Eds.). *Neuropsychology* . San Diego, CA.: Academic Press, Inc.

Corbetta, M., Shulman, G. L., Conturo, T. E., Snyder, A. Z., Akbudak, E., Peterson, S., Marcus E., Raichle, E. (1997). A functional magnetic resonance imaging (fMRI) study of visuospatial attention. *Neurology, 48,* (suppl) S62.006.

Corina, D., Kritchevsky, M., Bellugi, U. (1996). Visual language processing and unilateral neglect: Evidence from american sign language. *Cognitive Neuropsychology, 13(3),* 321–356.

Cornelius, J. R., Soloff, P. H., Perel, J. M., and Ulrich, R. F. (1993). Continuation pharmacotherapy of borderline personality disorder with haloperidol and phenelzine. *American Journal of Psychiatry, 150,* 1843–1848.

Cosgrove, F. (1994). Recent advances in paediatric psychopharmacology: A brief overview. *Human Psychopharmacology Clinical and Experimental, 9(5),* 381–382.

Coslett, B. (1997). Neglect in vision and visual imagery: a double dissociation, *Brain, 120,* 1163–1171.

Costa, G. (1988). Clinical neuropsychology: Prospects and problems. *Clinical Neuropsychology, 2,* 3–11.

Cowell, L. C. and Cohen, R. (1995). Amantadine: A potential adjuvant therapy following traumatic brain injury. *Journal of Head Trauma Rehabilitation, 10(6),* 91–94.

Cowen, T. D. and Meythaler, J. M. (1994). Hypotensive effects of thioridazine in an elderly patient with traumatic brain injury. *Brain Injury, 8,* 735–737.

Cowley, G. and Ramo, J. C. (1993). The not-young and the restless. *Newsweek Jul. 26,* 48–49.

Cramond, B. (1994). Attention deficit hyperactivity disorder and creativity: What is the connection? *Journal of Creative Behavior, 28(3),* 193–210.

Cremona-Meteyard, S. L., and Geffen, G. M. (1994). Event-related potential indices of visual attention following moderate to severe closed head injury. *Brain Injury, 8,* 541–558.

Crick, N. R. and Dodge, K. A. (1994). A review and reformulation of social information processing mechanisms in children's social adjustment. *Psychological Bulletin, 115,* 74–101.

Cronin-Golomb, A. and Braun, A. E. (1997). Visuospatial dysfunction and problem solving in Parkinson's disease. *Neuropsychology, 11(1),* 44–52.

Cuesta, M. J., Peralta, V., Caro, F., and Leon, J. de. (1995). Is poor insight in psychotic disorders associated with poor performance on the Wisconsin Card Sorting Test? *American Journal of Psychiatry, 152,* 1380–1382.

Cummings, J. L. and Kaufer, D. (1996). Neuropsychiatric aspects of Alzheimer's disease: The cholinergic hypothesis revisited. *Neurology, 47,* 876–883.

Cutler, N. R., Veroff, A. E., Frackiewicz, E. J., Welke, T.L., Kirtz, N. M., and Sramek, J. J. (1996). Assessing the Neuropsychological Profile of Stable Schizophrenic Outpatients. *Journal of Neuropsychiatry, 8,* 423–428.

Dagenbach, D. and Carr, T. H. (Eds.) (1994). *Inhibitory Processes in Attention, Memory, and Language.* New York: Academic Press.

Dahl, R. E, Pelham, W. E., and Wierson, M. (1991). The role of sleep disturbances in attention deficit disorder symptoms: A case study. *Journal of Pediatric Psychology, 16(2),* 229–239.

Dairiki Shortcliffe, L. M. (1993). Primary Nocturnal Enuresis: Introduction. *Clinical Pediatrics Special Edition,* 3–4.

Daugherty, T. K., Quay, H. C., and Ramos, L. (1993). Response perseveration, inhibitory control, and central dapaminergic activity in childhood behavior disorders.

Davidson, J. R., Potts, N., Richichi, E., Krishnan, K. R., et al. (1993). Treatment of social phobia with clonazepam and placebo. *Journal of Clinical Psychopharmacology, 13,* 423–428.

Davidson, M., Harvey, P., Welsh, K. A., Powchik, P., Putnam, K. M., and Mohs, R. C. (1996). Cognitive Functioning in Late-Life Schizophrenia: A Comparison of Elderly Schizophrenic Patients and Patients with Alzheimer's Disease. *American Journal of Psychiatry, 153,* 1274–1279.

Davila, M. D., Shear, P. K., Lane, B., Sullivan, E. V., and Pfefferbaum, A. (1994). Mammillary body and cerebellar shrinkage in chronic alcoholics: An MRI and neuropsychological study. *Neuropsychology, 8,* 433–444.

Davis, M. (1997). Neurobiology of fear responses: The role of the amygdala. *Journal of Neuropsychiatry, 9(3),* 338–402.

Dawson, P. (1992, June). Helping children with attention deficits survive in the classroom: What does the school psychologist have to offer? *Ch.A.D.D.er Box, 5(5)*, 1–7.

Deary, I. J., Ebmeier, K. P., MacLeod, K. M., and Dougall, N. (1994). PASAT performance and the pattern of uptake of – super (99m) Tc-exametazime in brain estimated with single photon emission tomography. *Biological Psychology, 38*, 1–8.

Deary, I. J., Langan, S. J., Hepburn, D. A., and Frier, B. M. (1991). Which abilities does PASAT test? *Personality and Individual Differences, 12*, 983–987.

Degos, J. D., da Fonseca, N., Gray, F., and Cesaro, P. (1993). Severe frontal syndrome associated with infarcts on the left anterior cingulate gyrus and the head of the right caudate nucleus. *Brain, 116*, 1541–1548.

de Groot, C. M., Yeates, K. O., Baker, G. B., and Bornstein, R. A. (1997). Impaired neuropsychological functioning in Tourette's syndrome subjects with co-occurring-compulsive and attention deficit symptoms, *The Journal of Neuropsychiatry and Clinical Neurosciences, 9(2)*, 267–272.

Dehaene, S. (1996). The organization of brain activations in number comparison: Event-related potentials and the additive-factors method. *Journal of Cognitive Neuroscience, 8(1)*, 47–68.

DeLeón, O. A., Blend, M. J., Jobe, T. H., and Pontón, M., and Gaviria, M. (1997). Application of Ictal brain SPECT for differentiating epileptic from non epileptic. *Neuropsychiatry and Clinical Neurosciences, 9*, 99–101.

Dellatolas, G., Luciani, S., Castresana, A., Remy, C., Jallon, P., Laplane, D., and Bancaud, J. (1993). Pathological left-handedness. *Brain, 116*, 1565–1574.

DeLuca, J. W., Moore, G. J., Mueller, R. A. Slovis, T. L., and Chugani, H. T. (1997). Right hemisphere learning disability syndrome: differential findings from PET and MRS. ANPA Abstracts, *Journal of Neuropsychiatry and Clinical Neurosciences, 9(1)*, 131, P3.

Demonet, J.-F., Price, C., Wise, R., and Frackowiak, R. S. J. (1994). A PET study of cognitive strategies in normal subjects during language tasks: Influence of phonetic ambiguity and sequence processing on phoneme monitoring. *Brain, 117*, 671–682.

Denckla, M. B. (1991). Attention deficit hyperactivity disorder—residual type. *Journal of Child Neurology, 6(Suppl.)*, S44–S50.

Denckla, M. B. (1993). The child with developmental disabilities grown up: Adult residua of childhood disorders. *Neurologic Clinics, 11(1)*, 105–125.

Denckla, M. B. (1996). Executive function in children with TS and TS/ADHD. *Journal of the International Neuropsychological Society, 2(4)*, 370.

Deonna, T. (1993). Annotation: Cognitive and behavioural correlates of epileptic activity in children. *Journal of Child Psychology and Psychiatry, 34*, 611–620.

de Quiros, G. B., Kinsbourne, M., Palmer, R. L., and Tocci Rufo, D. (1994). Attention deficit disorder in children: Three clinical varants. *Developmental and Behavioral Pediatrics, 15(5)*, 311–319.

des Rosiers, G. and Kavanagh. D. (1987). Cognitive assessment in closed head injury: Stability, validity, and parallel forms for two neurpsychological measures of recovery. *International Journal of Clinical Neuropsychology, 9*, 162–173.

D'Esposito, M., Onishi, K., Thompson, H., Robinson, K., Armstrong, C., and Grossman, M. (1996). Working memory impairments in multiple sclerosis: Evidence from a dual-task paradigm. *Neuropsychology, 10(1),* 51–56.

Deuschl, G., Krack, P., Lauk, M., and Timmer, J. (1996). Clinical neurophysiology of tremor. *Journal of Clinical Neurophysiology, 13(2),* 110–121.

Devinsky, O., Bear, D., Moya, K., and Benowitz, L. (1993). Perception of emotion in patients with Tourette's syndrome. *Neuropsychiatry, Neuropsychology, and Behavioral Neurology, 6,* 166–169.

Devor, E. J. (1994). A developmental-genetic model of alcoholism for genetic research. *Journal of Consulting and Clinical Psychology, 62(6),* 1108–1115.

de Wit, H. (1996). Priming effects with drugs and other reinforcers. *Experimental and Clinical Psychopharmacology, 4(1),* 5–10.

Digirolamo, G. J. and Posner, M. I. (1996). Attention and schizophrenia: A view from cognitive neuroscience. *Cognitive Neuropsychiatry, 1,* 95–102.

Diplock, A. T. (1991). Antioxidant nutrients and disease prevention: An overview. *American Journal of Clinical Nutrition, 53(1 Suppl.),* 189S–193S.

Dodge, K. A. (1986). A social information processing model of social competence in children. In M. Perlmutter (Ed.). *Cognitive Perspective on children's social and behavioral development.* Hillsdale, NJ. Lawrence Erlbaum Associates, Inc.

Dodrill, C. B. (1978). A neuropsychological battery for epilepsy. *Epilepsia, 19,* 619–623.

Dodson, E. Edwin, Leppik, Ilo E., and Slovis, Corey M. (1992). Status epilepticus, patient care, *The practical Journal for Primary Care Physicians, 26(18),* 100–117.

Domenico, D. and Windle, M. (1993). Intrapersonal and interpersonal functioning among middle-aged female adult children of alcoholics. *Journal of Consulting and Clinical Psychology, 61,* 659–666.

Doran, S. (1997). Fragile X syndrome and attention deficit hyperactive disorder. *ADHD Report, 5(1),* 8–11.

Douglas, V. L., Barr, R. G., Desilets, J., and Sherman, E. (1995). Do high doses of stimulants impair flexible thinking in attention-deficit hyperactivity disorder? *Journal of the American Academy of Child and Adolescent Psychiatry, 34(7),* 877–885.

Drake, D. D., Johnson, C., and Clark, M. (1997). Acute improvement in alertness and cognition following methylphenidate in attention-deficit hyperactivity disorder (ADHD) predicts chronic cognitive improvement. ANPA Abstracts *Journal of Neuropsychiatry and Clinical Neurosciences, 9(1),* 141, P37.

Drake, D. D., Johnson, C., and Clark, M. (1997). Pupillometry-predicted alerting methylphenidate dosage also predicts cognitive improvement in nonvigilant, inattentive attention deficit hyperactivity disorder (ADHD). ANPA Abstracts *Journal of Neuropsychiatry and Clinical Neurosciences, 9(1),* 141, P38.

Duane, D. D., Clark, M., and Gottlob, L. (1996). Right hemisphere dysfunction correlates with nonwakefulness in attention deficit disorder. *Neurology, 46(2, Suppl.),* A125.

Duchek, J. M. and Balota, D. A. (1993). Sparing activation process in older adults in *Adult Information Processing: Limits on Loss.* New York: Academic Press, Inc. 384–406.

Duffy, J. D. and Campbell, J. J., III. (1994). The regional prefrontal syndromes: A theoretical and clinical overview. *Journal of Neuropsychiatry and Clinical Neurosciences, 6,* 3379–3387.

Duncan, C. C., Rumsey, J. M., Wilkniss, S. M., and Denckla, M. B. (1994). Developmental dyslexia and Attention Dysfunction in adults: Brain potential indices of information processing. *Psychophysiology, 31,* 386–401.

Duncan, J. S. (1997). Imaging and epilepsy. *Brain, 120,* 339–377.

DuPaul, G. J., Barkley, R. A., and McMurray, M. B. (1991). Therapeutic effects of medication on ADHD: Implications for school psychologists. *School Psychology Review, 20(2),* 203–219.

DuPaul, G. J., Barkley, R. A., and McMurray, M. B. (1994). Response of children with ADHD to methylphenidate. Interaction with internalizing symptoms. *Journal American Academy Child Adolescent Psychiatry, 33(6),* 894–903.

DuPaul, G. J. and Henningson, P. N. (1993). Peer tutoring effects on the classroom performance of children with attention deficit hyperactivity disorder. *School Psychology Review, 22,* 134–143.

Dyche, G. M. and Johnson, D. A. (1991a). Development and evaluation of CHIPASAT an attention test for children: II. test-retest reliability and practice effect for a normal sample. *Perceptual and Motor Skills, 72,* 563–572.

Dyche, G. M. and Johnson, D. A. (1991b). Information processing rates derived from CHIPASAT. *Perceptual and Motor Skills, 73,* 720–722.

Dykman, R. A. and Ackerman, P. T. (1983). Behavioral subtypes of attention deficit disorder. Issues in the education of children with attention deficit disorder. *Exceptional Children, 60(2),* 132–141.

Dykman, R. A. and Ackerman, P. T. (1993). Cluster vs. dimensional analysis of attentional deficit disorders. In J. L. Matson (Ed). *Handbook of Hyperactivity in Children,* pp 11–34.

Dykman, R. A., Ackerman, P. I. (1993). Behavioral subtypes of attention deficit disorder. *Exceptional Children, 60(2),* 132–141.

Dykman, R. A., Oglesby, D. M., and Newton, J. E. (1994). EEG power spectra of children with dyslexia, slow learners, and normally reading children with ADD during verbal processing. *Journal of Learning Disabilities, 27,* 619–630.

Eberle, A. J. (1995). Hyperactivity and Graves' disease. *Journal of the American Academy of Child and Adolescent Psychiatry, 34(8),* 973.

Ebersbach, G., Trottenberg, T., Hattig, H., Schelosky, L., Schrag, A., and Poewe, W. (1996). Directional bias of initial visual exploration: A symptom of neglect in Parkinson's disease. *Brain, 119(1),* 79–87.

Edelstyn, N. M. J. and Riddoch, M. J., Oyebode, F., Humphreys, G. W. and Forde, E. (1996). Visual processing in patients with Fregoli syndrome. *Cognitive Neuropsychiatry, 1(2),* 103–124.

Eden, G. F., Stein, J. F., Wood, H. M., and Wood, F. B. (1995). Temporal and spatial processing in reading disabled and normal children. *Cortex, 31(3),* 451–468.

Edwards, G. (1993, June). Short-term treatment model for ADHD/ODD. *ADHD Report, 1(3),* 4–5.

Eidelberg, D., Moeller, J. R., Antonini, A., Kazumata, K., Dhawan, V., Budman, C., and Feigin, A. (1997). The metabolic anatomy of Tourette's syndrome. *Neurology, 48,* 927–934.

Eiraldi, R. B., Power, T. J., and Nezu, C. M. (1997). Patterns of comorbidity associated with subtypes of attention-deficit hyperactivity disorder among 6- to 12-year old children. *Journal of the American Academy of Child and Adolescent Psychiatry, 36(4),* 503–514.

Eisen, J. L., Beer, D. A., Pato, M. T., Venditto, T. A., and Rasmussen, S. A. (1997). Obsessive-compulsive disorder in patients with schizophrenia or schizoaffective disorder. *American Journal of Psychiatry, 154(2),* 271–273.

Eisenberg, J., Chazan-Gologorsky, S., Hattab, J., and Belmaker, R. H. (1984). A controlled trial of vasopressin treatment of childhood learning disorder. *Biological Psychology, 19(7),* 1137–1141.

Elble, R. J. (1996). Central mechanisms of tremor. *Journal of Clinical Neurophysiology, 13,* 133–144.

Elia, J., Gulotta, C., Rose, S. R., and Marin, G. (1994). Thyroid function and attention-deficit hyperactivity disorder. *Journal of the American Academy of Child and Adolescent Psychiatry, 33,* 169–172.

Elia, J. and Rapoport, J. L. (1991). Ritalin versus dextroamphetamine in ADHD: Both should be tried. In L. L. Greenhill, and B. B. Osman (Eds.), *Ritalin Theory and Patient Management,* (pp. 69–74). New York: Maryann Liebert, Inc.

Elias, M. J., Tobias, S. E., and Friedlander, B. S. (1994). Enhancing skills for everyday problem solving, decision making, and conflict resolution in special needs students with the support of computer-based technology. *Special Services in the Schools, 8(2),* 33–52.

Elovic, E. (1996). Pharmacology of attention and arousal in the low level patient. *NeuroRehabilitation, 6,* 57–67.

Elterman, R., Glauser, T., Ritter, F. J., Reife, R., Wu, Su-Chen, and Raritan, N. J. (1997). Efficacy and safety of topiramate in partial seizures in children. *Neurology, 48,* 1729.

Eppright, T. D., Kashani, J. H., Robinson, B. D., and Reid, J. C. (1993). Comorbidity on conduct disorder and personality disorders in an incarcerated juvenile population. *American Journal of Psychiatry, 150,* 1233–1236.

Erlenmeyer-Kimling, L., Cornblatt, B. A., Rock, D., Roberts, S., Bell, M., and West, A. (1993). The New York high risk project: Anhedonia, attentional deviance, and psychopathology. *Schizophrenia Bulletin, 19(1),* 141–153.

Erickson, R. J., Goldinger, S. D., and LaPointe, L. L. (1996). Auditory vigilance in aphasic individuals detecting nonlinguistic stimuli with full or divided attention. *Brain-Cognition, 30(2),* 244–253.

Ernst, M., Liebenauer, L. L., King A. C., Fitzgerald, G. A., et al. (1994a). Reduced brain metabolism in hyperactive girls. *Journal of the American Academy of Child and Adolescent Psychiatry, 33,* 858–868.

Ernst, M., Zametkin, A. J., Matochik, J. A., and Liebenauer, L. (1994b). Effects of intravenous dextroamphetamine on brain metabolism in adults with attention-deficit hyperactivity disorder (ADHD): Preliminary findings. *Psychopharmacology Bulletin, 30(2),* 219–225.

Eson, M. E., Yen, J. K., and Bourke, R. S. (1978). Assessment and recovery from serious head injury. *Journal of Neurology, Neurosurgery, and Psychiatry, 41,* 1036–1042.

Evans, G. W. and Bowman, T. D. (1992). Chromium picolinate increases membrane fluidity and rate of insulin internalization. *Journal of Inorganic Biochemistry, 46(4),* 243–250.

Evans, H. M. and Seymour, P. H. K. (1997). Genetic constraints on the development of alphabetic literacy: A cognitive study of two 48, XXXY cases. *Cognitive Neuropsychology, 14(2),* 255–291.

Evans, S. E., Pelham, W., and Grudberg, M. V. (1995). The efficacy of notetaking to improve behavior and comprehension of adolescents with attention deficit hyperactivity disorder. *Exceptionality, 5(1),* 1–17.

Evans, S. W., Vallano, G., and Pelham, W. (1994). Treatment of parenting behavior with a psychostimulant: A case study of and adult with attention-deficit hyperactivity disorder. *Journal of Child and Adolescent Psychopharmacology, 4(1),* 63–69.

Evans, W. J. and Schwartz, B. D. (1997). Attentional mechanisms of saccadic eye movements in Schizophrenia. *Journal of Clinical Neuroscience, 10,* 17–24.

Eyre, S., Rounsaville, B., and Kleber, H. (1982). History of childhood hyperactivity in a clinic population of opiate addicts. *Journal of Nervous and Mental Disease, 170,* 522–529.

Faigel, H. C. (1995). Attention deficit disorder in college students: Facts, fallacies, and treatment. *Journal of American College Health, 43(4),* 147–155.

Farah, M. J., Stowe, R. M., and Kevinson, K. L. (1996). Phonological dyslexia: Loss of a reading-specific component of the cognitive architecture? *Cognitive Neuropsychology, 13,* 849–868.

Faraone, S. V. (1996). Discussion of "Genetic influence on parent-reported attention-related problems in a Norwegian general population twin sample." *Journal of the American Academy of Child and Adolescent Psychiatry, 35(5),* 596–598.

Faraone, S. V., Biederman, J., Chen, W., Milberger, S., et al. (1995). Genetic heterogeneity in attention-deficit hyperactivity disorder (ADHD): Gender, psychiatric comorbidity and maternal ADHD. *Journal of Abnormal Psychology, 104,* 334–345.

Faraone, S. V., Biederman, J., Mennin, D., Gershon, J. et al. (1996). A prospective four-year follow-up study of children at risk for ADHD: Psychiatric, neuropsychological, and psychosocial outcome. *Journal of the American Academy of Child and Adolescent Psychiatry, 35(11),* 1449–1459.

Fastenau, P. S. and Fisk, J. L. (1997). Use of visual memory tests to discriminate between left and right temporal lobe epilepsy, ANPA Abstracts *Journal of Neuropsychiatry and Clinical Neurosciences, 9(1)* 160, P134.

Faust, M. E. and Balota, D. A. (1997). Inhibition or return and visuospatial attention in healthy older adults and individuals with dementia of the alzheimer type. *Brain, 11(1),* 13–29.

Favorov, O. V. and Kelly, D. G. (1994). Minicolumnar organization within somatosensory cortical segregates: II. Emergent functional properties. *Cerebral Cortex, 4,* 428–442.

Fee, V. E., Matson, J. L., and Benavidez, D. A. (1994). Attention deficit-hyperactivity disorder among mentally retarded children. *Research in Developmental Disabilities, 15(1),* 67–79.

Fee, V. E., Matson, J. L., Moore, L. A., and Benavidez, D. A. (1993). The differential validity of hyperactivity/attention deficits and conduct problems among mentally retarded children. *Journal of Abnormal Child Psychology, 21(1),* 1–11.

Feigin, A.,. Kurlan, R., McDermott, M. P., Beach, J., Dimitsopulos, T., Brower, C. A., Chapieskim, L., Trinidad, K., Como, P., and Jankovic, J. (1996). A controlled trial of deprenyl in children with Tourette's syndrome and attention deficit hyperactivity disorder. *Neurology, 46,* 965–968.

Feldman, E., Levin, B., Luds, H., Rabin, M., Lubs, M. L., Jallad, B., and Kusch, A. (1993). Adult family dyslexia: A retrospective developmental and psychological profile. *Journal of Neuropsychiatry and Clinical Neurosciences, 5,* 195–199.

Fenton, W. S., McGlashan, T. H., Victor, B. J., and Blyler, C. (1997). Symptoms, subtype and suicidality in patients with schizophrenia spectrum disorders. *American Journal of Psychiatry, 154(2),* 199–204.

Ferguson, H. B. and Rapoport, J. L. (1983). Nosological issues and biological validation, In Rutter, M. (Ed.). *Development Neuropsychiatry,* New York: The Guilford Press, 369–384.

Fergusson, D. M. and Horwood, L. J. (1995). Predictive validity of categorically and dimensionally scored measures of disruptive childhood behaviors. *Journal of the American Academy of Child and Adolescent Psychiatry, 34(4),* 477–485.

Fergusson, D. M., Horwood, L. J., and Lynskey, M. T. (1992). Family change, parental discord and early offending. *Journal of Child Psychology and Psychiatry, 33,* 1059–1075.

Fergusson, D. M., Horwood, L. J., and Lynskey, M. T. (1993). The effects of conduct disorder and attention deficit in middle childhood on offending and scholastic ability at age 13. *Journal of Child Psychology and Psychiatry, 34,* 899–916.

Fiez, J. A. (1997). Phonology, semantics, and the role of the left inferior prefrontal cortex. *Human Brain Mapping, 5,* 79–83.

Filoteo, J. V., Delis, D. C., Demadura, T. L., Salmon, D. P., Roman, M. J., and Shults, C. W. (1994). Abnormally rapid disengagement of covert attention to global and local stimulus levels may underlie the visuoperceptual impairment in Parkinson's patients. *Neuropsychology, 8,* 210–217.

Filipek, P. A., Semrud-Clikeman, M., Steingard, R. J., Renshaw, P. F., Kennedy, D. N., and Biederman, J. (1997). Volumeric MRI analysis comparing subject having attention-deficit hyperactivity disorder with normal controls. *Neurology, 48,* 589–601.

Fillmore, M. T. and Vogel-Sprott, M. (1997). Resistance to cogntive impairment under alcohol: The role of environment consequences. *Experimental and Clinical Psychopharmacology, 5(3),* 251–255.

Fiolteo, V. J., Delis, D. C., Salmon, D. P., Demadura, T., Roman, M. J., and Shults, C. W. (1997). An examination of the nature of attentional deficits in patients with parkinson's disease: Evidence from a spatial orienting task. *Journal of the International Neuropsychological Society, 3,* 337–347.

Findley, L. J. (1996). Classification of tremors. *Journal of Clinical Neurophysiology, 13,* 122–132.

Fischer, M., Barkley, R. A., Fletcher, K. E., and Smallish, L. (1993a). The stability of dimensions of behavior in ADHD and normal children over an 8-year followup. *Journal of Abnormal Child Psychology, 21(3),* 315.

Fischer, M., Barkley, R. A., Fletcher, K. E., and Smallish, L. (1993b). The adolescent outcome of hyperactive children: Predictors of psychiatric, academic, social and emotional adjustment. *Journal of the American Academy of Child and Adolescent Psychiatry, 32,* 324–332.

Fisher, N. J. and DeLuca, J. W. (1997). Verbal learning strategies of right hemisphere learning-disabled adolescents and adults. ANPA Abstracts *Journal of Neuropsychiatry and Clinical Neurosciences, 9(1),* 169, P135.

Fitzpatrick, P. A., Klorman, R., Brumaghim, J. T., and Borgstedt, A. D. (1992). Effects of sustained-release and standard preparations of methylphenidate on attention deficit disorder. *Journal of the American Academy of Child and Adolescent Psychiatry, 31,* 226–234.

Flicek, M. (1992). Social status of boys with both academic problems and attention-deficit hyperactivity disorder. *Journal of Abnormal Child Psychology, 20(4),* 353–366.

Foodman, A. (1996). ADD and soft signs. *Journal of the American Academy of Child and Adolescent Psychiatry, 35(7),* 841–842.

Foong, J., Rozewicz, L., Quaghebeur, G., Davie, C. A., Kartsounis, L. D., Thompson, A. J., Miller, D. H., Ron, M. A. (1997). Executive function in multiple sclerosis: The role of frontal lobe pathology. *Brain, 120,* 15–26.

Frankenburg, F. R. and Kanda, J. C. (1994). Sertraline treatment of attention deficit hyperactivity disorder and Tourette's syndrome. *Journal of Clinical Psychopharmacology, 14(5),* 359–360.

Franzen, M. D., Lovell, M. R., and Smith, S. S. (1997). Relative effects of CHI on forward and backward digit repetition. ANPA Abstracts *Journal of Neuropsychiatry and Clinical Neurosciences, 9(1),* 156, P92.

Frazer, A. (1997). Pharmacology of antidepressants. *Journal of Clinical Psychopharmacology, 17(2),* (Suppl. 1), 2S–18S.

Frederich, B. P. and Olmi, D. J. (1994). Children with attention-deficit/hyperactivity disorder: A review of the literature on social skills deficits. *Psychology in the Schools, 31(4),* 288–296.

Frick, P. J. (1993). Childhood conduct problems in a family context. *School Psychology Review, 22(3),* 376–385.

Frick, P. J., Lahey, B. B., Applegate, B., and Kerdyck L. (1994). DSM-IV field trials for disruptive behavior disorders: Symptom utility estimates. *Journal of the American Academy of Child and Adolescent Psychiatry, 33,* 529–539.

Fristoe, N. M., Salthouse, T. A., Woodard, J. L. (1997). Examination of age-related deficits on the Wisconsin Card Sorting Test. *Neuropsychology, 11(3),* 428–436.

Frost, J. A., Binder, J. R., Hammeke, T. A., Rao, S. M., and Cox, R. W. (1996). Arousal, attention, and auditory systems revealed with whole-brain functional magnetic resonance imaging. *Neurology, 46(2, Suppl.),* A125.

Fuentes, L. J. and Humphreys, G. W. (1996). On the processing of "extinguished" stimuli in unilateral Vvsual neglect: An approach using negative priming. *Cognitive Neuropsychology, 13,* 111–136.

Fuster, J. M. (1997). *The Prefrontal Cortex, Anatomy, Physiology, and Neuropsychology of the Frontal Lobe.* 3rd ed., Philadelphia, Lippincott-Raven.

Gadow, K. D., Nolan, E., Sprafkin, J., and Sverd, J. (1995a). School observations of children with attention-deficit hyperactivity disorder and comorbid tic disorder: Effects of methylphenidate treatment. *Journal of Developmental and Behavioral Pediatrics, 16(3),* 167–176.

Gadow, K. D., Sverd, J., Sprafkin, J., Nolan, E. E., et al. (1995b). Efficacy of methylphenidate for attention-deficit hyperactivity disorder in children with tic disorders: Correction. *Archives of General Psychiatry, 52(10),* 836.

Gahring, L. C., Rogers, S. W., and Twyman, R. E. (1997). Autoantibodies to glutamate receptor subunit Glu R2 in nonfamilial olivopontocerebellar degeneration. *Neurology, 48,* 494–500.

Galaburda, A. M. (1994). Cerebral lateralization: Structural basis. In Heilman, K. M., Ed., *Right Hemisphere Dominance and Unilateral Neglect,* The 20th Annual Course in Behavioral Neurology & Neuropsychology. Lake Buena Vista, FL: The Florida Society of Neurology & The Center for Neuropsychological Studies at The University of Florida.

Galynker, I., Ieronimo, C., Miner, C., Rosenblum, J. et al. (1997). Methylphenidate treatment of negative symptoms in patients with dementia. *The Journal of Neuropsychiatry and Clinical Neurosciences, 9(2),* 231–239.

Gammon, G. D. and Brown, T. E. (1993). Fluoxetine and methylphenidate in combination for treatment of attention deficit disorder and comorbid depressive disorder. *Journal of Child and Adolescent Psychopharmacology, 3(1),* 1–10.

Gangestad, S. W. and Yeo, R. A. (1994). Parental handedness and relative hand skill: A test of the developmental instability hypothesis. *Neuropsychology, 8,* 572–578.

Garber, S. W., Garber, M. D., and Spizman, R. F. (1995). *Is Your Child Hyperactive? Inattentive? Impulsive? Distractible? Helping the Add/Hyperactive Child.* New York: Villard Books.

Garth, J., Anderson, V., and Wrennall, J. (1997). Executive functions following moderate to severe frontal lobe injury: Impact of injury and age at injury. *Pediatric Rehabilitation, 1(2),* 99–108.

Gathercole, S. E. (1994). Neuropsychology and working memory: A review. *Neuropsychology, 8,* 494–505.

Gaub, M. and Carlson, C. L. (1996). Meta-analysis of gender differences in AD/HD. *Attention!, 2(4),* 25–30.

Gaub, M. and Carlson, C. L. (1997). Behavioral characteristics of DSM-IV ADHD subtypes in a school-based population. *Journal of Abnormal Child Psychology, 25(2),* 103–111.

Gazella, K. A. (1994). Attention deficit hyperactivity disorder: Focusing on alternative treatments. *Health Counselor, 6(1),* 24–29.

Gazzaniga, M. S. (Ed.) (1995). *The Cognitive Neurosciences.* Cambridge, MA: MIT Press.

Geldmacher, D. S. and Hills, E. C. (1997). Effect of stimulus number, target-to-distractor ratio, and motor speed on visual spatial search quality following traumatic brain injury. *Brain Injury, 11,* 59–66.

Geldmacher, D. S., Doty, L., and Heilman, K. M. (1994). Spatial performance bias in normal elderly subjects on a letter cancellation task. *Neuropsychiatry, Neuropsychology, and Behavioral Neurology, 7(4),* 274–280.

George, M. S., Ketter, T. A., Parekh, P. J., Rosinsky, N., King, H. A., Pazzaglia, P. J., Marangell, L. B., Callahan, L. B., and Post, R. M. (1997). Blunted left cingulate activation in mood disorder subjects during a response interference task (the stroop). *Neuropsychiatry and Clinical Neurosciences, 9,* 55–63.

George, M. S., Ketter, T. A., Parekh, P. J., Rosinsky, N., King, H., Casey, B. J., Trimble, M. R., Horwitz, B., Herscovitch, P., and Post, R. M. (1994). Regional brain activity, when selecting a response despite interference: An H2-50 PET study of the stroop and an emotional stroop. *Human Brain Mapping, 1,* 194–209.

Georgiuos, N., Bradshaw, J. L., Phillips, J. G., Bradshaw, J. A., and Chiv, E. (1995). The Simon effect and attention deficits in Gilles de la Tourette's syndrome and Huntington's disease. *Brain, 118,* 1305–1318.

Gerring, J. P., Brady, K., D., Miller, G., Christiansen, J., Bryan, R. N., and Denckla, M. B. (1997). Psychiatric disorders and MRI pathology after closed head injury in children, ANPA Abstracts. *Journal of Neuropsychiatry and Clinical Neurosciences, 9(1),* 135.

Giddan, J. J. (1991). Communication issues in attention-deficit hyperactivity disorder. *Child Psychiatry and Human Development, 22(1),* 45–51.

Giedd, J. N., Castellanos, F. X., Casey, B. J., and Kozuch, P. (1994). Quantitative morphology of the corpus callosum in attention deficit hyperactivity disorder. *American Journal of Psychiatry, 151,* 665–669.

Gillis, J. J., Gilger, J. W., Pennington, B. F., and DeFries, J. C. (1992). Attention deficit disorder in reading disabled twins: Evidence for a genetic etiology. *Journal of Abnormal Child Psychology, 20(3),* 303–315.

Girardi, N. L., Shaywitz, S. E., Shaywitz, B. A., Marchione, K., Fleischman, S. J., Jones, T. W. and Tamborlane, W. V. (1995). Blunted catecholamine responses after glucose ingestion in children with attention deficit disorder. *Pediatric Research, 38(4),* 529–542.

Girelli, M. and Luck, S. J. (1997). Are the same attentional mechanisms used to detect visual search targets defined by color, orientation, and motion? *Journal of Cognitive Neuroscience, 9(2),* 238–253.

Gitlin, M. J. (1990). *The Psychotherapist's Guide to Psychopharmacology.* New York: The Free Press.

Glitz, D. A. (1993, January). Anxiety and panic disorders in primary care practice. *Clinical Advances in the Treatment of Psychiatric Disorders, 7(1),* 4–6.

Glosser, G., Cole, L. C., French, J. A., Saykin, A. J., and Sprling, M. R. (1997). Predictors of intellectual performance in adults with intractable temporal lobe epilepsy. *Journal of the International Neuropsychological Society, 3,* 252–259.

Godefry, O., Lhullier, C., and Rousseaux, M. (1996). Non-spatial attention disorders in patients with frontal or posterior brain damage. *Brain, 119(1),* 191–202.

Gold, J. M., Goldberg, T. E., and Weinberger, D. R. (1992). Prefrontal function and schizophrenic symptoms. *Neuropsychiatry, Neuropsychology, and Behavioral Neurology, 5(4),* 253–261.

Goldberg, E., Podell, K., and Lovell, M. (1994). Lateralization of frontal lobe functions and cognitive novelty. *Journal of Neuropsychiatry and Clinical Neurosciences, 6,* 371–378.

Goldberg, I. K. (1995). Serzone appears to cause minimal sexual dysfunction, sleep problems. *Psychopharmacology Update, 6,* 1–4.

Golden, C. J. (1981). The Luria-Nebraska children's battery: Theory and formation. In G. Hynd and J. Obrzut (Eds). *Neuropsychological Assessment of the School Age Child.* New York: Grune & Stratton.

Golden, C. J. (1981). *Diagnosis and Rehabilitation in Clinical Neuropsychology.* Springfield, IL: Charles Thomas.

Goldhammer, N. M. (1991). The co-occurrence of attention deficit hyperactivity and dyslexia: rate, characteristics and inheritance. *Dissertation Abstracts International, Feb. 1991,* 51, 4073B.

Goldman, S. J., D'Angelo, E. J., and DeMaso, D. R. (1993). Psychopathology in the families of children and adolescents with borderline personality disorder. *American Journal of Psychiatry, 150,* 1832–1835.

Goldman-Rakic, P. S. (1990). Cellular and circuit basis of working memory in prefrontal cortex of nonhuman primates (Review). *Prog. Brain Res., 85,* 325–336.

Goldman-Rakic, P. S. (1994). Working memory dysfunction in schizophrenia. *The Journal of Neuropsychiatry and Clinical Neurosciences, 6(4),* 348–357.

Goldman-Rakic, P. S., Selemon, L. D., Schwartz, M. L. (1984). Dual pathways connecting the dorsolateral prefrontal cortex with the hippocampal formation and parahippocampal cortex in the rhesus monkey. *Neuroscience, 12,* 719–743.

Goldman-Rakic, P. S. and Friedman, H. R. (1991). The circuitry of working memory revealed by anatomy and metabolic imaging. In Levin, H. S., Eisenberg, H. M., and Benton, A. L., (Eds.), *Frontal Lobe Function and Dysfunction,* New York, Oxford University Press, 72–91.

Goldstein, P. C., Rosenbaum, G., and Taylor, M. J. (1997). Assessment of differential attention mechanisms in seizure disorders and schizophrenia. *Neuropsychology, 11(2),* 309–317.

Goldstein, S. (1991, January). Young children at risk: The early signs of attention-deficit hyperactivity disorder. *Chadder Box.*

Goldstein, S. (1993). Young children at risk: Recognizing the early signs of ADHD. *The ADHD Report, 1(2),* 7–8.

Goldstein, S. and Goldstein, M. (1990). *Managing Attention Disorders in Children: A Guide for Practitioners.* New York: John Wiley & Sons.

Goodyear, P. R. (1991). Attention deficit disorders with and without hyperactivity, neuropsychological processes, *Dissertation Abstracts International, 51, Feb.,* 2681-A.

Goodyear, P. and Hynd, G. W. (1992). Attention deficit disorder with (ADD/H) and without (ADD/WO) Hyperactivity: Behavioral and Neuropsychological Differentiation. *Journal of Clinical Child Psychology, 21(3),* 273–305.

Gordon, M. (1995). Certainly not a fad, but it can be over-diagnosed. *Attention!*, *2(2)*, 20–22.

Gordon, M., Mettleman, B. B., and Irwin, M. (1994). Sustained attention and grade retention. *Perceptual and Motor Skills*, *78*, 555–560.

Gorenstein, E. E., Mammato, C. A., and Sandy, J. M. (1989). Performance of inattentive-overactive children on selected measures of prefrontal-type function. *Journal of Clinical Psychology*, *45(4)*, 619–632.

Grados, M. A., Gerring, J. P., Bryan, R. N., and Denckla, M. B. (1997). Obsessive-compulsive disorder (OCD) in children and adolescents with moderate to severe injury, ANPA Abstracts. *Journal of Neuropsychiatry and Clinical Neurosciences*, *9(1)*, 135.

Granger, D. A., Whalen, C. K., and Henker, B. (1993). Perceptions of methylphenidate effects on hyperactive children's peer interactions. *Journal of Abnormal Child Psychology*, *21(5)*, 535–549.

Grant, D. A. and Berg, E. A. (1948). A behavioral analysis of the degree of reinforcement and ease of shifting to new responses in a Weigl-type card sorting problem. *Journal of Experimental Psychology*, *38*, 404–411.

Grattan, L. M., Bloomer, R. H., Archambault, F. X., Eslinger, P. J. (1994). Cognitive flexibilty and empathy after frontal lobe lesion. *Neuropsychiatry, Neuropsychology and Behavioral Neurology*, *1*, 251–259.

Gray, J. A. (1987). *The Psychology of Fear and Stress (2nd ed.)*. Cambridge: Cambridge University Press.

Green, B. L., Korol, M., Grace, M. C., Vary, M. G., Leonard, A. C., Gleser, G. C., and Smitson-Cohen, S. (1991). Children and disaster: Age, gender and parental effects on PTSD symptoms. *Journal of the American Academy of Child and Adolescent Psychiatry*, *30*, 954–951.

Greenberg, G. S. and Horn, W. F. (1991). *Attention Deficit Hyperactivity Disorder: Questions and Answers for Parents*. Champaign, IL: Research Press.

Greene, R. W., Biederman, J. F., Stephen, V., Ouellette, C. A. et al. (1996). Toward a new psychometric definition of social disability in children with attention-deficit hyperactivity disorder. *Journal of the American Academy of Child and Adolescent Psychiatry*, *35(5)*, 571–578.

Greenfield, B., Hechtman, L., and Weiss, G. (1988). Two subgroups of hyperactives as adults: Correlation of outcome. *Canadian Journal of Psychiatry*, *33*, 505–508.

Greenhill, L. L. and Osman, B. B. (Eds.) (1991). *Ritalin: Theory and Patient Management*. New York: Mary Ann Liebert, Inc.

Greenwood, P. M., Parasuraman, R., and Alexander, G. E. (1997), Controlling the focus of spatial attention during visual search: effects of advanced aging and Alzheimer disease. *Neuropsychology*, *11(1)*, 3–12.

Griffin, M. G., Resick, P. A., and Mechanic, M. B. (1997). Objective assessment of peritraumatic dissociation: Psychophysiological indicators. *American Journal of Psychiatry*, *154(8)*, 1081–1088.

Griffiths, T. D., Rees, A., Witton, C., Cross, P. M., Shakir, R. A., and Green, G. G. R. (1997). Spatial and temporal auditory processing deficits following right hemisphere infarction: A psychophysical study. *Brain*, *120*, 785–794.

Grinspoon, L. and Bakalar, J. B. (1985). Drug dependence: Nonnarcotic agents, In *Comprehensive Textbook of Psychiatry IV* 4th ed., Kaplan, H. I. and Sadock, B.J., Eds., Baltimore: Williams and Wilkins, 1003–1015.

Grinspoon, L. and Bakalar, J. B. (1995). Marijuana as medicine: A plea for reconsideration. *JAMA, 273(23),* 1875–1876.

Gronwall, D. and Wrightson, P. (1974). Delayed recovery of intellectual function after minor head injury. *Lancet,* 2, 605–609.

Gronwall, D. and Sampson, H. (1974). *The Psychological Effects of Concussion.* Auckland, NZ: Auckland University Press, Oxford University Press.

Gross, T. V., Shalev, R. S., Manor, O., and Amir, N. (1995). Developmental right-hemisphere syndrome: Clinical spectrum of the nonverbal learning disability. *Journal of Learning Disabilities, 28(2),* 80–86.

Grossman, M., Crino, P., Reivich, M., Stern, M. B., and Hurtig, H. I. (1992). Attention and sentence processing deficits in Parkinson's disease: The role of anterior cingulate cortex. *Cerebral Cortex,* 2, 513–525.

Grunhaus, L., Pande, A. C., Brown, M. B., and Greden, J. F. (1994). Clinical characteristics of patients with concurrent major depressive disorder and panic disorder. *American Journal of Psychiatry, 151,* 541–546.

Guevremont, D. C. (1992, Fall/Winter). The parents role in helping the ADHD child with peer relationships. *Ch.A.D.D.er, 6(2),* 17–18.

Guevremont, D. C. (1994, February). Getting ready for the Little League and other group activities. *Chadder Box,* 8–11.

Gulyas, B. and Roland, P. (1995). Cortical fields participating in spatial frequency and orientation discrimination: Functional anatomy by position emission tomography. *Human Brain Mapping, 3,* 133–152.

Gurvits, T. V., Lasko, N. B., Schachter, S. C., Kuhne, A. A., Orr, S. P., and Pitman, R. K. (1992). Neurological status of Vietnam veterans with chronic posttraumatic stress disorder. *Journal of Neuropsychiatry and Clinical Neurosciences, 5(2),* 183–188.

Haapasalo, J. and Tremblay, R. E. (1994). Physically aggressive boys from ages 6 to 12: Family background, parenting behavior, and prediction of delinquency. *Journal of Consulting and Clinical Psychology, 62,* 1044–1052.

Hackerman, F., Buccino, D. L., Gallucci, G., and Schmidt, C.W., Jr. (1996). The effect of a split in WAIS-R VIQ and PIQ scores on patients with cognitive impairment and psychiatric illness. *Journal of Clinical Neuropsychiatry, 8,* 85–87.

Hagoort, P., Brown, C. M., and Swaab, T. Y. (1966). Lexical-semantic event-related potential effects in patients with left hemisphere lesions and aphasia, and patients with right hemisphere lesions without apasia. *Brain, 119,* 627–649.

Hall, J., Hynd, G. W., Cohen, M. J., and Riccio, C. A. (1996). ADHD subtypes: MRI morphometric analysis of the corpus callosum. *Journal of the International Neuropsychological Society, 2(1),* 58.

Halliday, R., Naylor, H., Brandeis, D., Callaway, E., Yano, L., and Herzig, R. (1994). The affect of Damphetamine, Clonidine, and Yohimbine on human information processing. *Psychophysiology, 31,* 331–337.

Halligan, P. W. and Marshall, J. C. (1994). Toward a principled explanation of unilateral neglect. *Cognitive Neuropsychology, 11(2),* 167–206.

Halliwell, B. (1994). Free radicals, antioxidants, and human disease: Curiosity, cause, or consequence? *Lancet, 344(8924),* 721–725.

Hallowell, E. M. and Ratey, J. J. (1993). Suggested diagnostic criteria for ADD in adults. *ADDult News,* Winter.

Hallowell, E. M. and Ratey, J. J. (1994). *Driven to Distraction.* New York: Pantheon Books.

Hallowell, N. (1993, Spring/Summer). Living and loving with attention deficit disorder: Couples where one partner has ADD. *Ch.A.D.D.er.,* 13–19.

Halperin, J. M., Sharma, V., Siever, L. J., Schwartz, S. T., Matier, K., Wornell, G., and Newcorn, J. H. (1994). Serotonergic function in aggressive and nonaggressive boys with attention deficit hyperactivity disorder. *American Journal of Psychiatry, 151,* 243–248.

Haltiner, A. M., Temkin, N. R., Winn, H. R., and Dikmen, S. S. (1996). The impact of posttraumatic seizures on 1-year neuropsychological and psychosocial outcome of head injury. *Journal of the International Neuropsychological Society, 2,* 494–504.

Handen, B. L., Feldman, H., and Gosling, A. (1991). Adverse side effects of methylphenidate among mentally retarded children with ADHD. *Journal of the American Academy of Child and Adolescent Psychiatry, 30,* 241–245.

Handen, B. L., Janosky, J., McAuliffe, S., and Breaux, A. M. (1994). Prediction of response to methylphenidate among children with ADHD and mental retardation. *Journal of the American Academy of Child and Adolescent Psychiatry, 33,* 1185–1193.

Handen, B. L., McAuliffe, S., Janosky, J., Feldman, H. et al. (1995). Methylphenidate in children with mental retardation and ADHD: Effects on independent play and academic functioning. *Journal of Developmental and Physical Disabilities, 7(2),* 91–103.

Hanemann, C. O., Anneke, A., Gabreëls-Festen, W. M., Müller, H. W., and Stoll, G. (1996). Low affinity NGF receptor expression in CMT1A nerve biopsies of different disease stages. *Brain,* 119, 1461–1469.

Hanes, K. R., Andrews, D. G., and Pantelis, C. (1995). Cognitive flexibility and complex integration in Parkinson's disease, Huntington's disease, and schizophrenia. *Journal of the International Neuropsychological Society, 1,* 545–553.

Hans, W. H., Susser, E., Buck, K. A., Lumey, L. H., Lin, S. P., and Gorman, J. M. (1996). Schizoid personality disorder after prenatal exposure to famine. *American Journal of Psychiatry, 153,* 1637–1639.

Harris, E. L., Schuerholz, L. J., Singer, H. S., Reader, M. J., Brown, J. E., Cox, C., Mohr, J., Chase, G. A., and Denckla, M. B. (1995). Executive function in children with Tourette's syndrome and/or attention deficit hyperactivity disorder. *Journal of the International Neuropsychological Society, 1,* 511–516.

Harris, G. J., Hoehn-Saric, R., Lewis, R., Pearson, G. D., and Streeter, C. (1994).

Hartmann, T. (1993). *Attention Deficit Disorder: A Different Perception.* Lancaster, PA: Underwood-Miller.

Harvard Mental Health Letter (1992, October). Addiction—Part I. *Harvard Mental Health Letter, 9(4),* 1–3.

Harvard Mental Health Letter (1994, May). Borderline Personality—Part I. *Harvard Mental Health Letter, 10(11)*, 1–3.

Harvard Mental Health Letter (1993, May). Child Abuse—Part I. *Harvard Mental Health Letter, 9(11)*, 1–3.

Harvard Mental Health Letter (1993, July). Child Abuse—Part III. *Harvard Mental Health Letter, 10(1)*, 1–5.

Harvard Mental Health Letter (1992, December). Eating disorders—Part I. *Harvard Mental Health Letter, 9(6)*, 1–4.

Harvard Mental Health Letter (1993, December). Mood disorders in childhood and adolescence—Part II. *Harvard Mental Health Letter, 10(6)*, 1–3.

Harvard Mental Health Letter (1994, September). Sleep disorders—Part II. *Harvard Mental Health Letter, 11(3)*, 1–5.

Harvard Mental Health Letter (1994, October). Social phobia—Part I. *Harvard Mental Health Letter, 11(4)*, 1–3.

Harvard Mental Health Letter (1994, November). Social phobia—Part II. *Harvard Mental Health Letter, 11(5)*, 1–3.

Harvard Mental Health Letter (1994, December). Update on mood disorders—Part I. *Harvard Mental Health Letter, 11(6)*, 1–4.

Harvard Mental Health Letter (1995, January). Update on mood disorder—Part II. *Harvard Mental Health Letter, 11(7)*, 1–4.

Haslam, C., Batchelor, J., Fearnside, M. R., Haslam, S. A., Hawkins, S., and Kenway, E. (1994). Post-coma disturbance and post-traumatic amnesia as nonlinear predictors of cognitive outcome following severe closed head injury: Findings from the Westmead Head Injury Project. *Brain Injury, 8*, 519–528.

Haxby, J. V., Ungerleider, L. G., Horwitz, B., Rappoport, S. I., and Grady, C. L. (1995). Hemispheric differences in neural systems for face working memory: A PET-rCBF study. *Human Brain Mapping, 3*, 68–82.

Hauser, P., Zametkin, A. J., Martinez, P., Vitiello, B., Matochik, J. A., Mixson, A. J., and Weintraub, B. D. (1993). Attention deficit-hyperactivity disorder in people with generalized resistance to thyroid hormone. *New England Journal of Medicine, 32B(14)*, 997–1001.

Hawkins, K. A., Hoffman, R. E., Quinlan, D. M., Rakfeldt, J., Docherty, N. M., Sledge, W. H. (1997). Cognition, negative symptoms, and diagnosis: A comparison of schizophrenic, bipolar, and control samples. *Journal of Neuropsychiatry and Clinical Neurosciences, 9(1)*, 81–89.

Haznedar, M. M., Buchsbaum, M. S., Metzger, M., Solimando, A., Spiegel-Cohen, J., and Holander, E. (1997). Anterior cingulate gyrus volume and glucose metabolism in autistic disorder. *American Journal of Psychiatry, 154(8)*, 1047–1050.

Healey, J. M., Newcorn, J. H., Halperin, J. M., Wolf, L. E., Pascualvaca, D. M., Schmeidler, J., and O'Brien, J. D. (1993). The factor structure of ADHD items in DSM III-R: Internal consistency and external validation. *Journal of Abnormal Child Psychology, 21(4)*, 441–453.

Heaton, R. K. (1981). *Wisconsin Card Sorting Test Manual.* Odessa, FL: Psychological Assessment Resources.

Hécan, H. (1962). Clinical symptomatology in right and left hemisphere lesions. In Mountcastle, V. B., Ed., Inter-Hemispheric Relations and Cerebral Dominance. Baltimore: The John Hopkins Press, 215–243.

Hécan, H. and Albert, M. L. (1978). *Human Neuropsychology,* New York: Wiley.

Hechtman, L. (1994). Genetic and neurobiological aspects of attention hyperactivity disorder: A review. *Journal of Psychiatry and Neuroscience, 19(3),* 193–201.

Hechtman, L. (1996). Families of children with attention deficit hyperactivity disorder: A review. *Canadian Journal of Psychiatry, 41(6),* 350–360.

Heffelfinger, A., Craft, S., and Shyken, J. (1997). Visual attention in children with prenatal cocaine exposure. *Journal of the International Neuropsychological Society, 3,* 237–245.

Heilman, K. M. (1994). Right hemisphere dominance and unilateral neglect. The 20th Annual Course in Behavioral Neurology & Neuropsychology. Lake Buena Vista FL; The Florida Society of Neurology & The Center for Neuropsychological Studies at The University of Florida.

Heilman, K. M. (1994). Emotion and the brain: A distributed modular network mediating emotional experience, In. Zaidel, D. W., Ed., *Neuropsychology,* San Diego: Academic Press, 139–158.

Heilman, K. M. (1997). The neurobiology of emotional experience. *Journal of Neuropsychiatry, 9(3),* 439–438.

Heilman, K. M., Bowers, D., Coslett, H. B., Whelan, H., and Watson, R. T. (1985). Directional hypokinesia: Prolonged reaction times for leftward movements in patients with right hemisphere lesions and neglect. *Neurology, 35,* 855–860.

Heilman, K. M., Chatterjee, A., and Doty, L. C. (1995). Hemispheric asymmetries of near-far spatial attention. *Neuropsychology, 9(1),* 58–61.

Heilman, K. M. and Valenstein, E. (1972). Frontal lobe neglect in man. *Neurology, 22,* 660–664.

Heilman, K. M. and Valenstein, E. (Eds.) (1979). *Clinical Neuropsychology,* New York: Oxford University Press.

Heilman, K. M. and Valenstein, E. (Eds.) (1993). *Clinical Neuropsychology,* 3rd ed., New York: Oxford University Press.

Heilman, K. M., Chatterjee, A., and Doty, L. C. (1995). Hemispheric asymmetries of near-far spatial attention. *Neuropsychology, 9,* 58–61.

Heilman, K. M., Valenstein, E., and Watson, R. T. (1995). *Attentional and Intentional Disorders: Assessment of Behavioral Disorders.* The Florida Society of Neurology and the Center for Neuropsychological Studies at the University of Florida, Gainesville, FL.

Heilman, K. M., Watson, R. T., and Valenstein, E. (1998). Neglect and related disorders. In Heilman, K. M. and Valenstein, E., (Eds.). *Clinical Neuropsychology,* 3rd ed., Oxford: Oxford University Press.

Heilman, K. M., Voeller, K. K., and Nadeau, S. E. (1991). A possible pathophysiologic substrate of attention deficit hyperactivity disorder. *Journal of Child Neurology, 6(Suppl.),* S76–S81.

Heimer, L., Alheid, G. F., de Olmos, J. S., Groenewegen, H. J. et al. (1997). The accumbens: Beyond the core-shell dichotomy. *The Journal of Neuropsychiatry and Clinical Neurosciences, 9(3),* 354–381.

Heller, W. (1993). Neuropsychological mechanisms of individual differences in emotion, personality, and arousal. *Neuropsychology, 7,* 476–489.

Hellgren, L., Gillberg, C., and Gillberg, I. C. (1994). Children with deficits in attention, motor control and perception (DAMP) almost grown up: The contribution of various background factors to outcome at age 16 years. *European Child and Adolescent Psychiatry, 3(1),* 1–15.

Hendriks, A. W. and Kolk, H. H. J. (1997). Strategic control in developmental dyslexia. *Cognitive Neuropsychology, 14(3),* 321–366.

Henik, A. (1996). Paying attention to the Stroop effect. *Journal of the International Neurological Society, 2(5),* 467–470.

Hennekens, C. H. (1994). Antioxidant vitamins and cancer. *American Journal of Medicine, 97(3A),* 2S–4S.

Herbert, J. and Devinsky, O. (1995). Rehabilitation after brain injury: impact of posttraumatic epilepsy. *NeuroRehabilitation, 5,* 169–280.

Herman, B. P., Wyler, A. R., and Richey, E. T. (1988). Wisconsin Card Sorting Test performance in patient: with complex partial seizures of temporal lobe origin. *Journal of Clinical and Experimental Psychology, 10,* 467–476.

Hermann, D. and Parenté, (1994). The multimodal approach to cognitive rehabilitation. *NeuroRehabilitation, 4(3),* 133–142.

Hermans, H. J. M. (1966). Voicing the self: From information processing to dialogical interchange. *Psychological Bulletin, 119(1),* 31–50.

Hern, K. L. (1997). Plasticity in functional recovery: is it a question of all or none? ANPA Abstracts *Journal of Neuropsychiatry and Clinical Neurosciences, 9(1),* 139, P32.

Hernandez, T. D. and Naritoku, D. K. (1997). Seizures, epilepsy, and functional reovery after traumatic brain injury: A reappraisal. *Neurology, 48,* 803–806.

Hersh, N. A. and Treadgold, L. G. (1994). Neuropage: The rehabilitation of memory dysfunction by prosthetic memory and cueing. *NeuroRehabilitation, 4(3),* 187–197.

Hestad, K., Aukrust, P. Ellertsen, B., and Klove, H. (1996). Neuropsychological deficits in HIV-1 seropositive and seronegative intravenous drug users (IVDUs): A follow-up study. *Journal of the International Neuropsychological Society, 2,* 126–133.

Hillier, S. L., Sharpe, M. H. and Metzer, J. (1997). Outcomes 5 years post-traumatic brain injury (with further reference to neurophysical impairment and disability). *Brain Injury, 11(9),* 661–675.

Hillyard, S. A., Hinrichs, H., Tempelmann, C., Morgan, S. T., Hansen, J. C., Scheich, H., and Heinze, H. J. (1997). Combining steady-state visual evoked potentials and fMRI to localize brain activity during selective attention. *Human Brain Mapping, 5,* 287–292.

Hillyard, S. A., Mangun, G. R., Woldorff, M. G., and Luck, S. J. (1995). Neural Systems Mediating Selective Attention. In Gazzaniga, P. S., Ed., *The Cognitive Neurosciences,* Cambridge: Massachusetts Institute of Technology, 665–681.

Hilton, D. K., Martin, C. A., Heffron, W. M., Hall, B. D., and Johnson, G. L. (1991). Imipramine treatment of ADHD in a fragile X child. *Journal of American Academy of Child and Adolescent Psychiatry, 30(5),* 831–834.

Hinnant, C. A. (1994). Thromboembolic infarcts occurring after mild traumatic brain injury in a paediatric patient with Noonan's syndrome. *Brain Injury, 8,* 719–727.

Hinshaw, S. P. (1992a). Academic underachievement, attention deficits, and aggression: comorbidity and implications for intervention. *Journal of Consulting and Clinical Psychology, 60,* 893–903.

Hinshaw, S. P. (1992b). Externalizing behavior problems and academic underachievement in childhood and adolescence: Causal relationships and underlying mechanisms. *Psychological Bulletin, 111,* 127–155.

Hinshaw, S. P., Heller, T., and McHale, J. P. (1992). Covert antisocial behavior with attention-deficit hyperactivity disorder: External validation and effects of methylphenidate. *Journal of Consulting and Clinical Psychology, 60,* 274–281.

Hitri, A., Casanova, M. F., Kleinman, J. E., and Wyatt, R. J. (1994). Fewer dopamine transporter receptors in the prefrontal cortex of cocaine users. *American Journal of Psychiatry, 151,* 1074–1076.

Hittmair-Delazer, M., Semenza, C., and Denes, G. (1994). Concepts and facts in calculation. *Brain, 117,* 715–728.

Hoek, H. W., Susser, E., Buck, K. A., Lumey, L. H., Lin, S. P., and Gorman, J. M., (1996). Schizoid personality disorder after prenatal exposure to famine. *American Journal of Psychiatry, 153,* 1637–1639.

Hoffman, R. E., Buchsbaum, M. S., Jensen, R. V., Guich, S. M., Tsai, K., and Nuechterlein, K. H. (1996). Dimensional complexity of EEG waveforms in neuroleptic-free schizophrenic patients and normal control subjects. *Journal of Neuropsychiatry, 8,* 436–441.

Holcomb, P. J., Ackerman, P. T., and Dykman, R. A. (1985). Cognitive event related brain potentials in children with attention and reading deficits. *Psychophysiology, 22,* 656–66.

Holcomb, P. J., Ackerman, P. T., and Dykman, R. A. (1986). Auditory event related brain potentials in attention and reading disabled boys. *International Journal of Psychophysiology, 3,* 263–273.

Holdnack, J. A., Molberg, P. J., Arnold, S. E., Gur, R. C., and Gur, R. E. (1995). Speed of processing and verbal learning deficits in adults diagnosed with attention deficit disorder. *Neuropsychiatry, Neuropsychology and Behavioral Neurology, 8(4),* 282–292.

Hollander, E. and Wong, C. M. (1996). The relationship between executive function impairment and serotonergic sensitivity in obsessive-compulsive disorder. *Neuropsychiatry, Neuropsychology and Behavioral Neurology, 9,* 230–233.

Holmes, V. M. and Standish, J. M. (1996). Skilled reading with impaired phonology: A case study. *Cognitive Neuropsychology, 13(8),* 1207–1222.

Hooks, K., Milich, R., and Lorch, E. P. (1994). Sustained and selective attention in boys with attention deficit hyperactivity disorder. *Journal of Clinical Child Psychology, 23(1),* 69–77.

Hooten, W. M. and Lyketsos, C. G. (1996). Frontotemporal dementia: A clinicopathological review of four postmortem studies. *Journal of Clinical Neuropsychiatry, 8,* 10–19.

Hopkins, R. O., Gale, S. D., Johnson, S. C., Anderson, C. V., Bigler, E. D., Blatter, D.D., and Weaver, L. K. (1995). Severe anozia with and without concomitant brain atrophy and neuropsychological impairments. *Journal of the International Neuropsychological Society, 1,* 501–509.

Hoptman, M. J. and Davidson, R. J. (1994). How and why do the two cerebral hemispheres interact? *Psychological Bulletin, 116,* 195–219.

Horacek, H. J. (1994). Clonidine extended-release capsules as an alternative to oral tablets and transdermal patches. *Journal of Child and Adolescent Psychopharmacology, 4(3),* 211–212.

Horn, W. F., Ialongo, N. S., Pascoe, J. M., Greenberg, G., Packard, T., Lopez, M., Wagner, A., and Puttler, L. (1991). Additive effects of psychostimulants, parent training, and self-control therapy with ADHD children. *Journal of the American Academy of Child and Adolescent Psychiatry, 30,* 233–240.

Horner, B. R. and Scheibe, K. E. (1997). Prevalence and implications of attention-deficit hyperactivity disorder among adolescents in treatment for substance abuse. *Journal of the American Academy of Child and Adoles Psychiatry, 36,* 30–36.

Hornstein, A., Lennihan, L., Seliger, G., Lichtman, S., and Schroeder, K. (1996). Amphetamine in recovery from brain injury. *Brain Injury, 10(2),* 145–148.

Howard, D. and Best, W. (1996). Developmental phonological dyslexia: Real word reading can be completely normal. *Cognitive Neuropsychology, 13,* 887–934.

Hoza, B., Pelham, W. E., Milich, R., Pillow, D., and McBride, K. (1993). The self-perceptions and attributions of attention deficit hyperactivity disordered and nonreferred boys. *Journal of Abnormal Child Psychology, 21(3),* 271–286.

Hua, M. S., Huang, C. C., and Yang, Y. J. (1995). Chronic elemental mercury intoxication: Neuropsychological follow-up case study. *Brain Injury, 10(5),* 377–384.

Hubbard, K. (1994, October/November). Bringing Section 504 into the classroom. *Chadder Box,* 8–9.

Hublin, C., Kaprio, J., Partinen, M., Heikkilä, K., and Koskenvuo, M. (1997). Prevalence and genetics of sleepwalking: A population-based twin study. *Neurology, 48,* 177–181.

Hughes, J. R. (1997). Substance abuse and ADHD. *American Journal of Psychiatry, 154(1),* 132.

Humphreys, G. W., Boucart, M., Datar, V., and Riddoch, M. J. (1996). Processing fragmented forms and strategic control of orienting in visual neglect. *Cognitive Neuropsychology, 13,* 177–203.

Hunt, R. D., Harralson, P., Hoehn, R., and Turner, T. (1993, Fall/Winter). Neurobiological subtypes of ADHD: A clinical model based on a neurobiological hypothesis. *Ch.A.D.D.er, 7(2),* 7–10.

Hunt, R. D., Lau, S., and Ryu, J. (1991). Alternative therapies for ADHD. In Greenhill, L. L. and Osman, B. B., Eds., *Ritalin Theory and Patient Management.* New York: Maryann Liebert, 75–96.

Hunt, R. D., Mandel, L., Lau, S., and Hughes, M. (1991). Neurobiological theories of ADHD and ritalin. In Greenhill, L. L. and Osman, B. B., Eds., *Ritalin Theory and Patient Management.* New York: Maryann Liebert, 267–288.

Huntzinger, R. M. (1995). Neuropsychological functioning in two children diagnosed with Asperger's disorder. *Journal of Neuropsychiatry, 7(3),* Abstract No. 85.

Hynd, G. W., Hern, K. L., and Voeller, K. K. (1991). Neurobiological basis of attention-deficit hyperactivity disorder (ADHD). *School Psychology Review, 20,* 174–186.

Hynd, G. W., Lorys, A. R., Semrud-Clikeman, M., and Nieves, N. (1991). Attention deficit disorder without hyperactivity: A distinct behavioral and neurocognitive syndrome. *Journal of Child Neurology, 6(Suppl.),* S37–S43.

Hynd, G. W., Hiemenz, J., Hall, J., Vaughn, M., and Cody, H. (1996). Gyral morphology in the bilateral perisylvian cortex in dyslexia. *Journal of the International Neuropsychological Society, 2(3),* 185.

Hynd, G. W., Hern, K. L., Novey, E. S., Eliopulos, D. et al. (1993). Attention deficit disorder and asymmetry of the caudate nucleus. *Journal of Child Neurology, 8,* 339–347.

Hynd, G. W., Semrud-Clickeman, M., Lorys, A. P., Novey, E. S., Eliopulos, D. and Lyytinen, H. (1989). Corpus callosum morphology in attention deficit hyperactivity disorder (ADHD): Morphometric analysis of MRI. *Journal of Learning Disabilities, 24,* 141–146.

Hyperactivity: A review and research report. *Journal of Abnormal Child Psychology, 20,* 163–185.

Iaboni, F., Douglas, V. I., and Baker, A. G. (1995). Effects of reward and response costs on inhibition in ADHD children. *Journal of Abnormal Psychology, 104(1),* 232–240.

Ingersoll, B. (1995). ADD: Not just another fad. *Attention! 2(2),* 17–19.

Ionasescu, V. V., Shearby, C. H., Ionasescu, R., Neuhaus, I. M., and Werner, R. (1996). Mutations of the noncoding region of the connexin32 gene in X-linked dominant Charcot-Marie-tooth neuropathy. *Neurology, 47,* 541–544.

Ionescu, G., Kiehl, R., Ona, L., and Wichmannn-Kunz, F. (1990). Abnormal plasma catecholamines in hyperkinetic children. *Biological Psychiatry, 28,* 547–550.

Ishai, A. and Sagi, D. (1997). Visual imagery facilitates visual perception: psychophysical evidence. *Journal of Cognitive Neuroscience, 9(4),* 476–489.

Ivanusa, Z., Hécimović, H., and Demarin, V. (1997). Serotonin syndrome, neuropsychiatry. *Neuropsychology and Behavioral Neurology, 10(3),* 209–212.

Iverson, G. L., Iverson, A. M., and Barton, E. A. (1994). The children's orientation and amnesia test: Educational status is a moderator variable in tracking recovery from TBI. *Brain Injury, 8,* 685–688.

Jackson, C. W. and Bachman, D. L. (1996). Narcolepsy-related psychosis misinterpreted os schizophrenia. *Neuropsychiatry, Neuropsychology, and Behavioral Neurology, 9,* 139–140.

Jacobsen, L. K., Chappell, P., and Woolston, J. L. (1994). Bupropion and compulsive behavior. *Journal of the American Academy of Child and Adolescent Psychiatry, 33,* 143–144.

Jaffe, S. L. (1991). Intranasal abuse of prescribed methylphenidate by an alcohol and drug abusing adolescent with ADHD. *Journal of the American Academy of Child and Adolescent Psychiatry, 30,* 773–775.

Jankovic, J. (1993). Deprenyl in attention deficit associated with Tourette's syndrome. *Archives of Neurology, 50,* 286–288.

Jansen, J. H. M. and Andrews, J. S. (1994). The effects of serotonergic drugs on short-term spatial memory in rats. *Journal of Psychopharmacology, 8(3),* 157–163.

Janzen, T., Graap, K., Stephanson, S., Marshall, W., and Fitzsimmons, G. (1995). Differences in baseline EEG measures for ADD and normal achieving preadolescent males. *Biofeedback and Self Regulation, 20(1),* 65–82.

Jarrold, C. and Baddeley, A. D. (1997). Short-term memory for verbal and visuospatial information in down's syndrome. *Cognitive Neuropsychiatry, 2(2),* 101–122.

Javorsky, J. (1993). Language coding deficits in ADHD children and adolescents. *The ADHD Report, 1(2),* 8–9.

Javorsky, J. (1996). An examination of youth with ADHD and attention-deficit/hyperactivity disorder and language learning disabilities: A clinical study. *Journal of Learning Disabilities, 29(3),* 247–258.

Jeanmonod, D., Magnin, M., and Morel, A. (1966). Low-threshold calcium spike bursts in the human thalamus. *Brain, 119,* 363–375.

Jenike, M. A. and Rauch, S. L. (1994). Managing the patient with treatment-resistant obsessive-compulsive disorder: Current strategies. *Journal of Clinical Psychiatry, 55(3 Suppl.),* 11–17.

Jenkins, M., Malloy, P., Cohen, R., Salloway, S., Neeper, R., Penn, J., and Chang, K. (1996). Attentional and learning dysfunction among adults with history of childhood ADHD. *Journal of the International Neuropsychological Society, 2(3),* 185.

Jensen, P. S. (1995). Predictive validity of categorically and dimensionally scored measures of disruptive childhood behaviors: Comment. *Journal of the American Academy of Child and Adolescent Psychiatry, 34(4),* 485–487.

Jensen, P. S., Shervette, R. E. III, Xenakis, S. N., and Richters, J. (1993). Anxiety and depressive disorders in attention deficit disorder with hyperactivity: New findings. *American Journal of Psychiatry, 150,* 1203–1209.

Jerome, L. (1995). Comorbidity of central auditory processing disorder and attention-deficit hyperactivity disorder: Comment. *Journal of the American Academy of Child and Adolescent Psychiatry, 34(2),* 126–127.

Jeste, D. V., Heaton, S. C., Paulsen, J. S., Ercoli, L., Harris, J., and Heaton, R. K. (1996). Clinical and neuropsychological comparison of psychotic depression with nonpsychotic depression and schizophrenia. *American Journal of Psychiatry, 153(4),* 490–496.

Jibson, M. D. and Tandon, R. (1996). Special report: A summary of research findings on the new antipsychotic drugs. *The Psychiatry Forum, 16,* 1–6.

Johnson, C. R., Handen, B. L., Lubetsky, M. J., and Sacco, K. A. (1994). Efficacy of methylphenidate and behaviioral intervention on classroom behavior in children with ADHD and mental retardation. *Behavior Modification, 18(4),* 470–487.

Johnson, D. A., Roethig-Johnston, K., and Middleton, J. (1988). Development and evaluation of an attentional test for head injured children. 1. Information processing capacity in a normal sample. *Journal of Child Psychology and Psychiatry, 29,* 199–208.

Johnson, M. A. (1991). Cognitive differences in the attention deficit disorder differentiation of attention deficit disorder with and without hyperactivity. *Dissertation Abstracts International, 52,* 3297.

Johnson, M. J. (Ed.) (1992). *A.D.D. A Lifetime Challenge: Life Stories of Adults with Attention Deficit Disorder.* Toledo, OH: ADDult Support Network.

Johnson, S. C., Bigler, E. D., Burr, R. B., and Blatter, D. D. (1994). White matter atrophy, ventricular dilation, and intellectual functioning following traumatic brain injury. *Neuropsychology, 8,* 307–315.

Johnston, C. and Fine, S. (1993). Methods of evaluating methylphenidate in children with attention deficit hyperactivity disorder: Acceptability, satisfaction, and compliance. *Journal of Pediatric Psychology, 18,* 717–730.

Johnston, C. and Freeman, W. (1997). Attributions for child behavior in parents of children without behavior disorders and children with attention deficit-hyperactivity disorder. *Journal of Consulting and Clinical Psychology, 65(4),* 636–645.

Jones, C. B. (1993, Fall/Winter). The young and the restless: Helping the preschool child with attention deficit hyperactivity disorder. *Ch.A.D.D.er, 7(2),* 13–17.

Jones, C. B. (1994, Summer). The pleasure of their company: Building social skills. *Attention!, 1(1),* 17–20.

Jordan, B. K., Marmar, C. R., Fairbank, J. A., Schlenger, W. E., Kulka, R. A., Hough, R. L., and Weiss, D. S. (1992). Problems in families of male Vietnam vetrans with posttraumatic stress disorder. *Journal of Consulting and Clinical Psychology, 60,* 916–926.

Jordan, F. M., Cremona-Meteyard, S., and King, A. (1996). High-level linguistic disturbances subsequent to childhood closed head injury. *Brian Injury, 10,* 729–738.

Jordan, F. M. and Murdoch, B. E. (1994). Severe closed-head injury in childhood: Linguistic outcomes into adulthood. *Brain Injury, 8,* 501–508.

Journal of American Academy. 30(2), 246–256.

Journal of Clinical and Experimental Neuropsychology, 12, 247–264.

Journal of Genetic Psychology, 154(2), 177–188.

Kabadi, U. M. (1993). Subclinical hypothyroidism: Natural course of the syndrome during a prolonged follow-up study. *Archives of Internal Medicine, 153,* 957–961.

Kalivas, P. W. and Barnes, C. D. (1993). *Limbic Motor Circuits and Neuropsychiatry.* Boca Raton, FL: CRC Press.

Kaminer, Y. (1992). Clinical implications of the relationship between attention-deficit hyperactivity disorder and psychoactive substance use disorders. *American Journal Addictions, 1,* 257–264.

Kane, R. L., Gantz, N. M., and DiPino, R. K. (1996). Neuropsychological and Psychological Functioning in Chronic Fatigue Syndrome. *Journal of Clinical Neuroscience, 10,* 25–31.

Kaneko, M., Hoshino, Y., Hashimoto, S., Okano, T., and Kumashiro, H. (1993). Hypothalmic-pituitary-adrenal axis function in children with attention-deficit hyperactivity disorder. *Journal of Autism and Developmental Disorders, 23(1)*, 59–65.

Kant, R., Smith-Seemiller, L., Issac, G., and Duffy, J. (1997). Tc-HMPAO SPECT in persistent post-concussion syndrome after mild head injury: comparison with MRI/ CT. *Brain Injury, 11(2)*, 115–124.

Kaplan, B. J., McNicol, R. A., and Conte, R. A. (1987). Sleep disturbance in preschool-aged hyperactive and nonhyperactive children. *Pediatrics, 80(6)*, 839–844.

Kaplan, C. P. and Shachter, E. (1991). Adults with undiagnosed learning disabilities: Practice considerations. *Families in Society, 72(4)*, 195–201.

Kapur, S., Meyer, J., Wilson, A. A., Houle, S., et al. (1994). Modulation of cortical neuronal activity by a serotonergic agent. A PET study in humans. *Brain Research, 646(2)*, 292–294.

Kareken, D. A., Oberg, P. J., and Gur, R. C. (1966). Proactive inhibition and semantic organization: Relationship with verbal memory in patients with schizophrenia. *Journal of the International Neuropsychological Society, 2*, 486–493.

Karper, L. P., Freeman, G. K., Grillon, C., Morgan, C. A., Charney, D. S., and Krystal, J. H. (1996). Preliminary evidence of an association between sensorimotor gating and distractibility in psychosis. *Journal of Neuropsychiatry, 8(1)*, 60–66.

Kaste, A. M. and Sharna, S. (1996). Patients with traumatic brain injury referred to a rehabilitation and re-employment programme: social and professional outcome for 508 Finnish patients 5 or more years after injury. *Brain Injury, 10*, 883–899.

Kasper, S. (1997). Efficacy of antidepressants in the treatment of severe depression: The place of mirtazapine. *Journal of Clinical Psychopharmacology,17(2)*, (Suppl. 1), 19S–28S.

Kataria, S., Hall, C. W., Wong, M. M., and Keys, G. F. (1992). Learning styles of LD and NLD ADHD children. *Journal of Clinical Psychology, 48*, 371–378.

Katon, W., Sheehan, D. V., and Uhde, T. W. (1992). Panic disorder: A treatable problem. *Patient Care*, 81–90.

Katz, M. (1994, May). From challenged childhood to achieving adulthood: Studies in resilience. *Chadder Box*, 8–11.

Keck, P. E., Jr., McElroy, S. I., Vuckovic, A., and Friedman, L. M. (1992). Combined valproate and carbamazepine treatment of bipolar disorder. *The Journal of Neuropsychiatry and Clinical Neurosciences, 4*, 319–322.

Keck, P. E., Jr. and McElroy, S. L. (1996). Outcome in the pharmacologic treatment of bipolar disorder. *Journal of Clinical Psychopharmacology, 16(2)*, (Suppl. 1), 15S–23S.

Keenan, K. and Shaw, D. (1997). Developmental and Social Influences on young girl's early problem behavior. *Psychological Bulletin, 1*, 95–113.

Kelly, M. D. (1995). Neuropsychological assessment of children with hearing impairment on trail making tactual performance and category test. *Assessment, 2(4)*, 305–312.

Kelly, K. and Ramundo, P. (1993). *You mean I'm not lazy, stupid, or crazy?! A self-help book for adults with attention deficit disorder,* Cincinnati: Tyrell and Jerem Press.

Kendall-Tackett, K., Williams, L. M., and Finkelhor, D. (1993). Impact of sexual abuse on children: A review and synthesis of recent empirical studies. *Psychological Bulletin, 113,* 164–180.

Kendler, K. S., Walters, E. E., Truett, K. R., Heath, A. C., Neale, M. C., Martin, N. G., and Eaves, L. J. (1994). Sources of individual differences in depressive symptoms: Analysis of two samples of twins and their families. *American Journal of Psychiatry, 151,* 1605–1614.

Kennedy, P., Terdal, L., and Fusetti, L. (1993). *The Hyperactive Child Book.* New York: St. Martin's Press.

Kessali, M., Zemmouri, R., Guilbot, A., Maisonobe, T., Brice, A., LeGuern, E., and Grid, D. (1997). *Neurology, 48,* 867–873.

Kiernan, J. A. and Hudson, A. J. (1994). Frontal lobe atrophy in motor neuron diseases. *Brain, 117,* 747–757.

Kim, H. (1994). Distributions of hemispheric asymmetry in left-handers and right-handers: Data from perceptual asymmetry studies. *Neuropsychology, 8,* 148–159.

Kinsbourne, M. (1974). Lateral interactions in the brain. In M. Kinsbourne and W. L. Smith (Eds.), *Hemispheric Disconnection and Cerebral Function.* Springfield, MA: Thomas, 239–259.

Kinsbourne, M. (1994). Neuropsychology of attention. In Zaidel, D. W., Ed., *Neuropsychology,* San Diego, Academic Press, 105–123.

Kirby, M. Y. and Long, C. J. (1996). Minor head injury: Attempts at clarifying the confusion. *Brain Injury, 10(3),* 159–186.

Klein, R. G. and Mannuzza, S. (1991). Long-term outcome of hyperactive children: A review [Special Section: Longitudinal research]. *Journal of the American Academy of Child and Adolescent Psychiatry, 30,* 383–387.

Klorman, R., Brumashin, J. T., Fitzpatrick, P. A., Borgstedt, A. D. and Strauss, J. (1994). Clinical and cognitive effects of methylphenidate on children with attention deficit disorder as a funtion of aggression/oppositionality and age. *Journal of Abnormal Psychology, 103(2),* 206–221.

Klove, H., Troland, K., and Ellertsen, B. (1995). Children at risk: Diagnostic and treatment consideration. *Journal of the International Neuropsychological Society, 1(4),* 321.

Knight, R. T. (1991). Evoked potential studies of attentional capacity in human frontal lobe lesions. *Frontal Lobe Function and Dysfunction.* New York: Oxford University Press, 139–156.

Knight, R. T. (1997). Distributed cortical network for visual attention. *Journal of Cognitive Neuroscience, 9(1),* 75–91.

Knivsberg, A.-M. (1997). Urine patterns, peptide levels and IgA/lgG antibodies to food proteins in children with dyslexia. *Pediatric Rehabilitation, 1(1),* 25–23.

Koechlin, E. and Burnod, Y. (1996). Dual population coding in the neocortex: A model of interaction between representation and attention in the visual cortex. *Journal of Cognitive Neuroscience, 8(4),* 353–370.

Kolata, G. (1990). Advance in hyperactivity research. *The New York Times*, Thursday, November 15.

Koob, G. F. and Nestler, E. J. (1997). The neurobiology of drug addiction. *Journal of Neuropsychiatry, 9(3)*, 482–497.

Kopelowicz, A., Liberman, R. P., Mintz, J., and Zarate, R., (1997). Comparison of efficacy of social skills training for deficit and nondeficit negative symptoms in schizophrenia. *American Journal of Psychiatry, 154(3)*, 424–425.

Korkman, M. and Pesonen, A. E. (1994). A comparison of neuropsychological test profiles of chldren with attention deficit-hyperactivity disorder and/or learning disorder. *Journal of Learning Disabilities, 27(6)*, 383–392.

Kosslyn, S. M., Anderson, A. K., Hillger, L. A., and Hamilton, S. E. (1994). Hemispheric differences in sizes of receptive fields or attentional biases? *Neuropsychology, 8*, 139–147.

Kosslyn, S. M., Thompson, W. L., Kim, I. J., Rauch, S. L., and Alpert, N. M. (1996). Individual differences in cerebral blood flow in area 17 predict the time to evaluate visualized letters. *Journal of Cognitive Neuroscience, 8(1)*, 78–82.

Kranzler, H. R. and Anton, R. F. (1994). Implications of recent neuropsychopharmacologic research for understanding the etiology and development of alcoholism. *Journal of Consulting and Clinical Psychology, 62(6)*, 1116–1126.

Kraus, M. F. and Maki, P. (1977). The combined use of amantadine and L-dopa/carbidopa in the treatment of chronic brain injury. *Brain Injury, 11(6)*, 455–460.

Kravets, M. (1994, Summer). Choosing the best college when you have ADD. *Attention! 1(1)*, 22–25.

Kujala, P., Portin, R., Revonsuo, A., and Ruutiainen, J. (1994). Automatic and controlled information processing in multiple sclerosis. *Brain, 117*, 1115–1126.

Kujala, P., Portin, R., and Ruutiainen, J. (1997). The progress of cognitive decline in multiple sclerosis: A controlled 3-year follow-up. *Brain, 120*, 289–297.

Kulynych, J. J., Vladar, K., Jones, D. W., and Weinberger, D. R. (1994). Gender differences in the normal lateralization of the supratemporal cortex: MRI surface-rendering morphometry of heschl's gyrus and the planum temporale. *Cortex, 4(2)*, 107–118.

Kuperman, S., Johnson, B., Arndt, S., Lindgreen, S. et al. (1996). Quantitative EEG differences in a nonclinical sample of children with ADHD and undifferentiated ADD. *Journal of the American Academy of Child and Adolescent Psychiatry, 35(8)*, 1009–1017.

Kuppinger, H. E., Harrington, A., Kaczmerek, H. J., Panos, J. J., and Steinpreis, R. E. (1996). The effects of phencyclidine and amphetamine on social behavior in tether-restrained and freely moving rats. *Experimental and Clinical Psychopharmacology, 4(1)*, 77–81.

Kurlan, Roger, Daragjati, C., Como, P. G., McDermott, M., Trinidad, K. S., Roddy, S., Brower, C. A., and Robertson, M. M., (1996). Nonobscene complex socially inappropriate behavior in Tourette's syndrome. *The Journal of Neuropsychiatry and Clinical Neurosciences, 8*, 311–317.

Kusche, C. A., Cook, E. T., and Greenberg, M. T. (1993). Neuropsychological and cognitive functioning in children with anxiety, externalizing, and comorbid psychopathology. *Journal of Clinical Child Psychology, 22,* 172–195.

Kutcher, S. and Garner, D. (1996). Buspirone for generalized anxiety disorder in children and adolescents. *Child & Adolescent Psychopharmacology News, 1,* 1–2.

Kutja, K. S., Voeller, R., Bogoian, G., Geffken, C., Wilson, P., Edge, M., Garofalakis, P., and Mutch, J. (1997). Comorbidity of ADHD and dyslexia in adults. ANPA Abstracts *Journal of Neuropsychiatry and Clinical Neurosciences, 9(1),* 149, P64.

Kwasman, A., Tinsley, B. J., and Lepper, H. S. (1995). Pediatricians' knowledge and attitudes concerning diagnosis and treatment of attention deficit and hyperactivity disorders: A national survey approach. *Archives of Pediatric Adolescent Medicine, 149(11),* 1211–1216.

Làdavas, E., Farne, A., Carletti, M., and Zeloni, G. (1994). Neglect determined by the relative location of responses. *Brain, 117,* 705–714.

Làdavas, E., Zeloni, G., Zaccara, G., and Fangemi, P. (1997). Eye movements and orienting of attention in patients with visual neglect. *Journal of Cognitive Neuroscience, 9(1),* 67–74.

Lahey, B. B., Pelham, W. E., Schaughency, E. A., Atkins, M. S., Murphy, H. A., Hynd, G. W., Russo, M., Hartdagen, S., and Lorys-Vernon, A. (1988). Dimensions and types of attention deficit disorder. *Journal of American Academy of Child and Adolescent Psychiatry, 27,* 330–335.

Lahey, B. B. and Carlson, C. L. (1991). Validity of the diagnostic category of attention deficit disorder without hyperactivity: A review of the literature. *Journal of Learning Disabilities, 24(2),* 110–120.

Lahey, B. B., Hart, E. L., Pliszka, S., Applegate, B., and McBurnett, K. (1993). Neuropsychological correlates of conduct disorder: A rationale and a review of research. *Journal of Clinical Child Psychology, 22(2),* 141–153.

Lahey, B. B., Applegate, B., Barkley, R. A., Garfinkel, B., McBurnett, K., Kerdyk, L., Greenhill, L., Hynd, G. W., Frick, P. J., Newcorn, J., Biedreman, J., Ollendick, T., Hart, E. L., Perez, D., Waldman, I., and Shaffer, D. (1994a). DSM-IV field trials for oppositional defiant disorder and conduct disorder in children and adolescents. *American Journal of Psychiatry, 151,* 1163–1171.

Lahey, B. B., Applegate, B., McBurnett, K., Biederman, J., Greenhill, L., Hynd, G. W., Barkley, R. A., Newcorn, J., Jensen, P., Richters, J., Garfinkel, B., Kerdyk, L., Frick, P. J., Ollendick, T., Perez, D., Hart, E. L., Waldman, I., and Shaffer, D. (1994b). DSM-IV field trials for attention deficit hyperactivity disorder in children and adolescents. *American Journal of Psychiatry, 151,* 1673–1685.

Landau, S. and Moore, L. A. (1991). Social skill deficits in children with attention-deficit hyperactivity disorder. *School Psychology Review, 20,* 235–251.

Langdon, D. W. and Warrington, E. K. (1997). The abstraction of numerical relations: A role for the right hemisphere in arithmetic? *Journal of the International Neuropsychological Society, 3,* 260–268.

Latham, P. H., Latham, J. D., and Latham, P. S. (1995, Spring). Succeeding in the workplace with ADD. *Attention! 1(4),* 40–43.

Lavenstein, B. L. and Fore, C. (1997). Modification of the "on off" effect induced by stimulants in patients with ADHD utilizing propranolol. *Neurology, 48(3, Suppl),* P05.003.

Lavoie, M. E. and Charlebois, P. (1994). The discriminant validity of the Stroop Color and Word Test: Toward a cost-effective strategy to distinguish subgroups of disruptive preadolescents. *Psychology in the Schools, 31(2),* 98–107.

Laws, K. R., McKenna, P. J., and McCarthy, R. A. (1997). Reconsidering the gospel according to group studies: A neuropsychological case study approach to schizophrenia. *Cognitive Neuropsychiatry, 1(4),* 319–343.

Lazar, M. F. and Menaldino, S. (1995). Cognitive outcome and behavioral adjustment in children following traumatic brain injury: A developmental perspective. *Journal of Head Trauma Rehabilitation, 10(5),* 55–63.

Leach, J. P. and Bordie, M. J. (1995). Lamotrigine, clinical use. In Levy, R. H., Mattson, R. H., and Meldrum, B. S., Eds., *Antiepileptic Drugs,* 4th ed., New York, Raven Press, 889–896.

Leach, M. J., Lees, G., and Riddall, D. R. (1995). Lamotrigine, mechanisms of action. In Levy, R. H., Mattson, R. H., and Meldrum, B. S., Eds., *Antiepileptic Drugs,* 4th ed., New York, Raven Press, 861–870.

Leafhead, K. M., Young, A. W. (1996). Delusions demand attention. *Cognitive Neuropsychiatry, 1,* 5–16.

Leathem, J. M. and Body, C. M. (1997). Neuropsychological sequelae of head injury in a New Zealand adolescent sample. *Brain Injury, 11(8),* 565–575.

Leckman, J. F., Goodman, W., North, W. G., Chappell, P. B. (1994). Elevated cerebrospinal fluid levels of oxytocin in obsessive compulsive disorder comparison with tourette's syndrome and healthy controls. *Archives of General Psychiatry, 51(10),* 782–792.

Lee, G. P., Loring, D. W., Dahl, J. L., and Meador, K. J. (1993). Hemispheric specialization for emotional expression. *Neuropsychiatry, Neuropsychology, and Behavioral Neurology, 6,* 143–148.

Leibovitch, E. R. (1993, March). Thyroid tests: Help on sorting them out. *Modern Medicine, 61,* 58–69.

Lekwuwa, G. U. and Barnes, G. R. (1996). Cerebral control of eye movements I. The relationship between cerebral lesion sites and smooth pursuit deficits. *Brain, 119,* 473–490.

Leonard, C. (1995). Asymmetry of the human brain: Handedness and dyslexia. In *Syllabus for Neurobiology of Behavior and Cognition.* Chicago: North Western University Medical School.

Leonard, H. L., Topol, D., Bukstein, O., Hindmarsh, D. et al. (1994). Clonazepam as an augmenting agent in the treatment of childhood-onset obsessive-compulsive disorder. *Journal of the American Academy of Child and Adolescent Psychiatry, 33,* 792–794.

Leone, M. et al. (1997). Alcohol use is a risk factor for a first generalized tonic-clonic seizure. *Neurology, 48,* 614–620.

Levin, H. and Kraus, M. F. (1994). The frontal lobes and traumatic brain injury. *Journal of Neuropsychiatry and Clinical Neurosciences, 6,* 443–454.

Levin, H. S., Mendelsohn, D., Lilly, M. A., Fletcher, J. M., Culhane, K. A., Chapman, S. B., Harward, H., Kusnerik, L., Bruce, D., and Eisenberg, H. M. (1994). Tower of London performance in relation to magnetic resonance imaging following closed head injury in children. *Neuropsychology, 8,* 171–179.

Levine, B. K. and Pincus, H. (1996). Conduct disorder in attention deficit hyperactivity boys. *Neurology, 46(2, Suppl.),* A126.

Levinson, H. N. (1990). *Total Concentration: How to Understand Attention Deficit Disorders with Treatment Guidelines for You and Your Doctor.* New York: M. Evans and Company, Inc.

Levinson, H. N. (1991). Dramatic favorable responses of children with learning disabilities or dyslexia and attention deficit disorder to antimotion sickness medications: Four case reports. *Perceptual and Motor Skills, 73,* 723–738.

Levitt, J. L., O'Donnell, B. F., McCarley, R. W., Nestor, P. G., and Shenton, M. E. (1996). Correlation's of premorbid adjustment in schizophrenia with auditory event-related potential and neuropsychological abnormalities. *American Journal of Psychiatry, 153,* 1347–1349.

Levy, F. and Hobbes, G. (1988). The action of stimulant medication in attention deficit disorder with hyperactivity: Dopaminergic noradrenexgix of both? *Journal American Academy Child Adolescent Psychiatry, 27,* 802–805.

Levy, F. and Hobbes, G. (1989). Reading, spelling and vigilance in attention deficit and conduct disorder. *Journal of Abnormal Child Psychology, 17,* 291–298.

Lewine, R., Hudgins, P., Risch, S. C., and Walker, E. F. (1993). Lowered attention capacity in young, medically healthy men with magnetic resonance brain hyperintensity signals. *Neuropsychiatry, Neuropsychology, and Behavioral Neurology, 6(1),* 38–42.

Lezak, M. D. (1982). Tinker toy test: The problem of assessing executive functions. *International Journal of Psychology, 17,* 281–297.

Libon, D. J., Glosser, G., Malamut, B. L., Kaplan, E., Goldberg, E., Swenson, R., and Sands, L. P. (1994). Age executive functions, and visuospatial functioning in healthy older adults. *Neuropsychology, 8,* 38–43.

Lichter, D. G., Diegelman, N. M., and Jackson, L. A. (1997). The relationship between Tourette's syndrome and "childhood schizophrenia", ANPA Abstracts, *Journal of Neuropsychiatry and Clinical Neurosciences, 9(1),* 136.

Lie, N. (1992). Follow-ups of children with attention deficit hyperactivity disorder (ADHD): Review of literature. *Acta Psychiatrica Scandinavica, 85(368, Suppl.),* 40.

Lilienfeld, S. O. and Weldman, I. D. (1990). The relation between childhood attention-deficit hyperactivity disorder and adult antisocial behavior reexamined: The problem of hetergeneity. *Clinical Psychology Review, 10,* 699–725.

Lim, K. O., Tew, W., Kushner, M., Chow, K., Matsumoto, B., and DeLisi, L. E. (1996). Cortical gray matter volume deficit in patients with first-episode schizophrenia. *American Journal of Psychiatry, 153(12),* 1548–1553.

Lin, K. C., Cermack, S. A., Kinsbourne, M., and Trombly, C. A. (1996). Effects of left-sided movements on line bisection in unilateral neglect. *Journal of the International Neuropsychological Society, 2,* 404–411.

Lin, K. C., Tew, W., Kushner, M., Chow, K., Matsumoto, B., and DeLisi, L. E. (1996). Cortical gray matter volume deficit in patients with first-episode schizophrenia. *American Journal of Psychiatry, 153,* 1548–1553.

Liotti, M., Laberge, D., Jerabek, P. A., Martin, C. C., and Fox, P. T. (1995). A pet study of focused visual attention to letter shapes. *Human Brain Mapping, (Suppl. 1),* Abst., 271.

Lloyd, L. F. and Cuvo, A. J. (1994). Maintenance and generalization of behaviours after treatment of persons with traumatic brain injury. *Brain Injury, 8,* 529–540.

Lochman, J. E., Dunn, S. E., and Klimes-Dougan, B. (1993). An intervention and consultation model from a social cognitive perspective: A description of the anger coping program. *School Psychology Review, 33,* 458–468.

Loiseau, P. and Duché (1995). Carbamazepine, Clinical Use, In 4th ed., Levy, R. H., Mattson, R. H., and Meldrum, B. S., Eds., *Antiepileptic Drugs,* New York, Raven Press, 555–556.

Lombroso, P. J., Pauls, D. L., and Leckman, J. F. (1994). Genetic mechanisms in childhood psychiatric disorders. *Journal of the American Academy of Child and Adolescent Psychiatry, 33(7),* 921–938.

Lonigan, C. J., Carey, M. P., and Finch, A. J., Jr. (1994). Anxiety and depression in children and adolescents: Negative affectivity and the utility of self-reports. *Journal of Consulting and Clinical Psychology, 62,* 1000–1008.

Lorys, A. R., Hynd, G. W., and Lahey, B. (1990). Do neurocognitive measures differentiate attention deficit disorder (ADD) with and without hyperactivity? *Archives of Clinical Neuropsychology, 5,* 119–135.

Lou, H. C. (1991). Cerebral glucose metabolism in hyperactivity. *New England Journal of Medicine, 324,* 1216.

Lubar, J. F. (1991). Discourse on the development of EEG diagnostics and biofeedback for attention-deficit/hyperactivity disorders. *Biofeedback and Self-Regulation, 16(3),* 201–225.

Lubar, J. F., Swartwood, M. O., Swartwood, J. N., and O'Donnell, P. H. (1995). Evaluation of the effectiveness of EEG neurofeedback training for ADHD in a clinical setting as measured by changes in TOVA scores, behavioral ratings and WISC-R performance. *Biofeedback and Self-Regulation, 20,* 83–99.

Lubinski, R., Moscato, B. S., and Willer, B. S. (1997). Prevalence of speaking and hearing disabilities among adults with traumatic brain injury from a national household survey. *Brain Injury, 11(2),* 103–114.

Lubow, R. E. and Gewirtz, J. C. (1995). Latent inhibition in humans: Data, theory, and implications for schizophrenia. *Psychological Bulletin, 117(1),* 87–103.

Lubow, R. E. and Josman, Z. E. (1993). Latent inhibition deficits in hyperactive children. *Journal of Child Psychology and Psychiatry, 34(6),* 959–973.

Luciana, M. and Collins, P. F. (1997). Dopaminergic modulation of working memory for spatial but not object cues in normal humans. *Journal of Cognitive Neuroscience, 9(3),* 330–347.

Lufi, D. and Parish-Plass, J. (1995). Personality assessment of children wuth attention deficit hyperactivity disorder. *Journal of Clinical Psychology, 51(1),* 94–99.

Lyketsos, C. G., Baker, L., Warren, A., Steele, C. et al. (1997). Depression, delusions and hallucinations in alzehiemer's disease: No relationship to apoliproptein E. Geneotype. *The Journal of Neuropsychiatry and Clinical Neurosciences, 9(1),* 64–67.

Lynch, W. J., (1995). Achievement testing in traumatic brain injury: Two new approaches. *Journal Head Trauma Rehabilitation, 10(5),* 95–98.

Maag, J. W. and Reid, R. (1994). Attention-deficit hyperactivity disorder: A functional approach to assessment and treatment. *Behavioral Disorders, 20(1),* 5–23.

MacLeod, D. and Prior, M. (1996). Attention deficits in adolescents with ADHD and other clinical groups. *Child Neuropsychology, 2,* 1–10.

Maddocks, D. and Saling, M. (1996). Neuropsychological deficits following concussion. *Brain Injury, 10(2),* 99–103.

Madden, D. J. and Plude, D. J. (1993). *Selective Preservation of Selective Attention in Adult Information Processing: Limits on Loss.* Cerella, J., Rybash, J., Hoyer, W., and Commons, M. L. (Eds.). San Diego, CA: Academic Press, Inc.

Maddrey, A. M., Cullum, C. M., Weiner, M. F., and Filey, C. M. (1996). Premorbid intelligence estimation and level of dementia in Alzheimer's disease. *Journal of the International Neuropsychological Society, 2,* 551–555.

Maes, M., Bosmans, E., Meltzer, H. Y., Scharpe, S., and Suy, E. (1993). Interleukin-1B: A putative mediator of HPA axis hyperactivity in major depression. *American Journal of Psychiatry, 150,* 1189–1193.

Magee, R., Maier, D., and Reesal, R. T. (1992). Adult attention deficit hyperactivity disorder and desipramine. *Canadian Journal of Psychiatry, 37(2),* 148–149.

Malinosky-Rummell, R. and Hansen, D. J. (1993). Long-term consequences of childhood physical abuse. *Psychological Bulletin, 114,* 68–79.

Malone, M. A., Couitis, J., Kershner, J. R., and Logan, W. J. (1994). Right hemisphere dysfunction and methylphenidate effects in children with attention-deficit/hyperactivity disorder. *Journal of Child and Adolescent Psychopharmacology, 4(4),* 245–253.

Malone, M. A., Kershner, J. R., and Swanson, J. M. (1994). Hemispheric processing and methylphenidate effects in attention-deficit hyperactivity disorder. *Journal of Child Neurology, 9(2),* 181–189.

Manford, M., Fish, D. R., and Shorvon, S. D. (1996). An analysis of clinical seizure patterns and their localizing value in frontal and temporal lobe epilepsies. *Brain, 119(1),* 17–40.

Mann, C. A. (1991). Topographic brain mapping as a diagnostic of attention deficit hyperactivity disorder. *Dissertation Abstracts International, 52(3-B),* 1769–1770.

Mandoki, M. (1994). Buspirone treatment of traumatic brain injury in a child who is highly sensitive to adverse effects of psychotropic medications. *Journal of Child and Adolescent Psychopharmacology, 4(2),* 129–139.

Mannuzza, S., Klein, R. G., Banagura, N., Konig, P. H., and Shenker, R. (1988). Hyperactive boys almost grown up: II. Status of subjects without a mental disorder. *Archives of General Psychiatry, 45,* 13–18.

Mannuzza, S., Klein, R. G., Bessler, A., Malloy, P., LaPadula, M. (1993). Adult outcome of hyperactive boys educational achievement, occupational rank and psychiatric status. *Archives General Psychiatry, 50,* 565–576.

Manoach, D. S., Sandson, T. A., and Weintraub, S. (1995). The developmental social-emotional processing disorder is associated with right hemisphere abnormalities. *Neuropsychiatry, Neuropsychology and Behavioral Neurology, 8(2),* 99–105.

Mapping of SPECT regional cerebral perfusion abnormalities in obsessive-compulsive disorder. *Human Brain Mapping, 1(4),* 237–248.

Marangell, L. B., Ketter, T. A., George, M. S., Pazzaglia, P. J., Callahan, A. M., Parekh, P., Andreason, P. J., Horwitz, B., Herscovitch, P., and Post, R. M. (1997). Inverse relationship of peripheral thyrotropin-stimulating hormone levels to brain activity in mood disorders. *American Journal of Psychiatry, 154(2),* 224–230.

March, J. S., Wells, K., and Conners, C. K. (1995). Attention-deficit/hyperactivity disorder. I. Assessment and diagnosis. *Journal of Practical Psychiatry and Behavioral Health, 1(4),* 219–228.

March, J. S., Wells, K., and Conners, C. K. (1995). Attention-deficit/hyperactivity disorder. II. Treatment strategies. *Journal of Practical Psychiatry and Behavioral Health, 2(1),* 23–32.

Mardell-Czudmowski, C. (1995). Performance of Asian and White children on the K-ABC: Understanding information processing differences. *Assessment, 2(1),* 19–29.

Marshall, V. G., Longwell, L., Goldstein, M. J., and Swanson, J. M. (1990). Family factors associated with aggressive symptomatology in boys with attention deficit hyperactivity disorder: A research note. *Journal of Child Psychology Psychiatry, 31(4),* 629–636.

Martin, R. C. and Romani, C. (1994). Verbal working memory and sentence comprehension: A multiple-components view. *Neuropsychology, 8,* 506–523.

Masamitsu, S., Yamanaka, T., and Furuya, T. (1993). Attention state in electrodermal activity during auditory stimulation of children with attention-deficit hyperactivity disorder. *Perceptual and Motor Skills, 77,* 331–338.

Mateer, C. A. and Mapou, R. L. (1996). Understanding, evaluating, and managing attention disorders following traumatic brain injury. *Journal of Head Trauma Rehabilitation, 11,* 1–16.

Mateer, C. M., Sohlberg, N. M., and Youngman, P. K. (1990). The management of acquired attention and memory deficits. In Wood, R. L. I. and Fussey, I., *Cognitive Rehabilitation in Perspective,* New York: Taylor & Francis, pp. 68–95.

Matochik, J. A., Liebenauer, L. L., King, A. C., and Szymanski, H. V. (1994). Cerebral glucose metabolism in adults with attention deficit hyperactivity disorder after chronic stimulant treatment. *American Journal of Psychiatry, 151,* 658–664.

Mayberg, H. S. (1994). Frontal lobe dysfunction in secondary depression. *Journal of Neuropsychiatry and Clinical Neurosciences, 6,* 428–442.

Mayes, S. D., Crites, D. L., Bixler, E. O., Humphrey, F. J. et al. (1994). Methylphenidate and ADHD: Influence of age, IQ and neurodevelopmental status. *Developmental Medicine and Child Neurology, 36(12),* 1099–1107.

Max, J. E., Lindgren, S. D., Robin, D. A., Smith, W. L., Jr., Sato, Y., Mattheis, P. J., Castillo, C. S., and Stierwalt, J. A. G. (1997). Traumatic brain injury in children and adolescents: psychiatric disorders in the second three months. ANPA Abstracts. *Journal of Neuropsychiatry and Clinical Neurosciences, 9(1),* 137.

Max, J. P., Thystere, P., Chapleur-Chateau, M., and Buriet, A. (1994). Hypothalmic neuropeptides could mediate the anorectic effects of fenfluramine. *Neuroreport an International Journal for the Rapid Communications of Research in Neuroscience, 5(15)*, 1925–1929.

Mayes, S. D., Crites, D. L., Bixler, E. O., Humphrey, F. J. et al. (1994). Methylphenidate and ADHD: Influence of age, IQ and neurodevelopmental status.

McBurnett, K., Harris, S. M., Swanson, J. M., Pfiffner, L. J., Tamm, L., and Freeland, D. (1993). Neuropsychological and psychophysiological differentiation of inattention/overactivity and aggression/defiance symptom groups. *Journal of Clinical Child Psychology, 22(2)*, 165–171.

McCarney, S. B. (1989). *Attention Deficit Disorders Evaluation Scale Home Version.* Columbia, MO: Hawthorne Educational Services.

McCarthey, C., Kirk, U., and Goff, E. (1996). Contributions of visual-spatial functions to arithmetic skill in school-aged children. *Journal of the International Neuropsychological Society, 2(3)*, 185.

McCarty, M. F. (1993). Homologous physiological effects of phenformin and chromium picolinate. *Medical Hypotheses, 41(4)*, 316–324.

McConaughy, S. H. and Achenbach, T. M. (1988). *Practical Guide for the Child Behavior Checklist and Related Materials.* Burlington, VT: University of Vermont Department of Psychiatry.

McConaughy, S. H. and Skiba, R. J. (1993). Comorbidity of externalizing and internalizing problems. *School Psychology Review, 22*, 421–436.

McDermott, S. P., Spencer, T., and Wilens, T. E. (1995). For adults with ADD: Common sense about adult AD/HD. *Attention, 2(2)*, 36–41.

McGee, R. and Feehan, M. (1991). Are girls with problems of attention underrecognized? *Journal of Psychopathology and Behavioral Assessment, 13(3)*, 187–198.

McGee, R., Stanton, W. R., and Sears, M. R. (1993). Allergic disorders and attention deficit disorders in children. *Journal of Abnormal Child Psychology, 21(1)*, 79–87.

McGlinchey-Berroth, R., Bullis, D. P., Milberg, W. P., Verfaellie, M., Alexander, M., and D'Esposito, M. (1996). Assessment of neglect reveals dissociable behavior but not neuroanatomical subtypes. *Journal of the International Neuropsychological Society, 2*, 441–451.

McGlone, J., Losier, B. J., and Black, S. W. (1997). Are there sex differences in hemispatial visual neglect after unilatral stroke? *Neuropsychiatry, Neuropsychology, and Behavioral Neurology, 10(2)*, 125–134.

McGough J. J. and Cantwell, D. P. (1995, Winter). Current trends in the medication management of ADD. *Attention, 1(3)*, 16–23.

McGrath, J. (1997). Cognitive impairment associated with post-traumatic stress disorder and minor head injury: A case report. *Neuropsychological Rehabilitation, 7(3)*, 231–239.

McHugh, P. R. (1993). Multiple personality disorder. *The Harvard Mental Health Letter, 10(3)*, 4–6.

McKeith, I. G., Galasko, D. et al. (1996). Consensus guidelines for the clinical and pathologic diagnosis of dementia with Lewy bodies (DLB); Report of the consortium on DLB international workshop. *Neurology, 47*, 1113–1124.

McLachlan, R. S., Levin, S., and Blume, W. T. (1996). Treatment of Rasmussen's syndrome with ganciclovir. *Neurology, 47,* 925–928.

McLean, A., Cardenas, D., Haselkorn, J., and Peters, M. (1993). Cognitive psychopharmacology. *Neurorehabilitation, 3,* 1–14.

McLean, D. E., Kaitz, E. S., Keenan, C. J., Dabney, K., Cawley, M. F., and Alexander, M. A. (1995). Medical and surgical complications of pediatric brain injury. *Journal of Head Trauma Rehabilitation, 10(5),* 1–12.

McMahon, R. J. (1994). Diagnosis, assessment, and treatment of externalizing problems in children: The role of longitudinal data. *Journal of Consulting and Clinical Psychology, 62,* 901–917.

McMillan, T. M. (1996). Post-traumatic stress disorder following minor and severe closed head injury; 10 sing cases. *Brain Injury, 10,* 749–758.

McPherson, L. and Harvey, P. D. (1996). Discourse connectedness in manic and schizophrenic patients: associations with derailment and other clinical thought disorders. *Cognitive Neuropsychiatry, 1,* 41–53.

Meck, W. H. (1996). Clonidine-induced antagonism of norepinephrine modulates the attentional processes involved in peak-interval timing. *Experimental and Clinical Psychopharmacology, 4(1),* 82–92.

Mega, M. S. and Cummings, J. L. (1994). Frontal-subcortical circuits and neuropsychiatric disorders. *Journal of Neuropsychiatry and Clinical Neurosciences, 6,* 358–370.

Mega, M. S., Cummings, J. L., Salloway, S., and Malloy, P. (1997). The limbic system: An anatomic, phylogenetic, and clinical perspective. *Journal of Neuropsychiatry and Clinical Neurosciences, 9(3),* 315–330.

Mehta, Z. and Newcombe, F. (1996). Dissociable contributions of the two cerebral hemispheres to judgments of line orientation. *Journal of the International Neuropsychological Society, 2,* 335–339.

Melnyk, L. and Das, J. P. (1992). Measurement of attention deficit: Correspondence between rating scales and tests of sustained and selective attention. *American Journal on Mental Retardation, 96,* 599–606.

Meltzer, C. C., Zubieta, J. K., Brandt, J., Tune, L. E., Mayberg, H. S., and Frost, J. J., (1996). Regional hypometabolism in alzeimer's disease as measured by positron emission tomography after correction for effects of partial volume averaging. *Neurology, 47,* 454–461.

Mendez, M. F., Cherrier, M. M., and Cymerman, J. S. (1997). Hemispatial neglect on visual search tasks in Alzheimer's disease, *Neuropsychiatry, Neuropsychology and Behavioral Neurology, 10(3),* 203–208.

Mendez, M. F., Cherrier, M., Perryman, K. M., Pachana, N., Miller, B. L., and Cummings, J. L. (1996). Frontotemporal dementia versus Alzheimer's disease: Differential cognitive feature. *Neurology, 47,* 1189–1194.

Mendez, M. F., Engebrit, B., Doss, R., Miller, B. L., and Cummings, J. L. (1997). Clinical characteristics of epileptic aura with cognitive manifestations. ANPA Abstracts, *Journal of Neuropsychiatry and Clinical Neurosciences, 9(1),* 145, P51.

Mennemeier, M., Chatterjee, A., and Heilman, K. M. (1994). A comparison of the influences of body and enviroment centred reference frames on neglect. *Brain, 117,* 1013–1021.

Merlet, I., Garcia-Larrea, L., Gregoire, M. C., Lavenne, F., and Mauguiere, F. (1996). Source Propagation of interictal spikes in temporal lobe epilepsy. *Brain, 119*, 377–392.

Mertz, W. (1993). Chromium in human nutrition: A review. *Journal of Nutrition, 123(4)*, 626–634.

Mesulam, M.-M. (1981). A cortical network for directed attention and unilateral neglect [Review]. *Annals of Neurology, 10*, 309–25.

Mesulam, M.-M. (1985a). *Principles of Behavioral Neurology*. Philadelphia, PA: F. A. Davis Company.

Mesulam, M.-M. (1995b). Association cortex and networks. *Syllabus for Neurobiology of Behavior and Cognition*. Chicago: North Western University Medical School.

Mesulam, M.-M. (1995d). Limbic system and neurology of memory. *Syllabus for Neurobiology of Behavior and Cognition*. Chicago: North Western University Medical School.

Mesulam, M.-M. (Dec. 12–16, 1995). Right hemisphere specializations and spatial neglect. *Syllabus for Neurobiology of Behavior and Cognition*. Chicago: North Western University Medical School.

Michael and Hall (1994). 'Blunts' are more potent, more dangerous. *Psychopharmacology Update, 5(12)*, 6.

Milberger, S., Biederman, J., Faraone, S. V., Murphy, J., and Tsuang, M. T. (1995). Attention deficit hyperactivity disorder and comorbid disorders: Issues of overlapping symptoms. *American Journal of Psychiatry, 152*, 1793–1799.

Milberger, S., Biederman, J., Faraone, S. V., and Chen, L. et al. (1996). Is maternal smoking during pregnancy a risk factor for attention deficit disorder in children? *American Journal of Psychiatry, 153(9)*, 1138–1142.

Milberger, S., Biederman, J., Faraone, S. V., and Chen, L. (1997). ADHD is associated with early initiation of cigarette smoking children and adolescents. *Journal of the American Academy of Child and Adolescent Psychiatry, 36(1)*, 37–44.

Miller, D. and Blum, K. (1996). *Overload: Attention Deficit Disorder and the Addictive Brain*. Kansas City: Andrews and McMeel.

Millichap, G. J. (1997). Use of CNS stimulants for attention-deficit disorders. ANPA Abstracts *Journal of Neuropsychiatry and Clinical Neurosciences, 9(1)*, 150, P69.

Millichap, G. J. (1997). Temporal lobe arachnoid cyst-attention deficit disorder syndrome: Role of the electroencephalogram in diagnosis, *Neurology, 48*, 1435–1439.

Miller, K., Goldberg, S., and Atkin, B. (1989). Nocturnal enuresis: Experience with long-term use of intranasally administered desmopressin. *Journal of Pediatrics, 114(4)*, 723–726.

Milner, B. (1963). Effects of different brain lesion on card sorting: The role of the frontal lobes. *Archives of Neurology, 9*, 100–110.

Mimura, M., White, R. F., Albert, M. L. Mintzer, M. Z., Guarino, J., Kirk, T., Roache, J. D., and Griffiths, R. D. (1997). Ethanol and pentobarbital: Comparison of behavioral and subjective effects in sedative drug abusers. *Experimental and Clinical Psychopharmacology, 5(3)*, 203–215.

Mimura, M., White, R. F., and Albert, M. L., Corticobasal degeneration: Neuropsychological and clinical correltes. *The Journal of Neuropsychiatry and Clinical Neurosciences, 9(1),* 94–98.

Minshew, N. J., Goldstein, G., and Siegel, D. J. (1997). Neuropsychologic functioning in autism: Profile of a complex information processing disorder. *Journal of the International Neuropsychological Society, 3,* 303–316.

Miozzo, M. and Caramazza, A. (1997). On knowing the auxillary of a verb that cannot be named: Evidence for the independence of grammatical and phonological aspects of lexical knowledge. *Journal of Cognitive Neuroscience, 9(1),* 160–166.

Mitchell, P. B. et al. (1997). High level of Gsa in platelets of euthymic patients with bipolar affective disorder. *American Journal of Psychiatry, 154(2),* 218–223.

Mittenberg, W., Wittner, M. S., and Miller, L. J. (1997). Postconcussion Syndrome Occurs in Children. *Neuropsychology, 11(3),* 447–452.

Montague, M., McKinney, J. D., and Hocutt, A. (1994). Assessing students for attention deficit disorder. *Intervention in School and Clinic, 29(4),* 212–218.

Mooney, G. and Speed, J. (1997). Differential diagnosis in mild brain injury: understanding the role of non-organic conditions. *NeuroRehabilitation, 8,* 223–233.

Moore, A. D. and Stambrook, M. (1992). Coping strategies and locus of control following traumatic brain injury: relationship to long-term outcome. *Brain Injury, 6,* 89–94.

Moore, B. D., Slopis, J. M., Schomer, D., Jackson, E. F., and Levy, B. M. (1996). Neuropsychological significance of areas of high signal intensity on brain MRIs of children with neurofibromatosis. *Neurology, 46,* 161–1668.

Moore, L. A., Hughes, J. N., and Robinson, M. (1992). A comparison of the social information processing abilities or rejected and accepted hyperactive children. *Journal of Clinical Child Psychology, 2l(2),* 123–131.

Morgenson, G. J., Brudzynski, S. M., Wu, M., Yang, C. R., and Yim, C. C. Y. (1993). From motivation to action: A review of dopaminergic regulation of limbic → nucleus accumbens → ventral pallidum → pedunculopontine nucleus circuitries involved in limbic-motor integration, In Kalivas, P. W. and Barnes, C. D., Eds., *Limbic Motor Circuits and Neuropsychiatry,* Boca Raton, FL: CRC Press, 193–236.

Moriarty, M. B., Varma, A. R., Stevens, J., Fish, M., Trimble, M.R., and Robertson, M. M. (1997). A volumetric MRI study of Gilles de la Tourette's syndrome. *Neurology, 49,* 410–415.

Morris, M. E., Iansek, R., Matyas, T. A., and Summers, J. J. (1966). Stride length regulation in Parkinson's disease. *Brain, 119,* 551–568.

Morrow, L. A., Steinhauer, S. R., Condray, R., and Hodgson, M. (1997). Neuropsychological performance of journeymen painters under acute solvent exposure and exposure-free conditions. *Journal of the International Neuropsychological Society, 3,* 269–275.

Morrow, L. A., Steinhauer, S. R., and Condray, R. (1996). Differential associations of P300 amplitude and latency with cognitive and psychiatric function in solvent-exposed adults. *Journal of Neuropsychiatry, 8,* 446–449.

Morrow, L. A. (1994). Cueing attention: Disruptions following organic solvent exposure. *Neuropsychology, 8,* 471–476.

Morrow, L. A., Kamis, H., and Hodgson, M. J. (1993). Psychiatric symptomatology in persons with organic solvent exposure. *Journal of Consulting and Clinical Psychology, 61,* 171–174.

Morton, M. V. and Wehman, P. (1995). Psychosocial and emotional sequelae of individuals with traumatic brain injury: a literature review and recommendations. *Brain Injury, 9,* 81–92.

Moscovitch, M. (1994). Cognitive resources and dual-task interference effects at retrieval in normal people: The role of the frontal lobes and medial temporal cortex. *Neuropsychology, 8,* 524–534.

Moss, W. L. and Sheiffele, W. A. (1994). Can we differentially diagnose an attention deficit disorder without hyperactivity from a central auditory processing problem? *Child Psychiatry and Human Development, 25(2),* 85–96.

Murphy, K. (1994, October/ November). Interpersonal and social problems in adults with ADD. *Chadder Box,* 10–12.

Murphy, K. R. (1991). Biological parents of ADHD children: degree of attention deficit relative to the biological parents of normal children. *Dissertation Abstracts International, 52,* 524-B.

Murphy, K. and Barkley, R. A. (1996). Attention deficit hyperactivity disorder adults: Comorbidities and adaptive impairments. *Comprehensive Psychiatry, 37(6),* 393–401.

Murphy, D. A., Pelham, W. E., and Lang, A. R. (1992). Aggression in boys with attention deficit-hypyeractivity disorder: Methylphenidate effects on naturalistically observed aggression, response to provocation, and social information processing. *Journal of Abnormal Child Psychology, 20(5),* 451–465.

Murphy, T. K., Goodman, W. K., Fudge, M. W., William, R. C., Jr., Ayoub, E. M., Dalal, M., Lewis, M. H., and Zabriskie, J. B., (1997). B Lymphocyte antigen D8/17: A peripheral marker childhood-onset obsessive-compulsive disorder and tourette's syndrome? *American Journal of Psychiatry, 154(3),* 402–407.

Murray, P. K. (1994, January/February). Understanding and working with parents of hyperactive children: A guide for educators. *Challenge, 8(1),* 1–4.

Nada-Raja, S., Langley, J. D., McGee, R., Williams, S. M. et al. (1997). Inattentive and hyperactive behaviors and driving offenses in adolescence. *Journal of the American Academy of Child and Adolescent Psychiatry, 36(4),* 515–522.

Näätänen, R. (1992). *Attention and Brain Function.* Hillsdale, NJ: Lawrence Erlbaum Associates.

Nadeau, K. (1993). ADD in the workplace. *ADDult News, 4,* 1–7.

Nadeau, S. E. (1995). Phonology. The Florida Society of Neurology and the Center for Neuropsychological Studies at the University of Florida.

Nagahama, Y., Fukuyama, H., Yamauchi, S., Konishi, J. et al. (1996). Cerebral activation during performance of a card sorting test. *Brain, 119,* 1667–1675.

Nanson, J. L. and Hiscock, M. (1990). Attention deficits in children exposed to alcohol prenatally. *Alcoholism Clinical and Experimental Research, 14,* 656–661.

Neeper, R., Goldstein, S., Abuelo, D., Gascon, G., Huntzinger, R. (1995). Juvenile-onset Huntington's disease (HD) preceeded by attention-deficit-tic-obsessive-compulsive spectrum disease. *Journal of Neurophysychiatry, 7(3)*, Abstract No. 86.

Nettelbeck, T. and Wilson, C. (1994). Childhood changes inspeed of information processing and mental age: A brief report. *British Journal of Developmental Psychology, 12(3)*, 277–280.

Neumann, C. S., Baum, K. M., Walker, E. F., and Lewine, R. J. (1996). Childhood behavioral precursors of adult neuropsychological functioning in schizophrenia. *Neuropsychiatry, Neuropsychology, and Behavioral Neurology, 4*, 221–229.

Neve, J. (1992). Clinical implications of trace elements and endocrinology. *Biological Trace Element Research, 32*, 173–185.

Newcorn, J. H., Halperin, J. M., Schwartz, S., and Pascualvaca, D. (1994). Parent and teacher ratings of attention-deficit hyperactivity disorder symptoms: Implications for case identification. *Journal of Developmental and Behavioral Pediatrics, 15(2)*, 86–91.

Nickels, J. L., Schneider, W. N., Dombovy, M. L., and Wong, T. M. (1994). Clinical use of amantadine in brain injury rehabilitation. *Brain Injury, 8*, 709–718.

Nigg, J. T., Hindshaw, Stephen, P., and Halperin, J. M. (1996). Continuous performance test in boys with attention deficit hyperactivity disorder: Methylphenidate dose response and relations with observed behaviors. *Journal of Clinical Child Psychology, 25(3)*, 330–340.

Nigg, J. T. and Goldsmith, H. H. (1994). Genetics of personality disorders: Perspectives from personality and psychopathology research. *Psychological Bulletin, 115*, 346–380.

Nigg, J. T., Swanson, J. M., and Hinshaw, S. P. (1977). Covert visual spatial attention in boys with attention deficit hyperactivity disorder: Lateral effects, methylphenidate response and results for parents. *Neuropsychologia, 35(2)*, 165–176.

Nissen, M. J. (1986). Neuropsychology of attention and memory. *Journal of Head Trauma Rehabilitation, 1(3)*, 13–21.

Nobre, A. C., Sebestyen, G. N., Gitelman, D. R., Mesuam, M. M., Frackowiak, R. S. J., and Frith, C. D. (1997). Functional localization of the system for visuospatial attention using positron emission tomography. *Brain, 120*, 515–533.

Nolen-Hoeksema, S., Girgus, J. S., and Seligman, M. E. P. (1992). Predictors and consequences of childhood depressive symptoms: A 5-year longitudinal study. *Journal of Abnormal Psychology, 101*, 405–422.

Nuwer, M., (1997). Assessment of digital EEG, quantitative EEG, and EEG brain mapping: Report of the american academy of neurology and the american clinical neurophysiology society. *Neurology, 49*, 277–292.

O'Brien, T. E., Philips, W. H., and Rubinoff, A. (1994, July/August). ADD: Not just for boys. *Chadder Box*, 8–9.

O'Connor, M., Walbridge, M., Sandson, T., and Alexander, M. (1996). A Neuropsychological analysis of capgras syndrome. *Neuropsychiatry, Neuropsychology, and Behavioral Neurology, 9*, 265–271.

O'Donnell, B. F., Swearer, J. M., Smith, L. T., Nestor, P. G., Shenton, M. E., and McCarley, R. W. (1996). Selective deficits in visual perception and recognition in schizophrenia. *American Journal of Psychiatry, 153,* 687–692.

O'Donnell, B. F. and Cohen, R. A. (1993). Attention: A component of information processing. In Cohen, R. A., Ed., *The Neuropsychology of Attention.* New York: Plenum Press.

O'Donnell, J. P., MacGregor, L. A., Dabrowski, J. J., and Oestreicher, J. M. (1994). Construct validity of neuropsychological tests of conceptual and attentional abilities. *Journal of Clinical Psychology, 50,* 596–600.

O'Donnell, J. P. (1983). Neuropsychological test findings for naormal, learning disabled, and brain damaged young adults. *Journal of Consulting and Clinical Psychology, 51,* 726–729.

O'Leary, D. S., Andreasen, N. C., Hurtig, R. R., Watkins, G. L., Ponto, L. L. B., Rogers, M., Kirchner, P. T., and Hichwa, R. D. (1995) Language and attention in schizophrenics and normal controls: A positron emission tomography (PET) study of regional cerebral blood flow during binaural and dichotic tasks. *Journal of the International Neuropsychological Society, 1(4),* 371.

Ollendick, T. H. and King, N. J. (1994). Diagnosis, assessment, and treatment of internalizing problems in children: The role of longitudinal data. *Journal of Consulting and Clinical Psychology, 62,* 918–927.

O'Mara, S. and Walsh, V. (1994). *The Cognitive Neuropsychology of Attention: A Special Issue of Cognitive Neuropsychology.* East Sussex: Lawrence Erlbaum Associates.

Oshman, H. P. (1992, May/June). Evaluating the adult with ADD: Procedures and processes. *Challenge, May/June,* 1992.

O'Toole, K., Abramowitz, A., Morris, R., and Dulcan, M. (1996). Effects of methylphenidate on attention and nonverbal learning in children with attention deficit-hyperactivity disorder. *Journal of the International Neuropsychological Society, 2(1),* 24.

Ott, B. R., Noto, R. B., and Fogel, B. S., (1996). Apathy and Loss of Insight in Alzeheimer's Disease: A SPECT Imaging Study. *Journal of Clinical Neuropsychiatry, 8,* 41–46.

Owen, A. M., Roberts, A. C., Hodges, J. R., Summers, B. A., Polkey, C. E., and Robbins, T. W. (1993). Contrasting mechanisms of impaired attentional set-shifting in patients with frontal lobe damage or Parkinson's disease. *Brain, 116,* 1159–1175.

Owen, A. M., Milner, B., Petrides, M., and Evans, A. C. (1997). A specific role for the right parahippocampal gyrus in the retrieval of object-location: A positron emission tomography study. *Journal of Cognitive Neuroscience, 8(6),* 588–602.

Ozonoff, S. (1995). Reliability and validity of the Wisconsin Card Sorting Test in studies of autism. *Neuropsychology, 9(4),* 491–500.

Pachara, N. A., Boone, K. B., Miller, B. L., Cummings, J. L., and Berman, N. (1966). Comparison of neuropsychological functioning in Alzheimer's disease and frontotemporal dementia. *Journal of the International Neuropsychological Society, 2,* 505–510.

Palmer, B. W., Heaton, R., K., Paulsen, J. S., Kuck, J., Braff, D., Harris, M. J., Zisook, S., and Jeste, D. V. (1997). Is it possible to be schizophrenic yet neuropsychological normal? *Neuropsychology, 11(3),* 437–446.

Papatheodorou, G. (1996, February). A review of valproate in acute adolescent mania. *Child and Adolescent Psychopharmacology News, 1(1),* 10–11.

Paque, L. and Warrington, E. K. (1995). A longitudinal study of reading ability in patients suffering from dementia. *Journal of the International Neuropsychological Society, 1,* 517–524.

Paradiso, S., Andreasen, N. C., O'Leary, D. S., Arndt, S., and Robinson, R. G. (1997). Cerebellar size and cognition: Correlations with IQ, verbal membory and motor dexterity. *Journal of Clinical Neuroscience, 10,* 1–8.

Parasuraman, R. and Nestor, P. G. (1993). Preserved Cognitive Operations in Early Alzheimer's Disease. *Adult Information Processing: Limits on Loss,* (pp 77–111).

Parente, R., Stapleton, M. C., and Wheatley, C. J. (1991). Practical strategies for vocational reentry after traumatic brain injury. *Journal of Head Trauma Rehabilitation, 6(3),* 35–45.

Park, S., Lenzenweger, M. F., Puschel, J., and Holzman, P. S. (1996). Attentional inhibition in schizophrenia and schizotypy: A spatial negative priming study. *Cognitive Neuropsychiatry, 1,* 125–149.

Parker, H. C. (1988). *The ADD Hyperactivity Workbook for Parents, Teachers, and Kids.* Plantation, FL: Impact Publications Inc.

Parraga, H. C. and Cochran, M. K. (1992). Emergence of motor and vocal tics during imipramine administration in two children. *Journal of Child and Adolescent Psychopharmacology, 2(3),* 227–234.

Parraga, H. C., Kelly, D. P., Parraga, M. I., and Cochran, M. K. (1994). Combined psychostimulant and tricyclic antidepressant treatment of Tourette's syndrome and comorbid disorders in children. *Journal of Child and Adolescent Psychopharmacology, 4(2),* 113–122.

Paulesu, E., Frith, U., Snowling, M., Gallagher, A., Morton, J., Frackowiak, R. S. J., and Frith, C. D. (1996). Is developmental dyslexia a disconnection syndrome? Evidence from PET scanning. *Brain, 119(1),* 143–157.

Pauls, D. L. (1991). Genetic factors in the expression of attention-deficit hyperactivity disorder. *Journal of Child and Adolescent Psychopharmacology, 1(5),* 353–360.

Paus, T., Zatorre, R. J., Hofle, N., Caramanos, Z., Gotman, J., Petrides, M., and Evans, A. C. (1997). Time-related changes in neural systems underlying attention and arousal during the performance of an auditory vigilance task. *Journal of Cognitive Neuroscience, 9(3),* 392–408.

Pearsall, P. (1987). *Superimmunity,* New York: McGraw-Hill.

Pelham, W. E., Hoza, B., Kipp, H. L., Gnagy, E. M., and Trane, S. T. (1997). Effects of methylphenidate and expectancy on ADHD children's performance, self-evaluations, persistence, and attributions on a cognitive task. *Experimental and Clinical Psychopharmacology, 5(1),* 3–13.

Pelham, W. E., Jr. (1993a). Pharmacotherapy for children with attention-deficit hyperactivity disorder. *School Psychology Review, 22,* 199–227.

Pelham, W. E., Jr. (1993b). Recent developments in pharmacological treatment for child and adolescent mental health disorders [Annotated bibliography]. *School Psychology Review, 22,* 252–253.

Pelham, W. E., Jr., Murphy, D. A., Vannatta, K., Milich, R., Licht, B. G., Gnagy, E. M., Greenslade, K. E., Greiner, A. R., and Vodde-Hamilton, M. (1992). Methylphenidate and attributions in boys with attention-deficit hyperactivity disorder. *Journal of Consulting and Clinical Psychology, 60,* 282–292.

Pelham, W. E., Jr., Carlson, C., Sams, S. E., Vallano, G., Dixon, M. J., and Hoza, B. (1993). Separate and combined effects of methylphenidate and behavior modification on boys with attention deficit-hyperactivity disorder in the classroom. *Journal of Consulting and Clinical Psychology, 61,* 506–515.

Penn, I. V. and Salloway, S. (1995). Development of multiple sclerosis (MS) in a patient with attention-deficit hyperactivity disorder (ADHD). ANPA Abstracts, P32, *The Journal of Neuropsychiatry and Clinical Neurosciences, 7(3),* 406–407.

Penny, T. B., Holder, M. D., and Meck, W. H. (1996). Clonidine-induced antagonism of norepinephrine modulates the attentional processes involved in peak-interval timing. *Experimental and Clinical Psychopharmacology, 4(1),* 82–92.

Peresleni, L. I. and Rozhkova, L. A. (1994). Psychophysiological mechanisms of attention deficit in children of different ages with learning disabilities. *Human Physiology, 19(4),* 255–260.

Perry, W. and Braff, D. L. (1994). Information-processing deficits and thought disorder in schizophrenia. *American Journal of Psychiatry, 151(3),* 363–367.

Peterson, B. S. (1995). Neuroimaging in child and adolescent neuropsychiatric disorders. *Journal of the American Academy of Child and Adolescent Psychiatry, 34(12),* 1560–1576.

Pettit, G. S., Bates, J. E., and Dodge, K. A. (1993). Family interaction patterns and children's conduct problems at home and school: A longitudinal perspective. *School Psychology Review, 22(3),* 403–420.

Ph.D. (1997) Corticobasal degeneration: Neuropsychological and clinical correlates. *Neuropsychiatry and Clinical Neurosciences, 9,* 94–98.

Phares, V. and Compas, B. E. (1992). The role of fathers in child and adolescent psychopathology: make room for daddy. *Psychological Bulletin, 111(3),* 387–412.

Phône-Poulenc Rorer Pharmaceuticals Inc. (1995). DDAVP Nasal Spray, Collegeville, PA.

Pickworth, W. B., Rohrer, M. S., and Fant, Reginald V. (1997). Effects of abused drugs on psychomotor performance. *Experimental and Clinical Psychopharmacology, 5(3),* 233–241.

Pietrini, P. et al. (1997). Low glucose metabolism during brain stimulation in older Down's syndrome subjects at risk for Alzheimer's disease prior to dementia. *American Journal of Psychiatry, 154(8),* 1063–1069.

Pihl, R. O. and Peterson, J. B. (1991). Attention-deficit hyperactivity disorder, childhood conduct disorder, and alcoholism: Is there an association? *Alcohol Health and Research World, 15(1),* 25–31.

Pine, D. S., Kelin, R. G., Lindy, D. C., and Marshall, R. D. (1993). Attention-deficit hyperactivity disorder and comorbid psychosis: A review and two clinical presentations. *Journal of Clinical Psychiatry, 54(4),* 140–145.

Pineda, D., Rosselli, M., Cadavid, C., and Ardila, A. (1997a). Neurobehavioral characteristics of 10 to 12 year old children with attention deficit hyperactivity disorder (ADHD). ANPA Abstracts *Journal of Neuropsychiatry and Clinical Neurosciences, 9(1),* 138, P27.

Pineda, D., Roselli, M., Cadavid, C., and Ardila, A. (1997b). Neurobehavioral characteristics of 7 to 9 year old children with attention deficit hyperactivity disorder (ADHD), ANPA Abstracts, *Journal of Neuropsychiatry and Clinical Neurosciences, 9(1),* 137, P26.

Pisternman, S., McGrath, P., Firestone, P., Goodman, J. T., Webster, I., and Mallory, R. (1989). Outcome of parent-mediated treatment of preschoolers with attention deficit disorder with hyperactivity. *Journal of Consulting and Clinical Psychology, 57,* 628–635.

Piven, J., Bailey, J., Ranson, B. J., and Arndt, S. (1997). An MRI study of the corpus callosum in autism. *American Journal of Psychiatry, 154(8),* 1051–1056.

Piven, J., Palmer, P., Jacobi, Dinah, B. A., Childress, D., and Arndt, S. (1997). Broader autism phenotype: Evidence from a family history study of multiple-incidence autism families. *American Journal of Psychiatry, 154(2),* 185–190.

Platz, T. (1996). Tactile agnosia, casuistic evidence and theoretical remarks on modality-specific meaning representations and sensorimotor integration. *Brain, 119,* 1565–1574.

Pleak, R. R. (1995). Adverse effects of chewing methylphenidate. *American Journal of Psychiatry, 152(5),* 811.

Plioplys, A. V. (1997). Antimuscle and anti-CNS circulating antibodies in chronic fatigue syndrome. *Neurology, 48,* 1717–1719.

Pliskin, N. H., Hamer, D. P., Goldstein, D. S., Towle, V. L., Reder, A. T., Noronha, A., and Arnason, B. G. W. (1996). Improved delayed visual reproduction test performance in multiple sclerosis patients receiving interferon B-1b. *Neurology, 47,* 1463–1468.

Pliszka, S. R. (1990). Effect of anxiety on cognition, behavior, and stimulant response in ADHD. *Annual Progress in Child Psychiatry and Child Development,* 454–466.

Plizka, S. R. (1992). Comorbidity of attention-deficit hyperactivity disorder and overanxious disorder. *Journal of American Academy of Child and Adolescent Psychiatry, 31(2),* 197–203.

Pliszka, S. R. (1993, September/October). Differential and dual diagnosis in behavioral disorders. *Challenge, 7(5),* 6–7.

Pliszka, S. R., Maas, J. W., Javors, M. A., and Rogeness, G. A. (1995). Urinary catecholamines in attention-deficit hyperactivity disorder with and without comorbid anxiety. *Journal of the American Academy of Child and Adolescent Psychiatry, 33(8),* 1165–1173.

Plizka, S. R., McCracken, J. T., and Maas, J. W. (1996). Catecholamines in attention-deficit hyperactivity disorder: Current perspectives. *Journal of the American Academy of Child and Adolescent Psychiatry, 35(3),* 264–272.

Poillion, M. J. (1991). A comparison of characteristics and causes of attention deficit hyperactivity disorder identified by social defining groups. *Dissertation Abstracts International, 52,* 1695, p. 149.

Polich, J., Pollock, V. E., and Bloom, F. E. (1994). Meta-analysis of P300 amplitude from males at risk for alcoholism. *Psychological Bulletin, 115,* 55–73.

Pontius, A. A. and Yudowitz, B. S. (1980). Frontal lobe system dysfunction in some criminal actions as shown in the Narratines text. *Journal of Nervous and Mental Disorder, 168,* 111–117.

Pope, H. G., Jr. and Yurgelun-Todd, D. (1996). The residual cognitive effects of heavy marijuana use in college students. *Journal of the American Medical Association, 275(7),* 521–527.

Portius, A. A. (1973). Dysfunctional patterns analogous to frontal lobe system and caudate nucleus syndromes in some groups of minimal brain dysfunction. *Journal of American Medical Womens Association, 28,* 285–292.

Posner, M. I. and Synder, C. R. R. (1975). Attention and cognitive control. In Solso, R. L. (Ed). Information processing and cognition: The Loyola Symposium. Hillsdale, NJ: Erlbaum.

Posner, M. I. (1989). *Foundations of Cognitive Science.* Cambridge, MA: MIT Press.

Posner, J. B. (1995). Paraneoplastic syndromes involving the nervous system. *Neurology and General Medicine,*401–420.

Post, R. B. et al. (1997). Carbmazepine in bipolar disorder. *Child and Adolescent Psychopharmacology News, 2(3),* 6.

Post, R. B., Chaderjian, M. R., Lott, L. A., and Maddock, R. J. (1997). Effects of lorazepam on the distribution of spatial attention. *Experimental and Clinical Psychopharmacology, 5(2),* 143–149.

Potolicchio, S. J., Jr. (1994). Disorders of excesssive sleepiness. In Fairbanks, D. N. F. and Fujita, S., Eds., *Snoring and Obstructive Sleep Apnea,* 2nd ed., New York: Raven Press.

Pouget, A. and Sejnowski, T. J. (1997). Spatial transformations in the parietal cortex using basis functions. *Journal of Cognitive Neuroscience, 9(2),* 222–237.

Powell, A. L., Yudd, A., Zee, P., and Mandelbaum, D. E. (1997). Attention deficit hyperactivity disorder associated with orbitofrontal epilepsy in a father and a son. *Neuropsychiatry, Neuropsychology, and Behavioral Neurology, 10(2),* 151–154.

Powell, J. H., Al-Adawi, S., Morgan, J., and Greenwood, R. J. (1996). Motivational Deficits after brain injury: effects of bromocriptine in 11 patients. *Journal of Neurology, Neurosurgery and Psychiatry, 60,* 416–421.

Prather, P., Brownell, H., and Alexander, A. (1996). Contributions of the left versus right hemisphere to selective attention. *Journal of the International Neuropsychological Society, 2(1),* 10.

Prather, P., Brownell, H., Alexander, A., Estin, A., and Aram, D. (1996). Developmental trends and right hemisphere contributions to anticipation. *Journal of the International Neuropsychological Society, 2(1),* 10.

Pribor, E. F., Yutzy, S. H., Dean, T., and Wetzel, R. D. (1993). Briquet's syndrome, dissociation, and abuse. *American Journal of Psychiatry, 150,* 1507–1511.

Psychiatric dispatches: Noteworthy briefs from the field. (1994, November/December). *Primary Psychiatry,* 12–13.

Puente, A. E. and McCaffrey, R. J. (Eds.) (1992). *Handbook of Neuropsychological Assessment: A Biopsychological Perspective.* New York: Plenum Press.

Pulsifer, M. B. (1996). The Neuropsychology of mental retardation. *Journal of the International Neuropsychological Society, 2,* 159–176.

Quinn, P. O. and Stern, J. M. (1991). *Putting on the Brakes: Young People's Guide to Understanding Attention Deficit Hyperactivity Disorder (ADHD).* New York: Magination Press.

Quintana, J. and Fuster, J. M. (1993). Spatial and temporal factors in the role of prefrontal and parietal cortex in visuomotor integration. *Cerebral Cortex, 3,* 122–132.

Rafal, R. and Robertson, L. (1995). The neurology of visual attention, In Michael S. Gazzaniga, Ed., *The Cognitive Neurosciences,* Cambridge, MA: MIT Press, 625–648.

Rafal, R. and Henik, A. (1994). The neurology of inhibition: Integrating controlled and automatic processes. In D. Dagenbach and T. A. H. Carr (Eds). *Inhibitory Processes in Attention, Memory, and Language.* San Diego, CA: Academic Press.

Raine, A., Venables, P. H., and Williams, M. (1995). High autonomic arousal and electrodermal orienting at age 15 years as protective factors against criminal behavior at age 29 years. *American Journal of Psychiatry, 152(11),* 1595–1600.

Rajkowska, G. and Goldman-Rakic, P. S. (1995). Cytoarchitectonic definition of prefrontal areas in the normal human cortex: II. Variability in locations of areas 9 and 46 and relationship to the Talairach Coordinate System. *Cerebral Cortex, 5(4),* 232–337.

Rajkowska, G. and Goldman-Rakic, P. S. (1995). Cytoarchitectonic definition of prefrontal areas in the normal human cortex: II. Variability in locations of areas 9 and 46 and relationship to the Talairach Coordinate System. *Cerebral Cortex, 5(4),* 323–337.

Ramsey, J. M., Horwitz, B., Donohue, B. C., Nace, K., Maisog, J. M., and Andreason, P. (1997) Phonological and orthographic components of word recognition: A PET-rCBF study. *Brain, 120,* 739–759.

Randolph, C. (1995). The neuropsychology of schizophrenia. *Syllabus for Neurobiology of Behavior and Cognition.* Chicago: North Western University Medical School.

Rao, M. D., Tuski, P. A., Polcyn, R. E. et al. (1984). F positron emission computed tomography in closed head injury. *Archives in Physical Medicine Rehabilitation, 65,* 780–785.

Rapoport, J. L. and Elia, J. (1994). Thyroid function and attention-deficit hyyperactivity disorder: Reply. *Journal of the American Academy of Child and Adolescent Psychiatry, 33(7),* 1058.

Rapport, M. D., Denney, C., DuPaul, G. J., and Gardner, M. J. (1994). Attention deficit disorder and methylphenidate: Normalization rates, clinical effectiveness, and response prediction in 76 children. *Journal of the American Academy of Child and Adolescent Psychiatry, 33(6),* 882–893.

Raskin, S. A. (1997). The relationship between sexual abuse and mild traumatic brain injury. *Brain Injury, 11(8),* 587–603.

Rasmussen and R. Marino (Eds). (1993). *Functional Neurosurgery.* New York: Raven Press.

Ratey, J. J. (1991). Paying attention to attention in adults. *Chadder, Fall/Winter,* 13–14.

Ratey, J. J., Greenberg, M. S., Bemporad, J. R., and Lindem, K. J. (1992). Unrecognized attention-deficit hyperactivity disorder in adults presenting for outpatient psychotherapy. *Journal of Child and Adolescent Psychopharmacology, 2(4),* 267–275.

Ratey, J. J., Hallowell, E. M., and Miller, A. C. (1995). Relationship dilemmas for adults with ADD: The biology of intimacy (Ed.) Nadeau, K. G., In *A Comprehensive Guide to Attention Deficit Disorder in Adults, Research, Diagnosis and Treatment,* New York: Brunner/Mazel Publishers, 218–235.

Ratey, J. J. and Hallowell, E. M. (1993). 50 Tips on the management of adult attention deficit disorder. *The CH.A.D.D.ER Box, 6(1),* 1–8.

Raymond, M. J., Bennett, T. L., Malia, K. B., and Bewick, K. C. (1996). Rehabilitation of visual processing deficits following brain injury. *NeuroRehabilitation, 6,* 229–240.

Raz, S., Foster, M. S., Briggs, S. D., Shah, F., Baertschi, J. C., Lauterbach, M. D., Riggs, W. W., Magill, L. H., and Sander, C. J. (1994). Lateralization of perinatal cerebral insult and cognitive asymmetry: Evidence from neuroimaging. *Neuropsychology, 8,* 160–170.

Reeves, L. M. and Weisberg, R. W. (1994). The role of content and abstract information in analogical transfer. *Psychological Bulletin, 115,* 381–400.

Reid, R. and Katsiyannis, A. (1995). Attention-deficit/hyperactivity disorder and Section 504. *Remedial and Special Education, 16(1),* 44–52.

Reimer, W., van Patten, K., Templer, D. I., Schuyler, B., Gross, A., and Yanovsky, A. (1995). The neuropsychological spectrum in traumatically head-injured persons. *Brain Injury, 9,* 55–60.

Reitan, R. M. and Davidson, L. A. (Eds). (1974). *Clinical Neuropsychology: Current Status and Applications.* Washington, DC; Hemisphere Publishing Corp.

Reitan, R. M. and Wolfson, D. (1985). *The Halstead-Reitan Neuropsychological Test Battery: Theory and Clinical Interpretation.* Tucson, AZ: Neuropsychology Press.

Reitan, R. M. and Wolfson, D. (1986). *Traumatic Brain Injury, Vol. I. Pathophysiology and Neuropsychological Evaluation,* Tucson, AZ; Neuropsychology Press.

Reitan, R. M. and Wolfson, D. (1988). *Traumatic Brain Injury, Vol. II. Recovery and Rehabilitation,* Tucson, AZ; Neuropsychology Press.

Reitan, R. M. and Wolfson, D. (1992). *Neuroanatomy and Neuropathology: A Clinical Guide for Neuropsychologists* (2nd ed), Tucson, AZ; Neuropsychology Press.

Reitan, R. M. and Wolfson, D. (1992). *Neuropsychological Evaluation of Older Children,* Tucson, AZ; Neuropsychology Press.

Reitan, R. M. and Wolfson, D. (1993). *The Haldstead-Reitan Neuropsychological Test Battery: Theory and Clinical Interpretation* (2nd ed.). S. Tucson, AZ: Neuropsychology Press.

Reitan, R. M. and Wolfson, D. (1994). *Aphasia and Sensory-Perceptual Deficits in Children* (2nd ed), Tucson, AZ; Neuropsychology Press.

Reitan, R. M. and Wolfson, D. (1994a). A selective and critical review of neuropsychological deficits and the frontal lobes. *Neuropsychology Review, 4,* 161–198.

Reitan, R. M. and Wolfson, D. (1995). The category test and the trail making test as measures of frontal lobe functions. *The Clinical Neuropsychologist, 9,* 50–56.

Reitan, R. M. and Wolfson, D. (1996a). Can WISC-R IQ values be computed validly for learning disabled children? *Applied Neuropsychology, 3,* 15–20.

Reitan, R. M. and Wolfson, D. (1996b). Differential relationships of age and education to WAIS subtest scores among brain-damaged and control groups. *Archives of Clinical Neuropsychology, 11,* 303–311.

Reitan, R. M. and Wolfson, D. (1996c). The diminished effect of age and education on neuropsychological performances of learning-disabled children. *Child Neuropsychology, 2,* 11–16.

Reitan, R. M. and Wolfson, D. (1996d). Relationships between specific and general tests of cerebral functioning. *The Clinical Neuropsychologist, 10,* 37–42.

Reitan, R. M. and Wolfson, D. (1996e). Relationships of age and education to Wechsler Adult Intelligence Scale IQ values in brain-damaged and non-brain-damaged groups. *The Clinical Neuropsychologist, 10,* 293–304.

Remington, G. (1997). Selecting a neuroleptic and the role of side effects. *Child and Adolescent Psychopharmacology News, 2(2),* 1–9.

Resta, S. P. and Eliot, J. (1994). Writtten expression in boys with attention deficit disorder. *Perceptual and Motor Skills, 79,* 1131–1138.

Reuter-Lorenz, P. A., Drain, M., and Hardy-Morais, C. (1997). Object centered attentional biases in the intact brain. *Journal of Cognitive Neuroscience, 8(6),* 540–550.

Revesz, T., Kidd, D., Thompson, A. J., Barnard, R. O., and McDonald, W. I. (1994). A comparison of the pathology of primary and secondary progressive multiple sclerosis. *Brain, 117,* 759–765.

Rey, A. (1941). L'Examen Psychologique dans le cas d'encephalopathie traumatique. *Archives de Psychologie, 28,* 286–340.

Rey, J. M. (1993). Oppositional defiant disorder. *American Journal of Psychiatry, 150,* 1769–1778.

Riccio, C. A., Gonzalez, J. J., and Hynd, G. W. (1994). Attention deficit hyperactivity disorder (ADHD) and learning disabilities. *Learning Disability Quarterly, 17(4),* 311–322.

Riccio, C. A., Hynd, G. W., Cohen, M. J., Hall, J., and Molt, L. (1994). Comorbidity of central auditory processing disorder and attention-deficit hyperactivity disorder. *Journal of the American Academy of Child and Adolescent Psychiatry, 33,* 849–857.

Richters, J. E. and Cicchetti, D. (1993). Toward a developmental perspective on conduct disorder [Special Issue]. *Development and Psychopathology, 5,* 1–3.

Rickels, K., Derivan, A., Kunz, N., Pallay, A., and Schweizer, E. (1996). Zalospirone in major depression: A placebo-controlled multicenter study. *Journal of Clinical Psychopharmacology, 16,* 212–217.

Riddle, M. A., King, R. A., Hardin, M. T., and Scahill, L. (1991). Behavioral side effects of fluoxetine in children and adolescents. *Journal of Child and Adolescent Psychopharmacology, 1(3),* 193–198.

Ried, S., Strong, G., Wright, L., Wood, A., Goldman, A., and Bogen, D. (1995). Computers, assistive devices, and augmentative communication aids: Technology for social inclusion. *Journal of Head Trauma Rehabilitation, 10(5),* 80–90.

Robaey, P., Breton, F., Dugas, M., and Renault, B. (1992). An event-related potential study of controlled and automatic processes in 6 to 8-year-old boys with attention deficit hyperactivity disorder. *Electroencephalography and Clinical Neurophysiology, 82(5),* 330–340.

Robbins, T. W. and Everitt, B. J. (1995). Arousal systems and attentions. *The Cognitive Neurosciences,* Cambridge, MA. Massachusetts Institute of Technology, 703–720.

Roberts, M. A., Verduyn, W. H., Manshadi, F. F., and Hines, M. E. (1996). Episodic symptoms in dysfunctioning children and adolescents following mild and severe traumatic brain injury. *Brain Injury, 10(10),* 739–747.

Robertson, I. H., Ward, T., Ridgeway, V., and Nimmo-Smith, I. (1996). The structure of normal human attention: The Test of Everyday Attention. *Journal of the International Neuropsychological Society, 2,* 525–534.

Robertson, I. H., Ridgeway, V., Greenfield, E., and Parr, A. (1997). Motor recovery after stroke depends on intact sustained attention: A 2-year follow-up study. *Neuropsychology, 11(2),* 290–295.

Robertson, L., Treisman, A., Friedman-Hill, S., and Grabowecky, M. (1997). The interaction of spatial and object pathways: Evidence from Balint's Syndrome. *Journal of Cognitive Neuroscience, 9(3),* 295–317.

Robin, A. L. (1994, January). Talking with your teen: Communication tips from an expert. *Chadder Box,* 8–9.

Roelfsema, P. R., Engel, A., König, P., and Singer, W. (1997). The role of neuronal synchronization in response selection: A biologically plausible theory of structured representations in the visual cortex. *Journal of Cognitive Neuroscience, 8(6),* 603–625.

Roitman, S. E. L., Cornblatt, B. A., Bergman, A., Obuchowski, M., Mitropoulou, V., Keefe, R., Silverman, J. M., and Siever, L. J. (1997). Attentional functioning in schizotypal personality disorder. *American Journal of Psychiatry, 154(5),* 655–660.

Roman, D., Edwall, G., Buchanan, R., and Patton, J. (1991). Extended norms for the Paced Auditory Serial Addition Task. *The Clinical Neuropsychologist, 5,* 33–40.

Rose, F. D., Johnson, D. A., and Attree, E. A. (1997). Rehabilitation of the head-injured child: basic research and new technology. *Pediatric Rehabilitation, 1(1),* 3–7.

Ross, E. (1995). Neurological perspectives on human aggression, In *Neurology of Behavior and Cognition,* Seminar held at the Knickerbocker Hotel, Chicago, Illinois, December 12–16, 1995.

Ross, E. D. (1995a). Aprosodias, Presented at December 12–16, 1995 Conference, *Neurology of Behavior and Cognition,* 131–135.

Ross, E. D. (1995b). Neurology of affect. *Syllabus for Neurobiology of Behavior and Cognition.* Chicago: North Western University Medical School.

Ross, R. G., Hommer, D., Breiger, D., Varley, C., and Radant, A. (1994). Eye movement task related to frontal lobe functioning in children with attention deficit disorder. *Journal of the American Academy of Child and Adolescent Psychiatry, 33,* 869–874.

Rosselli, M. and Ardila, A. (1993). Developmental norms for the Wisconsin Card Sorting Test in 5- to 12-year-old children. *The Clinical Neuropsychologist, 7(2)*, 145–154.

Roth, A. S., Ostroff, R. B., and Hoffman, R. E. (1996). Naltrexone as a treatment for repetitive self-injurious behavior: An open-label trial. *Journal of Clinical Psychiatry, 57*, 233–237.

Rothstein, J. D. (1996). Excitotoxicity hypothesis. *Neurology, 47*, S19–S26.

Rozewicz, L., Langdon, D. W., Davie, C. A., Thompson, A. J., and Maria ron Institute of Neurology and National Hospital for Neurology and Neurosurgery, London, UK. (1996). Resolution of left hemisphere cognitive dysfunction in multiple sclerosis with magnetic resonance correlates: A case report. *Cognitive Neuropsychiatry, 1*, 17–25.

Rubinstein, S., Silver, L. B., and Licamele, W. L. (1994). Clonidine for stimulant-related sleep problems. *Journal of the American Academy of Child and Adolescent Psychiatry, 33*, 281–282.

Rugle, L. and Melamed, L. (1993). Neuropsychological assessment of attention problems in pathological gamblers. *Journal of Nervous and Mental Disease, 181(2)*, 107–112.

Ryan, N. D. (1990). Heterocyclic antidepressants in children and adolescents. Special Issue: The safe and effective use of psychotropic medications in adolescents and children. *Journal of Child and Adolescent Psychopharmacology, 1(1)*, 21–31.

Sabatino, D. A. and Vance, H. B. (1994). Is the diagnosis of attention deficit/hyperactivity disorders meaningful? *Psychology in the Schools, 31*, 188–196.

Sabelli, H., Fink, P., Fawcett, J., and Tom, C. (1996). Sustained antidepressant effect of PEA replacement. *Journal of Neuropsychiatry, 8(2)*, 168–171.

Safer, D. J. (1992). Relative cardiovascular safety of psychostimulants used to treat attention-deficit hyperactivity disorder. *Journal of Child and Adolescent Psychopharmacology, 2(4)*, 279–290.

Saffran, E. M. and Coslett, H. B. (1996). "Attentional dyslexia" in Alzheimer's disease: A case study. *Cognitive Neuropsychology, 13*, 205–228.

Salanova, V., Andermann, F., Rasmussen, T., Olivier, A., and Quesney, L. F. (1995). Parietal lobe epilepsy, clinical manifestations and outcome in 82 patients treated surgically between 1929 and 1988. *Brain, 118*, 607–627.

Sallee, F. R., Stiller, R. L., and Perel, J. M. (1992). Pharmacodynamics of pemoline in attention deficit disorder with hyperactivity. *Journal of the American Academy of Child and Adolescent Psychiatry, 31*, 244–251.

Salloway, S. P. (1994). Diagnosis and treatment of patients with frontal lobe syndromes. *Journal of Neuropsychiatry and Clinical Neurosciences, 6*, 388–398.

Sarkar, M. and Kornetsky, C. (1995). Methamphetamine's action on brain-stimulation reward threshold and stereotype. *Experimental and Clinical Psychopharmacology, 3(2)*, 112–117.

Sathian, K., Zangaladze, A., Green, J., Vitek, V. L., and DeLong, M. R. (1997). Tactile spatial acuity and roughness discrimination: Impairments due to aging and Parkinson's disease. *Neurology, 49*, 168–177.

Salthouse, T. A. (1994). The aging of working memory. *Neuropsychology, 8,* 535–543.

Sandler, A. D. (1995). *Attention Deficits and Neurodevelopmental Variation in Older Adults: A Comprehensive Guide to Attention Deficit Disorder in Adults Research, Diagnosis, Treatment,* Nadeau, K. (Ed.), New York: Brunner/Mazel, 58–73.

Satterfield, J. H., Schell, A. M., and Nicholas, T. (1994). Preferential neural processing of attended stimuli in attention-deficit hyperactivity disorder and normal boys. *Psychophysiology, 31(1),* 1–10.

Satz, P., Zaucha, K., McCleary, C., Light, R., and Becker, D. (1997). Mild head injury in children and adolescents: A review of studies (1970–1995). *Psychological Bulletin, 122(2),* 107–131.

Savage, C. R., Keuthen, N. J., Jenike, M. A., Brown, H. D., Baer, L., Kendrick, A. D., Miguel, E. C., Rauch, S. L., and Albert, M. S., (1996). Recall and recognition memory in obsessive-compulsive disorder. *Journal of Clinical Neuropsychiatry, 8,* 99–103.

Schachar, R. (1991). Childhood hyperactivity. *Journal of Child Psychology and Psychiatry, 32(1),* 155–191.

Schachar, R. and Logan, G. (1990). Are hyperactive children deficient in attentional capacity? *Journal of Abnormal Child Psychology, 18(5),* 493–513.

Schaughency, E., McGee, R., Shyamala, N., and Feehan, M. (1994). Self-reported inattention, impulsivity, and hyperactivity at ages 15 and 18 years in the general population. *Journal of the American Academy of Child and Adolescent Psychiatry, 33,* 173–184.

Schaughency, E. A., Vannatta, K., and Mauro, J. In Matson, J. L., (Eds.), *Handbook of Hyperactivity in Children.* Neeham Heights, MA: Allyn and Bacon, 256–281.

Scheffer, I. E., Bhatia, K. P., Lopes-Cendes, I., Fish, D. R., Marsden, C. D., Andermann, E., Andermann, F., Desbiens, R., Keene, D., Cendes, F., Manson, J. I., Constantinou, J. E. C., McIntosh, A., and Berkovic, S. F. (1995). Autosomal dominant nocturnal frontal lobe epilepsy: A distinctive clinical disorder. *Brain, 118,* 61–73.

Scheffer, I. E. and Berkovic, S. F. (1997) Generalized epilepsy with febrile seizures plus, A genetic disorder with heterogeneous clinical phenotypes. *Brain, 120,* 479–490.

Schlaepfer, T. E., Pearlson, G. D., Wong, D. F., Marenco, S., and Dannals, R. F. (1997). PET study of competition between intravenous cocaine and [11C] raclopride at dopamine receptors in human subjects. *American Journal of Psychiatry, 154(9),* 1209–1213.

Schlaug, G., Antke, C., Holthausen, H., Arnold, S., Ebner, A., Tuxhorn, I., Jäncke, L., Lüders, H., Witte, O. W., and Seitz, R. J. (1997). Ictal motor signs and interictal regional cerebral hypometabolism. *Neurology, 49,* 341–348.

Schmitter-Edgecombe, M. (1996). The effects of divided attention on implicit and explicit memory performance. *Journal of the International Neurological Society, 2(2),* 111–125.

Schneider, W. and Shiffrin, R. M. (1977). Controlled and automatic information processing: I. Detection, search, and attention. *Psychological Review, 84,* 1–66.

Schnitzer, P. G., Olshan, A. F., Savitz, D. A., and Erickson, J. D. (1995). Validity of mother's report of father's occupation in a study of paternal occupation and congenital malformations. *American Journal of Epidemiology, 141(9),* 872–877.

Schröger, E. (1996). A neural machanism for involuntary attention shifts to changes in auditory stimulation. *Journal of Cognitive Neuroscience, 8(6),* 527–539.

Schubiner, H., Tzelepis, A., Isaacson, J. H., Warbasse, L. H., et al. (1995). The dual diagnosis of attention-deficit/hyperactivity disorder and substance abuse: Case reports and literature review. *Journal of Clinical Psychiatry, 56(4),* 146–150.

Schuckit, M. A., Klein, J., Twitchell, G., and Smith, T. (1994). Personality test scores as predictors of alcoholism almost a decade later. *American Journal of Psychiatry, 151,* 1038–1042.

Schuerholz, L. J., Baumgardner, T. L., Singer, H. S., Reiss, A. L., and Denckla, M. B. (1996). Neuropsychological status of children with Tourette's syndrome with and without attention deficit hyperactivity disorder. *Neurology, 46,* 958–965.

Schuerholz, L. J., Harris, E. L., Baumgardner, T. L., Reiss, A. L., Freund, L. S., Church, R. P., Mohr, J., and Denckla, M. B. (1995). An analysis of two discrepancy-based models and a processing-deficit approach in identifying learning disabilities. *Journal of Learning Disabilities, 28(1),* 18–29.

Schwartz, R. L., Adair, J. C., D. Na, Williamson, D. J. G., and Heilman, K. M. (1997). Spatial bias: Attentional and intentional influence in normal subjects. *Neurology, 48,* 234–242.

Schweizer, K. (1994). Structural diversity of the speed-ability relationship due to information processing skills. *Personality and Individual Differences, 17,* 607–616.

Segalowitz, S. J., Dywan, J., and Unsal, A. (1997). Attentional factors in response time variability after traumatic brain injury: An ERP study. *Journal of the International Neuropsychological Society, 3,* 95–107.

Seger, C. A. (1994). Implicit learning. *Psychological Bulletin, 115,* 163–196.

Seidman, L. J., Faraone, S. V., Biederman, J., Weber, W., and Ouellette, C. (1997). Toward defining a neuropsychology of attention deficit-hyperactivity disorder: Performance of children and adolescents from a large clinically referred sample. *Journal of Consulting and Clinical Psychology, 65(1),* 150–160.

Seidman, L. J., Biederman, J., Faraone, S. V., and Weber, W. (1997). A pilot study of neuropsychological function in girls with ADHD. *Journal of the American Academy of Child and Adolescent Psychiatry, 36(3),* 366–373.

Seidman, L. J., Biederman, J., Faraone, S. V., and Milberger, S. et al. (1995). Effects of family history and comorbidity on the neuropsychological performance of children with ADHD: Preliminary findings. *Journal of the American Academy of Child and Adolescent Psychiatry, 34(8),* 1015–1024.

Sergeant, J. A. and Schotten, C. A. (1985). On resource strategy limitations in hyperactivity: Cognitive impulsivity reconsidered. *Journal of Child Psychology and Psychiatry, 26,* 97–110.

Sergent, J., Zuck, E., Levesque, M., and MacDonald, B. (1992). Positron emission tomography study of letter and object processing: Empirical findings and methodolical considerations. *Cerebral Cortex, 2,* 68–80.

Seutin, V., North, R. A., and Johnson, S. W. (1993). Transmitter regulation of mesencephalic dopamine cells. In Kalivas, P. W. and Barnes, C. D. (Eds.). *Limbic Motor Circuits and Neuropsychiatry.* Boca Raton, Fl: CRC Press, ch. 3.

Shaffer, D. (1994). Attention deficit hyperactivity disorder in adults. *American Journal of Psychiatry, 151,* 633–638.

Shah, M. R., Seese, L. M., Abikoff, H., and Klein, R. G. (1994). Pemoline for children and adolescents with conduct disorder: A pilot investigation. *Journal of Child and Adolescent Psychopharmacology, 4(4),* 255–261.

Shallice, T. (1982). Specific impairments in planning. *Phils. Trans. R. Soc. Lond., 298,* 199–209.

Shallice, T. (1994). Multiple levels of control processes, In Umiltà, Carlo and Moscovitch, Morris, *Attention and Performance* XV, MIT Press, Cambridge, MA: MIT Press, 395–420.

Shallice, T. and Burgess, P. (1991). Higher-order cognitive impairments and frontal lobe lesions in man. In Levin, H. S., Eisenberg, H. M., and Benton, A. L., Eds., Frontal lobe function and dysfunction. New York: Oxford University Press, 125–138.

Shallice, T., Burgess, P. W., Schon, F., and Baxter, D. (1989). The origins of utilization behavior. *Brain, 112,* 1587–1598.

Shapiro, E. G., Hughes, S. J., August, G. J., and Bloomquist, M. L. (1993). Processing of emotional information in children with attention deficit hyperactivity disorder. *Developmental Neuropsychology, 9(3,4),* 207–224.

Shapiro, S. K. and Hynd, G. W. (1993). Psychobiological basis of conduct disorder. *School Psychology Review, 22(3),* 386–402.

Shaw, G. A. and Giambra, L. M. (1993). Task-unrelated thoughts of college students diagnosed as hyperactive in childhood. *Developmental Neuropsychology, 9(1),* 17–30.

Shaywitz, B. A., Fletcher, J. M., and Shaywitz, S. E. (1995). Defining and classifying learning disabilities and attention-deficit/hyperactivity disorder. *Journal of Child Neurology, 10(Suppl. 1),* S20–S57.

Shaywitz, B. A. and Shaywitz, S. E. (1991). Comorbidity: A critical issue in attention deficit disorder. *Journal of Child Neurology, 6,* S13–S21.

Shaywitz, S. E. and Shaywitz, B. A. (1991). Attention deficit disorder: diagnosis and role of Ritalin in management. In Greenhill, L. L. and Osman, B. B., (Eds.). *Ritalin Theory and Patient Management,* New York: Maryann Liebert, Inc., 267–288.

Shaywitz, S. E., Shaywitz, B. A., Cohen, D. J., and Young, J. G. (1991). Monaminergic mechanisms in hyperactivity. *Ritalin Theory and Patient Management,* New York: Mary Ann Liebert, Inc., 267–288.

Shaywitz, S. E., Shaywitz, B. A., Cohen, D.J., and Young, J. G. (1983). Monoaminergic Mechanisms in Hyperactivity. *Developmental Neuropsychiatry,* 330–347.

Shaywitz, S. E., Schnell, C., Shaywitz, B. A., and Towle, V. R. (1986). Yale Children's Inventory: An Instrument of Assessing Children with Attentional Deficit and Learning Disabilities. *Journal of Abnormal Child Psychology, 14,* 347–364.

Shekim. W. O. (1990). Adult attention deficit hyperactivity disorder, residual state (ADHD,RS). *Chadder, Spring/Summer,* 16–18.

Sher, A. E. (1994). Obstructive sleep apnea: Diagnosis by history, physical examination, and special studies. In Fairbanks, D. N. F. and Frjita, S., Eds., *Snoring and Obstructive Sleep Apnea*, 2nd ed., New York: Raven Press.

Sher, K. J., Martin, E. D., Wood, P. K., and Rutledge, P. C. (1997). Alcohol use disorders and neuropsychological functioning in first-year undergraduates. *Experimental and Clinical Psychopharmacology, 5(3),* 304–315.

Sherman, D. K., McGue, M. K., and Iacono, W. G. (1997). Twin concordance for attention deficit hyperactivity disorder: A comparison of teachers' and mothers' reports. *American Journal of Psychiatry, 154(4),* 532–535.

Sherman, E. M. S., Janzen, L., and Joschko, M. (1996). Sustained attention and social functioning in children with Tourette's syndrome. *Journal of the International Neuropsychological Society, 2(1),* 41.

Shibagaki, M., Yamanaka, T., and Furuya, T. (1993). Attention state in electrodermal activity during auditory stimulation of children with attention-deficit hyperactivity disorder. *Perceptual and Motor Skills, 77,* 331–338.

Shiffrin, R. M. and Schneider, W. (1977). Controlled automatic human information processing: II perceptual learning, automatic attending, and a general theory. *Psychology Review, 84,* 127–190.

Short, R. J. and Shapiro, S. K. (1993). Conduct disorders: A framework for understanding and intervention in schools and communities. *School Psychology Review, 22(3),* 362–371.

Shortliffe, L. M. D. (1993). Primary nocturnal enuresis: Introduction. *Clinical Pediatrics, July,* 3–4.

Shue, K. L. and Douglas, V. I. (1989). Attention deficit hyperactivity disorder, normal development, and the frontal lobe syndrome. *Canadian Psychology, 30,* 498.

Shum, D. H. K., McFarland, K., Bain, J. D., and Humphreys, M. S. (1990). Effects of closed head injury on attentional processes: An information-processing stage analysis.

Siegel, B. A., Buchsbaum, M. S., Bunney, W. E., Gottschalk, L. A., Haier, R. J., Lohr, J. B., Lottenberg, S., Najafi, A., Nuechterlein, K. H., Potkin, S. G., and Wu, J. C. (1993a). Cortical-striatal-thalamic circuits and brain glucose metabolic activity in 70 unmedicated male schizophrenic patients. *American Journal of Psychiatry, 150,* 1325–1336.

Siegel, B. V., Asarnow, R., Tanguay, P., Call, J. D., Abel, L., Ho, A., Lott, I., and Buchsbaum, M. S. (1993b). Regional cerebral glucose metabolism amd attention in adults with a history of childhood autism. *Journal of Neuropsychiatry and Clinical Neurosciences, 4,* 406–414.

Silver, J. M. and McAllister, T. W. (1997). *Journal of Neuropsychiatry and Clinical Neurosciences, 9(1),* 102–113.

Silveri, M. C., Misciagna, S., Leggio, M. G., and Molinari, M. (1997). Spatial dysgraphia and cerebellar lesion: a case report. *Neurology, 48,* 1529–1532.

Silverman, I. W. and Ragusa, D. M. (1993). A short-term longitudinal study of the early development of self-regulation: Erratum. *Journal of Abnormal Child Psychology, 21(2),* 231.

Silverstein, J. M. and Allison, D. B. (1994). The comparative efficacy of antecendent exercise and methylphenidate: A single-case randomized trial. *Child Care Health and Development, 20(1),* 47–60.

Silverstein, S. M., Coma, P. G., Palumbo, D. R., West, L. L., and Osborn, L. M. (1995). Multiple sources of attentional dysfunction in adults with Tourette's Syndrome: Comparison with attention deficit-hyperactivity disorder. *Neuropsychology, 9,* 157–164.

Simeon, D., Gross, S., Guralnik, O., Stein, D. J., Schmeidler, J., and Hollander, E. (1997). Feeling unreal: 30 cases of DSM-III-R Depersonalization Disorder. *American Journal of Psychiatry, 154(8),* 1107–1113.

Simeon, J. G. (1997). Propranolol in aggressive children and adolescents, Ed., Kutcher, S. P., M.D., *Child and Adolescent Psychopharmacology News, 2(3),* 11–12.

Sirven, J. I., Liporace, J. D., French, J. A., O'Connor, M. J., and Sperling, M. R. (1997). Seizures in temporal lobe epilepsy: I. Reliability of scalp/sphenoidal ictal recording. *Neurology, (48),* 1041–1046.

Sisodiya, S. M., Free, S. L., Stevens, J. M., Fish, D. R., and Shorvon, S. D. (1995). Widespread cerebral structural changes in patients with cortical dysgenesis and epilepsy. *Brain, 118,* 1039–1050.

Sloane, M. S., Assadi, L., and Linn, L. (1991). *Attention Deficit Disorder in Teenagers and Young Adults.* Waterford, MI: Minerva Press Inc.

Slomkowski, C., Klein, R. G., and Mannuzza, S. (1995). Is self-esteem an important outcome in hyperactive children? *Journal of Abnormal Child Psychology, 23,* 303–315.

Smid, H. G. O. M. et al. (1997). Differentiation of hypoglycemia induced cognitive impairments: An electrophysiological approach. *Brain, 120,* 1041–1056.

Smith, G. P. (1976). The arousal function of central catecholamine neurons. *Annual New York Academy Science, 270,* 45–55.

Smith, I. M. and Bryson, S. E. (1994). Imitation and action in autism: A critical review. *Psychological Bulletin, 116,* 259–273.

Smith, P. T. (1994). Measuring visual neglect. *Neuropsychological Rehabilitation, 4(2),* 203–206.

Snow, P., Douglas, J., and Ponsford, J. (1997). Conversational asesment following traumatic brain injury: a comparison across two control groups. *Brain Injury, 11(6),* 409–429.

Sohlberg, M. M. and Raskin, S. A. (1996). Principles of Generalization Applied to Attention and Memory Interventions. *Journal of Head Trauma Rehabilitation, 11,* 65–78.

Sohlberg, M. M. and Mateer, C. A. (1987). Effectiveness of an attention training program. *Journal of Experimental and Clinical Neuropsychology, 19,* 117–130.

Solanto, M. V. and Wender, E. H. (1989). Does methylphenidate constrict cognitive functioning? *Journal of the American Academy of Child and Adolescent Psychiatry, 28,* 897–902.

Solomon, Z., Neria, Y., Ohry, A., Waysman, M., and Ginzburg, K. (1994). PTSD among Israeli former prisoners of war and soldiers with combat stress reaction: A longitudinal study. *American Journal of Psychiatry, 151,* 554–559.

Solyom, L. (1994). Controlling panic attacks with fenfluramine. *American Journal of Psychiatry, 151(4),* 621–622.

Sonneville, L. M. J. de, Njiokiktjien, C., and Hilhorst, R. C. (1991). Methylphenidate-induced changes in ADDH information processors. *Journal of Child Psychology and Psychiatry, 32(2),* 285–295.

Sonneville, L. M. J. de, Njiokiktjien, C., and Bos, H. (1994). Methylphenidate and information processing: I. Differentiation between responders and nonresponders. II. Efficacy in responders. *Journal of Clinical and Experimental Neuropsychology, 16(6),* 877–897.

Sorensen, D. J., Martin, E. M., and Robertson, L. C. (1994). Visual attention in HIV-1 infection. *Neuropsychology, 8,* 424–432.

Spanos, N. P. (1994). Multiple identity enactments and multiple personality disorder: A sociocognitive perspective. *Psychological Bulletin, 116,* 143–165.

Speech, T. J., Rao, S. M., Osmon, D. C., and Sperry, L. T. (1993). A double-blind controlled study of methylphenidate treatment in closed head injury. *Brain Injury, 7,* 333–338.

Spencer, T. J., Biederman, J., Harding, M., O'Donnell, D. et al. (1996). Growth deficits in ADHD children revisited: Evidence for disorder-associated growth delays? *Journal of the American Academy of Child and Adolescent Psychiatry, 35(11),* 1460–1469.

Spencer, T J., Biederman, J., and Wilens, T. (1994). Tricyclic antidepressant treatment of children with ADHD and tic disorders. *Journal of the American Academy of Child and Adolescent Psychiatry, 33,* 1203–1204.

Spencer, T., Biederman, J., Kerman, K., and Steingard, R. (1993a). Desipramine treatment of children with attention-deficit hyperactivity disorder and tic disorder or Tourette's syndrome. *Journal of the American Academy of Child and Adolescent Psychiatry, 32,* 354–360.

Spencer, T. J., Biederman, J., Steingard, R., and Wilens, T. (1993b). Bupropion exacerbates tics in children with attention-deficit hyperactivity disorder and Tourette's syndrome. *Journal of the American Academy of Child and Adolescent Psychiatry, 32,* 211–214.

Spencer, T. J., Biederman, J., Wilens, T., and Steingard, R. (1993c). Nortriptyline treatment of children with attention-deficit hyperactivity disorder and tic disorder or Tourette's syndrome. *Journal of the American Academy of Child and Adolescent Psychiatry, 32,* 205–210.

Spencer, T., Biederman, J., Harding, M., Wilens, T. et al. (1995). The relationship between tic disorders and Tourette's syndrome revisited. *Journal of the American Academy of Child and Adolescent Psychiatry, 34(9),* 1133–1139.

Sprengelmeyer, R., Lange, H., and Homberg, V. (1995). The pattern of attentional deficits in Huntington's disease. *Brain, 18,* 145–152.

Sramek, J. J., Mack, R. J., Awni, W., Hourani, J. O. (1997). Two rapid-dose titrations of sertindole in patients with schizophrenia. *Journal of Clinical Psychopharmacology, 17(5),* 419–422.

Sriram, S. and Rodriguez, M.D. (1997). Indictment of the microglia as the villain in multiple sclerosis. *Neurology, 48,* 464–470.

Stam, C. J., Visser, S. L., Op de Coul, A. A. W., Sonneville, L. M. J., Schellens, R. L. L. A., Brunia, C. H. M., de Smet, J. S., and Gielen, G. (1993). Disturbed frontal regulation of attention in Parkinson's disease. *Brain, 116,* 1139–1168.

Stanford, L. D. and Hynd, G. W. (1994). Congruence of behavioral symptomatology in children with ADD/H, ADD/WO, and learning disabilities. *Journal of Learning Disabilities, 27(4),* 243–253.

Starbuck, V., Bleiberg, J., and Kay, G. C. (1995). D-Amphetamine-mediated enhancement of the P300 ERP: A placebo-crossover double-blid case study. *Neuropsychiatry, Neuropsychology, and Behavioral Neurology, 8(3),* 189–192.

Stark, M., Coslett, H. B., and Saffran, E. M. (1996). Impairment of an Egocentric Map of Locations: Implications for Perception and Action. *Cognitive Neuropsychology, 13,* 481–523.

Steere, J. C. and Arnstein, A. F. T. (1995). Corpus callosum morphology in ADHD. *American Journal of Psychiatry, 152(7),* 1105.

Steigerwald, E. S., Anderson D. W., and Young A. M., (1994). Tolerance to discriminative stimulus effects of d-amphetamine. *Experimental and Clinical Psychopharmacology, 2(1),* 13–24.

Stein, B. E., Wallace, M. T., and Meredith, M. A. (1995). Neural mechanisms mediating attention and orientation to multisensory cues. In *The Cognitive Neurosciences.* Cambridge, MA: Massachusetts Institute of Technology, 683–702.

Stein, D. J., Trestman, R. L., Mitropoulou, V., Coccaro, E. F., Hollander, E., and Siever, L. J. (1996). Impulsivity and serotonergic function in compulsive personality disorder. *Journal of Neuropsychiatry, 8,* 393–398.

Stein, D. J., Hollander, E., and Liebowitz, M. R. (1993). Neurobiology of impulsivity and the impulse control disorders. *Journal of Neuropsychiatry and Clinical Neurosciences, 5,* 9–17.

Stein, M. B., Baird, A., and Walker, J. R. (1996). Social phobia in adults with stuttering. *American Journal of Psychiatry, 153,* 278–283.

Stein, M. B., Walker, J. R., Hazen, A. L., and Forde, D. R. (1997). Full and partial posttraumatic stress disorder: findings from a community survey. *American Journal of Psychiatry, 154(8),* 1114–1119.

Stein, M., Krasowski, M., Leventhal, B. L., Phillips, W., and Bender, B. G. (1996). Behavioral and cognitive effects of methylxanthines. *Archives of Pediatric Adolescent Medicine, 150(3),* 284–288.

Stein, M. B., Chartier, M. J., Hazen, A. L., Kroft, C. D. L., Chale, R. A., Cote, D., and Walker, J. R. (1996). Paroxetine in the treatment of generalized social phobia: open-label treatment and double-blind pacebo-controlled discontinuation. *Journal of Clinical Psychopharmacology, 16,* 218–222.

Steingard, R., Biederman, J., Spencer, T., and Wilens T. E. (1993). Comparison of clonidine response in the treatment attention-deficit hyperactivity disorder with and without comorbid tic disorders. *Journal of the American Academy of Child and Adolescent Psychiatry, 32,* 350–353.

Steingard, R. J., Goldberg, M., Lee, D., and DeMaso, D. R. (1994). Adjunctive clonazepam treatment of tic symptoms in children with comorbid tic disorders and ADHD. *Journal of the American Academy of Child and Adolescent Psychiatry, 33,* 394–399.

Stenberg, A. and Lackgren, G. (1993, July). Treatment with oral desmopressin in adolescents with primary nocturnal enuresis. *Clinical Pediatrics,* 25–27.

Stephens, R. S., Roffman, R. A., and Simpson E. E. (1994). Treating adult marijuana dependence: A test of the relapse prevention model. *Journal of Consulting and Clinical Psychology, 62,* 92–99.

Stern, Y., Liu, X., Marder, K., Todak, G., Sano, M., Malouf, R., Joseph, M., El Sadr, W., Ehrhardt, A., Williams, J. B. W., and Gorman, J. (1996). Neuropsychological changes in a prospectively followed cohort of intravenous drug users with and without HIV. *Neuropsychiatry, Neuropsychology, and Behavioral Neurology, 9,* 83–90.

Stern, R. A., Robinson, B., Thormer, A. R., Arruda, J. E., Prohaska, M. L., and Prange, A. J. (1996). A survey study of neuropsychiatric complaints in patients with Graves' disease. *Journal of Neuropsychiatry, 8(2),* 181–185.

Sterzi, R., Placentini, S., Polimeni, M., Liverani, F., and Bisiach, E. (1996). Perceptual and premotor components of unilateral auditory neglect. *Journal of the International Neuropsychological Society, 2,* 419–425.

Stich, S. (1993, September). Why can't your husband sit still? *Ladies Home Journal,* 74–77.

Stine, J. J. (1994). Psychosocial and psychodynamic issues affecting noncimpliance with psychostimulant treatment. *Journal of Child and Adolescent Psychopharmacology, 4(2),* 75–76.

Stoller, B. E., Garber, H. J., Tishler, T. A., and Oldendorf, W. H. (1994). Methylphenidate increases rat cerebral cortex levels of N-acetyl-aspartic acid and N-acetyl-aspartyl-glutamic acid. *Biological Psychiatry, 36,* 633–636.

Stoner, G., Carey, S. P., Ikeda, M. J., and Shinn, M. R. (1994). The utility of curriculum-based measurement for evaluating the effects of methylphenidate on academic performance. *Journal of Applied Behavior Analysis, 27,* 101–113.

Storrie-Baker, H. J., Segalowitz, S. J., Black, S. E., McLean, J. A. G., Sullivan, N. (1997). Improvement of hemispatial neglect with cold-water calorics: An electrophysiological test of the arousal hypothesis of neglect. *Journal of the International Neuropsychological Society, 3,* 394–402.

Stothard, S. E., Snowling, M. J., and Hulme, C. (1996). Deficits in phonology but not dyslexic? *Cognitive Neuropsychology, 13(3),* 641–672.

Stratta, P., Rossi, A., Mancini, F., Cupillari, M., Mattei, P., and Casacchia, M. (1993). Wisconsin Card Sorting Test performance and educational level in schizophrenic and control samples. *Neuropsychiatry, Neuropsychology, and Behavioral Neurology, 6,* 149–153.

Strauss, E., Spellacy, F., Hunter, M., and Berry, T. (1994). Assessing believable deficits on measures of attention and information processing capacity. *Archives of Clinical Neuropsychology, 9(6)*, 483–490.

Strayhorn, J. M. and Weidman, C. S. (1989). Reduction of attention deficit and internalizing symptoms in preschoolers through parent-child interaction training. *Journal of the American Academy of Child Adolescence Psychiatry, 28*, 888–896.

Stringer, A. Y. and Cooley, E. L. (1994). Divided attention performance in multiple personality disorder. *Neuropsychiatry, Neuropsychology, and Behavioral Neurology, 7(1)*, 51–56.

Sturm, W., Willmes, K., Orgass, B., and Hartje, W. (1997). Do specific attention deficits need specific training? *Neuropsychological Rehabilitation, 7(2)*, 81–103.

Stuss, D. T., Gow, C. A., and Hetherington, C. R. (1992). No longer gage. Frontal Lobe changes and emotional changes. *Journal of Consulting and Clinical Psychology, 60*, 349–359.

Stuss, D. T., Benson, D., and Frank, M. D. (1986). *The Frontal Lobes*, New York: Raven Press.

Stuss, D. T., Stethem, L. L., and Pelchat, G. (1988). Tests of attention and rapid information processing an extension. *Clinical Neuropsychologist, 2*, 246–250.

Sutker, P. B., Uddo, M., Brailey, K., Vasterling, J. J., and Errara, P. (1994). Psychopathology in war-zone deployed and nondeployed operation desert storm troops assigned graves registration duties. *Journal of Abnormal Psychology, 103(2)*, 383–390.

Swartz, B. E., Simpkins, F., Halgren, E., Mandelkern, M., Brown, C., Krisdakumtorn, T., and Gee, M. (1996). Visual working memory in primary generalized epilepsy: An FDG-PET study. *Neurology, 47*, 1203–1212.

Szabo, C. A., Rankman, M., and Stagno, S. (1996). Postictal psychosis: A review. *Neuropsychiatry, Neuropsychology, and Behavioral Neurology, 9*, 258–264.

Szatmari, P., Bremner, R., and Nagy, J. (1989). Asperger's syndrome: A review of clinical features. *Canadian Journal of Psychiatry, 34*, 554–560.

Szatmari, P., Boyle, M. H., and Offord, D. R. (1993). Familial aggregation of emotional and behavioral problems of childhood in the general population. *American Journal of Psychiatry, 150*, 1398–1403.

Tamminga, C. A., Kane, J., and Lahti, R. (1996). New antipsychotic treatments will soon hit the market. *Psychopharmacology Update, 7(5)*, 1–5.

Tannock, R. and Schachar, R. (1992). Methylphenidate and cognitive perseveration in hyperactive children. *Journal of Child Psychology and Psychiatry and Allied Disciplines, 33*, 1217–1228.

Tannock, R., Purvis, K. L., and Schachar, R. J. (1993). Narrative abilities in children with attention deficit hyperactivity disorder and normal peers. *Journal of Abnormal Child Psychology, 21(1)*, 103–116.

Tannock, R., Ickowicz, A., and Schachar, R. (1995). Differential effects of methylphenidate in working memory in ADHD children with and without comorbid anxiety. *Journal of the American Academy of Child and Adolescent Psychiatry, 34*, 886–896.

Tannock, R., Schachar, R., and Logan, G. (1995). Methylphenidate and cognitive flexibility: Dissociated dose effects in hyperactive children. *Journal of Abnormal Child Psychology, 23(2),* 235–266.

Tannock, R. (1997). Television, videogames, and ADHD: Challenging a popular belief. *ADHD Report, 5(3),* 3–7.

Taylor, E. (1979). Food additives, allergy, and hyperkineses. *Journal of Child Psychology and Psychiatry, 20,* 357–363.

Taylor, L. B. (1979). Psychological assessment of neurological patients. In The Florida Society of Neurology and The Center for Neuropsychological Studies at The University of Florida.

Tedeschi, G., Bertolino, A., Lundbom, N., Bonavita, S., Patronas, N. J., Duhn, J. H., Verhagen Metman, L., Chase, T. N., and Di Chiro, G. (1996). Cortical and subcortical chemical pathology in alzeheimer's disease as assessed by multislice proton magnetic resonance spectroscopic imaging. *Neurology, 47,* 696–704.

Thapar, A., Hervas, A., and McGuffin, P. (1985). Childhood hyperactivity scores are highly heritable and show sibling competition effects: Twin study evidence. *Behavior Genetics, 25,* 537–544.

Thapar, A., Hervas, A., and McGuffin, P. (1995). Childhood hyperactivity scores are highly heritable and show sibling competition effects: Twin study evidence. *Behavioral Genetics, 25(6),* 537–544.

Thase, M. E., Reynolds, C. F., Frank, E., Simons, A. D., McGeary, J., Fasiczka, A. L., Garamoni, G. G., Jennings, J. R., and Kupfer, D. J. (1994). Do depressed men and women respond similarly to cognitive behavior therapy? *American Journal of Psychiatry, 151,* 500–505.

Theodore, W. H., Jensen, P. K., and Kwan, R. M. F. (1995). Felbamate, clinical use, In Levy, R. H., Mattson, R. H., and Meldrum, B. S., Eds., *Antiepileptic Drugs, 4h ed.,* New York: Raven Press.

Thompson, N. M., Francis, D. J., Stuebing, K. K., Fletcher, J. M., Ewing-Cobbs, L., Miner, M. E., Levin, H. S., and Eisenberg, H. M. (1994). Motor, visual-spatial, and somatosensory skills after closed head injury an children and adolescents: A study of change. *Neuropsychology, 8,* 333–342.

Thompson, W. and Gottesman, I. (1994). Comparison of neuropsychological test performance in PTSD. Generalized anxiety disorder and control Vietnam Veterans. *Assessment, 1(2),* 133–142.

Timmerman, V., De Jonghe, P., Spoelders, P., Simmokovic, S., Lofgren, S., Nelis, E., Vance, J., Martin, J. J., and Van Broeckhoven, C. (1996). Linkage and mutation analysis of Charcot-Marie-Tooth neuropathy type 2 families with chromosomes 1p35-p36 and Xq13. *Neurology, 46,* 1311–1317.

Tingelstad, J. B. (1991). The cardiotoxicity of tricyclics. *Journal of the American Academy, 30(5),* 845–846.

Todd, J. A., Anderson, V., and Lawrence, J. A. (1996). Planning skills in head-injured adolescents and their peers. *Neuropsychological Rehabilitation, 6(2),* 81–99.

Tohen, M., Zarate, C. A., Jr., Centorrino, F., Hegarty, J. I., Froeschl, M., and Zarate, S. B. (1996). Risperidone in the treatment of mania. *Journal of Clinical Psychiatry, 57,* 249–253.

Tomporowski, P. D., Tinsley, V., and Hager, L. D. (1994). Visuospatial attentional shifts and choice responses of adults and ADHD and non-ADHD children. *Perceptual and Motor Skills, 79,* 1479–1490.

Toren, P., Silbergeld, A., Eldar, S., Laor, N. et al. (1997). Lack of effect of methylphenidate on serum growth hormone (GH), GH-binding protein and insulin-like growth factor I. *Clinical Neuropharmacology, 20(3),* 264–269.

Townsend, J., Harris, N. S., and Courchesne, E. (1996). Visual attention abnormalities in autism: Delayed orienting to location. *Journal of the International Neuropsychological Society, 2,* 541–550.

Tran, P., Hamilton, S. H., Kuntz, A. J., Potvin, J. H. L. (1997). Double-blind comparison of olanzapine versus risperidone in the treatment of schizophrenia and other psychotic disorders. *Journal of Clinical Psychopharmacology, 17(5),* 407–418.

Trenerry, M. R., Crosson, B., DeBoe, J., and Leber, W. R. (1990). *Visual Search and Attention Test: Professional Manual.* Odessa, FL: Psychological Assessment Resources, Inc.

Troland, K., Sommerfelt, K., and Ellertsen, B. (1995). Personality and behavior in ADHD children and low birth weight (LBW) children. *Journal of the International Neuropsychological Society, 1(4),* 321.

Trommer, B. L., Hoeppner, J. B., Lorber, R., and Armstrong, K. J. (1988). The go-no-go paradigm in attention deficit disorder. *Annals of Neurology, 24,* 610–614.

Trzepacz, P., Mahlab, R., Butters, M., and Soety, E. (1997). Weintraub-Mesulam cancellation tests (WMCT). ANPA Abstracts *Journal of Neuropsychiatry and Clinical Neurosciences, 9(1),* 168, P131.

Tucker, D. M. and Derryberry, D. (1992). Motivated attention: Anxiety and the frontal executive functions. *Neuropsychiatry, Neuropsychology, and Behavioral Neurology, 5(4),* 233–252.

Turkstra, L. S., McDonald, S., and Kaufmann, P. M. (1995). Assessment of pragmatic communication skills in adolescents after traumatic brain injury. *Brain Injury, 10,* 329–349.

Twum, M. (1994). Maximizing generalization of cognitions and memories after traumatic brain injury. *NeuroRehabilitation, 4(3),* 157–167.

Uitti, R. J., Rajput, A. H., Ahlskog, J. E., Offord, K. P., Schroeder, D. R., Ho, M. M., Prasad, M., Rajput, A., and Basran, P. (1996). Amantadine treatment is an independent predictor of improved survival in Parkinson's disease. *Neurology, 46,* 1551–1556.

Ullmann, R. K., Sleator, E. K., and Sprague, R. L. (1991). *Manual for the ADD-H Comprehensive Rating Scale* (2nd ed.). Champaign, IL: MetriTech.

Umansky, W. and Smalley, B. S. (1994). *ADD: Helping Your Child Untying the Knot of Attention Deficit Disorders.* New York: Warner Books.

Umilta, C. and Moscovitch, M. (Eds.) (1994). *Attention and Performance XV: Conscious and Nonconscious Information Processing.* Cambridge, MA: MIT Press.

Vaeth, J. M., Horton, A. M., and Ahadpour, M. (1992). Attention deficit disorder, alcoholism, and drug abuse: MMPI correlates. *International Journal of Neuroscience, 63(1–2),* 115–124.

Vakil, E. and Sigal, J. (1997). The effect of level of processing on perceptual and conceptual priming: Control versus closed-head-injured patients. *Journal of the International Neuropsychological Society, 3,* 327–336.

van Domburg, P. H. M. F., Gabreëls-Festen, A. A. W. M., Gabreëls, F. J. M., deCoo, R., Ruitenbeek, W., Wesseling, P., and ter Laak, H. (1996). Mitochondrial cytopathy presenting as hereditary sensory neuropathy with progressive external ophthalmoplegia, ataxia and fatal myoclonic epileptic status. *Brain, 119,* 991–1010.

van Dyck, C. H., McMahon, T. J., Rosen, M. I., O'Malley, S. S. et al. (1997). Sustained-release methylphenidate for cognitive impairment in HIV-1-infected drug abusers: A pilot study. *The Journal of Neuropsychiatry and Clinical Neurosciences, 9,* 29–36.

van Kammen, D. P., Kelley, M. E., Gilbertson M. W., Gurklis, J., and O'Connor, D. T. (1994). CSF dopamine B-hydroxylase in schizophrenia: Associations with premorbid functiong and brain computerized tomography scan measures. *American Journal of Psychiatry, 151,* 372–378.

van Reekum, R. and Links, P. S. (1994). N of 1 study: Methylphenidate in a patient with borderline personality disorder and attention deficit hyperactivity disorder. *Canadian Journal of Psychiatry, 39(3),* 186–187.

van Reekum, R., Bayey, M., Gardner, S., Burke, I. M., Gawcett, S., Hart, A., and Thompson, W. (1995). N of 1 study:amantadine for the amotivational syndrome in a patient with traumatic brain injury. *Brain Injury, 9,* 49–53.

van Reekum, R., Bolago, I., Finlayson, M. A. J., Garners, S., and Links, P. S. (1996). Psychiatric disorders after traumatic brain injury. *Brain Injury, 10,* 319–327.

van Vliet, I. M., DenBoer, J. A., Westenberg, H. G. M., and Slaap, B. R. (1996). A Double-Blind Comparative Study of Brofaromine and Fluvoxamine in Outpatients with Panic Disorder. *Clinical Psychopharmacology, 16,* 299–306.

van Zomeren, A. H., and Brouwer, W. H. (1994). *Clinical Neuropsychology of Attention.* Oxford: Oxford University Press. 250 pages.

Vargha-Khadem, F., Carr, L. J., Isaacs, E., Brett, E., Adams, C., and Mishkin, M. (1997). Onset of speech after left hemispherectomy in a nine-year-old boy. *Brain, 120,* 159–182.

Varley, C. K. (1984). Attention deficit disorder (the hyperactivity syndrome): A review of selected issues. *Developmental and Behavioral Pediatrics, 5(5),* 254–258.

Venkataraman, S., Naylor, M. W., and King, C. A. (1992). Mania associated with fluoxetine treatment in adolescents. *Journal of the American Academy of Child and Adolescent Psychiatry, 31,* 276–281.

Verbaten, M. N., Overtoom, C. C. E., Koelega, H. S., and Swaab-Barneveld, H. (1994). Methylphenidate influences on both early and late ERP waves of ADHD children in a continuous performance test. *Journal of Abnormal Child Psychology, 22(5),* 561–578.

Voeller, K. S. (1991). What can neurological models of attention, intention, and arousal tell us about ADHD? *Journal of Neuropsychiatry, 3(2),* 209–216.

Voeller, K. S., Edge, P., and Mann, L. (1996). Dyslexia modifies cancellation task performance in children with attention-deficit hyperactivity disorder. *Neurology, 46(2, Suppl.),* A114.

Vogt, B. A., Finch, D. M., and Olson, C. R. (1992). Functional heterogeneity in cingulate cortex: The anterior executive and posterior evaluative regions. *Cerebral Cortex, 2,* 435–443.

Volkow, N. D., Wang, G. J., Hitzemann, R., Fowler, J. S., Overall, J. E., Burr, G., and Wolf, A. P. (1994). Recovery of brain glucose metabolism in detoxified alcoholics. *American Journal of Psychiatry, 151,* 178–183.

Voller, K. K. (1991). Toward a neurobiologic nosology of attention deficit hyperactivity disorder. *Journal of Child Neurology, 6(suppl),* 52–58.

Waldrop, R. D. (1994). Selection of patients for management of attention deficit hyperactivity disorder in a private practice setting. *Clinical Pediatrics, 33(2),* 83–87.

Walker, R., Findlay, J. M., Young, A. W., and Lincoln, N. B. (1996). Saccadic eye movements in object-based neglect. *Cognitive Neuropsychology, 13,* 529–615.

Wallace, D. J. (1995). *The Lupus Book, A Guide for Patients and their Families,* New York: Oxford University Press.

Wallander, J. L. (1988). The relationship between attention problems in childhood and antisocial behavior 8 years later. *Journal of Child Psychology and Psychiatry, 29(1),* 53–61.

Walsh, K. (1994). *Neuropsychology: A Clinical Approach* (3rd ed.). New York: Churchill Livingstone.

Walsh, V. and Perrett, D. I. (1994). Visual attention in the occipitotemporal processing stream of the macaque. *Cognitive Neuropsychology, 2(2),* 243–263.

Walters, A. S., Hickey, K., Maltzman, J., Verrico, T., Joseph, D., Hening, W., Wilson, V., and Chokroverty, S. (1996). A questionnaire study of 138 patients with restless legs syndrome: The 'night-walkers' survey. *Neurology, 46(1),* 92–95.

Ward, A. S., Kelly, T. H., Foltin, R. W., and Fischman, M. W. (1997). Effects of d-Amphetamine on task performance and social behavior of humans in a residential laboratory. *Experimental and Clinical Psychopharmacology, 5(2),* 130–136.

Warden, D. L., Labbate, L. A., Salazar, A. M., Nelson, R., Sheley, E., Staudenmeier, J., and Martin, E., (1997). *Journal of Neuropsychiatry and Clinical Neurosciences, 9(1),* 18–22.

Warren, R. P., Odell, J. D., Warren, W. L., Burger, R. A. et al. (1995). Is decreased blood plasma concentration of the complement C4B protein associated with attention-deficit hyperactivity disorder? *Journal of the American Academy of Child and Adolescent Psychiatry, 34(8),* 1009–1014.

Warren, R. P., Odell, J. D., Warren, W. L., Burger, R. A. et al. (1995). Reading disability, attention-deficit hyperactivity disorder, and the immune system. *Science, 286(5212),* 786–787.

Warschausky, S., Cohen, E. H., Parker, J. G., Levendosky, A. A., and Okun, A. (1997). Social problem-solving skills of children with traumatic brain injury. *Pediatric Rehabilitation, 1(2),* 77–81.

Warshaw, M. G., Fierman, E., Pratt, L., Hunt, M., Yonkers, K. A., Massion, A. O., and Keller, M. B. (1993). Quality of life and dissociation in anxiety disorder patients with histories of trauma or PTSD. *American Journal of Psychiatry, 150,* 1512–1516.

Watson, F. L. and Tipper, S. P. (1997). Reduced negative priming in schizotypal subjects does reflect reduced cognitive inhibition. *Cognitive Neuropsychiatry, 2(1),* 67–79.

Watson, R. T., Valenstein, E., and Hedman, K. M. (1981). Thalamus neglect possible role of the medial thalamus and nucleus reticulant in behavior. *Archives of Neurology, 38,* 501–506.

Weber, A. M. (1990). A practical clinical approach to understanding and treating attentional problems. *Journal of Head Trauma-Rehabilitation, 5(1),* 73–85.

Webster-Stratton, C. (1993). Strategies for helping early school-aged children with oppositional defiant and conduct disorders: The importance of home-school partnerships. *School Psychology Review, 22,* 437–457.

Weiden, P. J. (1995). Using depot therapy for schizophrenia. *Journal of Practical Psychiatry and Behavioral Health, 1(4),* 247–250.

Weinberg, H. A. (1995). Generic bioequivalence. *Journal of the American Academy of Child and Adolescent Psychiatry, 34(7),* 834–835.

Weinberg, W. A. and Harper, C. R. (1993). Vigilance and its disorders. *Neurologic Clinics, 11(1),* 59–78.

Weinstein, C. S. (1994). Cognitive remediation strategies: An adjunct to the psychotherapy of adults with attention-deficit hyperactivity disorder. *Journal of Psychotherapy Practice and Research, 3(1),* 44–57.

Weintraub, S. and Mesulam, M. M. (1985). Mental state assessment of young and elderly adults in behavioral neurology. In M. M. Mesulam (Ed.). *Principles of Behavioral Neurology,* Philadelphia, PA: F.A. Davis Company.

Weiss, G. (1983). Long-term outcome: Findings, concepts, and practical implications, In Rutter, M. (Ed.). *Developmental Neuropsychiatry,* New York: The Guilford Press, 422–436.

Weiss, G., Hechtman, L., Perlman, T., Hopkins, J., and Wener, A. (1979). Hyperactives as young adults. A controlled prospective ten-year follow-up of 75 children. *Archives of General Psychiatry, 36,* 675–681.

Weiss, G. and Hechtman, L. T. (1986). *Hyperactive Children Grown Up.* New York: Guilford Press.

Weiss, G. and Hechtman, L. T. (1993). *Hyperactive Children Grown Up* (2nd ed.). *ADHD in Children, Adolescents, and Adults,* New York: Guilford Press.

Weiss, G. (1990). Hyperactivity in childhood. *New England Journal of Medicine, 323,* 1413–1415.

Weiss, L. (1992). *Attention Deficit Disorder in Adults.* Dallas, TX: Taylor Publishing Company.

Weiss, M. (1996, February). Changes in the approach to pharmacotherapy for ADHD. *Child and Adolescent Psychopharmacology News, 1(1),* 5–9.

Weiss, M. and Walkup, J. T. (1997). Clinically applied pharmacokinetics of the SSRI's and SNRI's, Kutcher, S. P., Ed., *Child and Adolescent Psychopharmacology News*, *2(3)*, 1–9.

Weitzner, M. A., Meyers, C. A., and Valentine, A. D. (1995). Methylphenidate in the treatment of neurobehavioral slowing associated with cancer and cancer treatment. *The Journal of Neuropsychiatry and Clinical Neurosciences, 7(3)*, 347–349.

Wender, P. H. (1971). *Minimal Brain Dysfunction in Children*, New York: Wiley.

Wender, P. H. (1978). Minimal brain dysfunction: An overview. In Lipton, M. A., DiMascio, A., and Killan, K. F., (Eds). *Psychopharmacology: A Generation of Progress*, New York: Raven Press.

Wender, P. H. (1995). *Attention-Deficit Hyperactivity Disorder in Adults*, New York: Oxford University Press.

Wender, P. H., Wood, D. R., and Reimher, F. W. (1991). Pharmacological treatment of attention deficit disorder, residual type (ADD-RT) in adults. *Ritalin (Methyphenidate) Theory and Patient Management*, New York: Mary Ann Liebert, Inc., 267–288.

Werry, J. S. (1995). Resolved: Cardiac arrhythmias make desipramine and unacceptable choice in children. *Journal of the American Academy of Child and Adolescent Psychiatry, 34(9)*, 1239–1231.

West, S. A., McElroy, S. L., Strakowski, S. M., and Keck, P. E. (1995a). Attention deficit hyperactivity disorder in adolescent mania. *American Journal of Psychiatry, 152*, 271–273.

West, S. A., Strakowski, D. M., Sax, K. W., Minnery, K. L., McElroy, S. L., and Keck, P. E., Jr. (1995b). The comorbidity of attention-deficit hyperactivity disorder in adolescent mania: Potential diagnostic and treatment implications. *Psychopharmacological Bulletin, 31(2)*, 347–351.

West, R. and Bell, M. A. (1997). Stroop color-word interference and electroencephalogram activation: Evidence for age-related decline of the anterior attention system. *Neuropsychology, 11(3)*, 421–427.

Westerveld, M., Marchione, K. E., Holahan, J. M., Schneider, A. E., Shaywitz, S. E., Shaywitz, J. M., Fletcher, J. M., and Shay, B. A. (1996). Wisconsin Card Sorting test performance in ADD versus ADHD children. *Journal of the International Neuropsychological Society, 2(4)*, 378.

Wexler, H. K. and McClelland, M. (1996). AD/HD substance abuse and crime. *Attention!, 2(3)*, 27–31.

Whalen, C. K. and Henker, B. (1991). Therapies for hyperactive children: Comparisons, combinations, and compromises. *Journal of Consulting and Clinical Psychology, 59*, 126–137.

Whalen, J., McCloskey, M., Lesser, R. P., and Gordon, B. (1997). Localizing arithmetic processes in the brain: evidence from a transient deficit during cortical stimulation. *Journal of Cognitive Neuroscience, 9(3)*, 409–417.

Wheeler, J. and Carlson, C. L. (1994). The social functioning of children with ADD with hyperactiviy and ADD without hyperactivity: A comparison of their peer relations and social deficits. *Journal of Emotional and Behavioral Disorders, 2(1),* 2–12.

When a Habit Isn't Just a Habit: A Guide to Obsessive–Compulsive Disorder. (1991). CIBA-GEIGY Corporation.

Wherry, J. N., Paal, N., Jolly, J. B., Adam, B., Holloway, C., Everett, B., and Vaught, L. (1993). Concurrent and discriminant validity of the Gordon Diagnostic System: A preliminary study. *Psychology in the Schools, 30,* 29–35.

Whyte, J. (1994). Attentional processes and dyslexia. *Cognitive Neuropsychology, 2(2),* 99–116.

Whyte, J., Polansky, M., Cavallucci, C., Fleming, M., Lhulier, J., and Coslett, B. H. (1996). Inattentive behavior after traumatic brain injury. *Journal of the International Neuropsychological Society, 2,* 274–281.

Wickens, C. D. (1981). *Engineering Psychology and Human Performance,* Columbus, OH: Charles E. Merril.

Wickens, C. D. (1984). Processing resources in attention. In Parasuraman and Davies, D. R., (Eds). *Varieties of Attention,* New York: Academic Press.

Wilder, B. J. (1995). Phenytoin, clinical use, In *Antiepileptic Drugs,* 4th ed., Levy, R. H., Mattson, R. H., and Meldrum, B. S., Eds., New York: Raven Hill, 339–344.

Wilens, T. E. and Lineham, C. E. (1995, Winter). ADD and substance abuse: An intoxicating combination. *Attention!, 1(3),* 25–31.

Wilens, T. E., Biederman, J., and Spencer, T. J. (1994). Clonidine for sleep disturbances associated with attention-deficit hyperactivity disorder. *Journal of the American Academy of Child and Adolescent Psychiatry, 33,* 424–426.

Wilens, T. E., Spencer, T. J., and Biederman, J. (1995). Pharmacotherapy of adult ADHD: A comprehensive guide to attention deficit disorder in adults. *Pharmacotherapy of Adult Attention Deficit.*

Wilens, T. E., Biederman, J., Geist, D. E., and Steingard, R. (1993). Nortriptyline in the treatment of ADHD: A chart review of 58 cases. *Journal of the American Academy of Child and Adolescent Psychiatry, 32,* 343–349.

Wilens, T. E., Biederman, J., Kiely, K., Bredin, E. et al. (1995). Pilot study of behavioral and emotional disturbances in the high-risk children of parents with opioid dependence. *Journal of the American Academy of Child and Adolescent Psychiatry, 34(6),* 779–785.

Wilens, T. E., Biederman, J., Mick, E., and Spencer, T. J. (1995). A systematic assessment of tricyclic antidepressants in the treatment of adult attention-deficit hyperactivity disorder. *Journal of Nervous and Mental Disease, 183(1),* 48–50.

Wilens, T. E., Biederman, J., Kiely, K., Bredin, E., et al. (1995a). Pilot study of behavioral and emotional disturbances in the high-risk children of parents with opioid dependence. *Journal of the American Academy of Child and Adolescent Psychiatry, 34(6),* 779–785.

Wilens, T. E., Biederman, J., Mick, E., and Spencer, T. J. (1995b). A systematic assessment of tricyclic antidepressants in the treatment of adult attention-deficit hyperactivity disorder. *Journal of Nervous and Mental Disease, 183(1),* 48–50.

Wilens, T. E., Prince, J. B., Biederman, J., Spencer, T. J. (1995). Pharmacotherapy of adult attention-deficit/hyperactivity disorder: A review. *Journal of Clinical Psychopharmacology, 15,* 270–279.

Wilkniss, S. M., Jones, M., Korol, D. L., Gold, P. E., and Manning, C. A. (1997). Age–related differences in an ecologically based study of route learning. *Psychology and Aging, 12(2),* 372–375.

Williams, M. C., Littell, R. R., Reinoso, C., and Greve, K. (1994). Effect of wavelength on performance of attention-disordered and normal children on the Wisconsin Card Sorting Test. *Neuropsychology, 8,* 186–193.

Willinck, L. (1996). Right hemisphere/afferent dysgraphia. Abstract. *Journal of the International Neuropsychological Society, 2(4),* 326.

Winokur, G., Coryell, W., Endicott, J., and Akiskal, H. (1993). Further distinctions between manic-depressive illness (bipolar disorder) and primary depressive disorder (unipolar depression). *American Journal of Psychiatry, 150,* 1176–1181.

Wirrell, E. C., Camfield, C. S., Camfield, P. R., Gordon, K. E., and Dooley, J. M. (1997). Long-term prognosis of typical childhood absence epilepsy: Remission or progression to juvenile myoclonic epilepsy. *Neurology, 47,* 912–918.

de Wit, H. (1996). Priming effects with drugs and other reinforcers. *Experimental and Clinical Psychopharmacology, 4(1),* 5–10.

Wiznitzer, M. (1995, Spring). Medication use in autism: When is it appropriate? *MIRA Reporter, 2(1),* 6–8.

Woldorff, M. G., Fox, P. T., Matzke, M., Lancaster, J. L., Veeraswamy, S., Zamarripa, F., Seabolt, M., Glass, T., Gao, J. H., Martin, C. C., and Jerabek, P. (1997). Retinotopic organization of early visual spatial attention effects as revealed by PET and ERPs. *Human Brain Mapping, 5,* 280–286.

Wolkenberg, F. (1987, October 1). Out of a Darkness. *New York Times.*

Wong, P. P., Dornan, J., Keating, A. M., Schentag, C. T., and Ip, R. Y. (1994). Re-examining the concept of severity in traumatic brain injury. *Brain Injury, 8,* 509–518.

Woodrum, D. T., Henderson, J. M., and Linger, B. (1994, Mar. 23–26). ADHD training modules for rural health care providers, educators, and parents. *Proceedings of the Annual National Conference of the American Council on Rural Special Education,* 381–189.

Worthington, A. D. (1996). Cueing strategies in neglect dyslexia. *Neuropsychological Rehabilitation, 6(1),* 1–17.

Wozniak, J., Biederman, J., Mundy, E., Mennin, D., and Faraone, S. V. (1995). A pilot family study of childhood-onset mania. *Journal of the American Academy of Child and Adolescent Psychiatry, 34(12),* 1577–1583.

Wright, J. V. and Beale, B. (1995). Multicultural AD/HD: A review of Ch.A.D.D.'s multicultural panel. *Attention!, 2(1),* 20–22.

Wroblewski, B. A. and Glenn, M. B. (1994). Pharmacological treatment of arousal and cognitive deficits. *Journal of Head Trauma Rehabilitation, 9(3),* 19–42.

Yeates, K. O. and Bornstein, R. A. (1994). Attention deficit disorder and neuropsychological functioning in children with Tourette's syndrome. *Neuropsychology, 8(1),* 65–74.

Young, G. B., Chandarana, P. C., Blume, W. T., McLachlan, R. S., Munoz, D. G., and Girvin, J. P. (1995). Mesial temporal lobe seizures presenting as anxiety disorders. *Journal of Neuropsychiatry, 7(3),* 352–357.

Young, L. T., Li, P. P., Kamide, A., She, K. P., Warsh, J. J. (1994). Mononuclear leukocyte levels of G proteins in depressed patients with bipolar disorder or major depressive disorder. *American Journal of Psychiatry, 151(4),* 594–599.

Zaidel, D. W. (Ed.) (1994). *Neuropsychology.* New York: Academic Press.

Zald, D. H. and Kim, S. W. (1996). Anatomy and function of the orbital frontal cortex, I: Anatomy, neurocircuitry, and obsessive-compulsive disorder. *The Journal of Neuropsychiatry and Clinical Neurosciences, 8(2),* 125–138.

Zald, D. H. and Kim, S. W. (1996). Anatomy and function of the orbital frontal cortex, II: Function and relevance to obsessive-compulsive disorder. *The Journal of Neuropsychiatry and Clinical Neurosciences, 3,* 249–261.

Zalewski, C., Thompson, W., and Gottesman, I. (1994). Comparison of neuropsychological test performance in PTSD, generalized anxiety disorder, and control Vietnam veterans. *Assessment, 1,* 133–142.

Zametkin, A. J. and Rapoport, J. (1987). The neurobiology of attention deficit disorder: Where have we come in 50 years? *Journal of the American Academy of Child and Adolescent Psychiatry, 26,* 676–686.

Zametkin, A. (1992). The neurobiology of attention deficit hyperactivity disorder. *Challenge.*

Zametkin, A. J., Nordahl, T. E., Gross, M., and King, A. C. (1990). Cerebral glucose metabolism in adults with hyperactivity of childhood onset. *New England Journal of Medicine, 323,* 1361–1366.

Zanarini, M. C. et. al. (1997). Reported pathological childhood experiences associated with the development of borderline personality disorder.

Zasler, N. D. (1992). Advances in neuropharmacological rehabilitation for brain dysfunction [Review]. *Brain Injury, 6,* 1–14.

Zasler, N. D. (1995). Bromocriptine: Neuropharmacology and clinical caveats. *Journal of Head Trauma Rehabilitation, 10(4),* 101–104.

Zatorre, R. J., Halpern, A. R., Perry, D. W., Meyer, E., and Evans, A. C. (1996). Hearing in the mind's ear: A PET investigation of musical imagery and perception. *Journal of Cognitive Neuroscience, 8(1),* 29–46.

Zelko, F. A. J., Strite, D., and Brill, W. (1996). Perceptual and visuographic skills in attention deficit disorder. *Journal of the International Neuropsychological Society, 2(4)*, 378.

Ziemann, U., Paulus, W., and Rothenberger, A., (1997). Decreased motor inhibition in tourette's disorder: evidence from transcranial magnetic stimulation. *American Journal of Psychiatry, 154(9)*, 1277–1284.

Zohar, A. H., Pauls, D. L., Ratzoni, G., Apter, A., Dycian, A., Binder, M., King, R., Leckman, J. F., Kron, S., and Cohen, D. J. (1997). Obsessive-compulsive disorder with and without tics in an epidemiological sample of adolescents. *American Journal of Psychiatry, 154(2)*, 274–276.

Index